DIGITAL HEALTH

Sociology of Health and Illness Monograph Series
Edited by Professor Karen Lowton
Department of Sociology
University of Sussex
Brighton, UK
BN1 9RH

Current titles

Digital Health: Sociological Perspectives (2019)
edited by *Flis Henwood and Benjamin Marent*

Materialities of Care: Encountering Health and Illness Through Artefacts and Architecture (2018)
edited by *Christina Buse, Daryl Martin and Sarah Nettleton*

Ageing, Dementia and the Social Mind (2017)
edited by *Paul Higgs and Chris Gilleard*

The Sociology of Healthcare Safety and Quality (2016)
edited by *Davina Allen, Jeffrey Braithwaite, Jane Sandall and Justin Waring*

Children, Health and Well-being: Policy Debates and Lived Experience (2015)
edited by *Geraldine Brady, Pam Lowe and Sonja Olin Lauritzen*

From Health Behaviours to Health Practices: Critical Perspectives (2014)
edited by *Simon Cohn*

Pandemics and Emerging Infectious Diseases: The Sociological Agenda (2013)
edited by *Robert Dingwall, Lily M Hoffman and Karen Staniland*

The Sociology of Medical Screening: Critical Perspectives, New Directions (2012)
edited by *Natalie Armstrong and Helen Eborall*

Body Work in Health and Social Care: Critical Themes, New Agendas (2011)
edited by *Julia Twigg, Carol Wolkowitz, Rachel Lara Cohen and Sarah Nettleton*

Technogenarians: Studying Health and Illness Through an Ageing, Science, and Technology Lens (2010)
edited by *Kelly Joyce and Meika Loe*

Communication in Healthcare Settings: Policy, Participation and New Technologies (2009)
edited by *Alison Pilnick, Jon Hindmarsh and Virginia Teas Gill*

Pharmaceuticals and Society: Critical Discourses and Debates (2009)
edited by *Simon J. Williams, Jonathan Gabe and Peter Davis*

Ethnicity, Health and Health Care: Understanding Diversity, Tackling Disadvantage (2008)
edited by *Waqar I. U. Ahmad and Hannah Bradby*

The View From Here: Bioethics and the Social Sciences (2007)
edited by *Raymond de Vries, Leigh Turner, Kristina Orfali and Charles Bosk*

The Social Organisation of Healthcare Work (2006)
edited by *Davina Allen and Alison Pilnick*

Social Movements in Health (2005)
edited by *Phil Brown and Stephen Zavestoski*

Health and the Media (2004)
edited by *Clive Seale*

Partners in Health, Partners in Crime: Exploring the boundaries of criminology and sociology of health and illness (2003)
edited by *Stefan Timmermans and Jonathan Gabe*

Rationing: Constructed Realities and Professional Practices (2002)
edited by *David Hughes and Donald Light*

Rethinking the Sociology of Mental Health (2000)
edited by *Joan Busfield*

Sociological Perspectives on the New Genetics (1999)
edited by *Peter Conrad and Jonathan Gabe*

The Sociology of Health Inequalities (1998)
edited by *Mel Bartley, David Blane and George Davey Smith*

The Sociology of Medical Science (1997)
edited by *Mary Ann Elston*

Health and the Sociology of Emotion (1996)
edited by *Veronica James and Jonathan Gabe*

Medicine, Health and Risk (1995)
edited by *Jonathan Gabe*

DIGITAL HEALTH

Sociological Perspectives

Edited by
Flis Henwood and Benjamin Marent

WILEY Blackwell

Contents

Notes on contributors

Margunn Aanestad   Department of Informatics, University of Oslo, Oslo, Norway

Helen Atherton   Department of Sociology, University of Warwick, UK

Rebecca Barnes   Department of Primary Care, University of Bristol, UK

Laura Hall   Research Department of Primary Care and Population Health, University College London, UK

Flis Henwood   School of Applied Social Science, University of Brighton, Brighton, UK

Eva Hilberg   Sheffield Institute for International Development, University of Sheffield, Sheffield, UK

Kelly Joyce   Sociology Department, Center for Science, Technology and Society, Drexel University, Philadelphia, PA, USA

Anna Lavis   Institute of Applied Health Research, Birmingham University, Birmingham, UK

Sarah Lewis   Department for Health, University of Bath, Bath, UK

Geraldine Leydon   Primary Care and Population Science, University of Southampton, UK

Alena Macková   Faculty of Social Sciences, Charles University, Prague, Czech Republic And Faculty of Social Studies, Masaryk University, Brno, Czech Republic

Benjamin Marent   School of Applied Social Science, University of Brighton, Brighton, UK

Enrico Maria Piras   Centre for Information and Communication Technology, Bruno Kessler Foundation, Trento, Italy

Andy Miah   School of Environment and Life Sciences, University of Salford, Salford, UK

Francesco Miele   Centre for Information and Communication Technology, Bruno Kessler Foundation, Trento, Italy

China Mills   School of Health Sciences, City, University of London, London, UK

Megan Munsie   Department of Anatomy and Neuroscience, Centre for Stem Cell Systems, School of Biomedical Sciences, University of Melbourne, Melbourne, Vic, Australia

Elizabeth Murray   Research Department of Primary Care and Population Health, University College London, UK

Dino Numerato   Faculty of Social Sciences, Charles University, Prague, Czech Republic

Alan Petersen   Sociology and Gender Studies, School of Social Sciences, Monash University, Melbourne, Vic, Australia

Martyn Pickersgill   Centre for Biomedicine, Self and Society, Edinburgh Medical School, University of Edinburgh, Edinburgh, UK

Jeannette Pols   Section of Medical Ethics, Amsterdam University Medical Centre, and Department of Anthropology, University of Amstrdam, Amsterdam, The Netherlands And Section of Medical Ethics, Amsterdam University Medical Centre, University of Amsterdam, Amsterdam, The Netherlands

Catherine Pope   Primary Care and Population Science, University of Southampton, UK

Emma Rich   Department for Health, University of Bath, Bath, UK

Nete Schwennesen   Department of Anthropology & Centre for Medical Science and Technology Studies And Department of Public Health, Copenhagen University, Copenhagen, Denmark

Maureen Seguin   Research Department of Primary Care and Population Health, University College London, UK

Fiona Stevenson   Research Department of Primary Care and Population Health, University College London, UK

Václav Štětka   Faculty of Social Sciences, Charles University, Prague, Czech Republic And School of Social Sciences, Loughborough University, Loughborough, UK

Claire Tanner   Department of Anatomy and Neuroscience, Centre for Stem Cell Systems, School of Biomedical Sciences, University of Melbourne, Melbourne, Vic, Australia

Ian M. Tucker   School of Psychology, University of East London, London, UK

Lenka Vochocová   Faculty of Social Sciences, Charles University, Prague, Czech Republic

Lucy van de Wiel   Department of Sociology, University of Cambridge, Cambridge, UK

Dick Willems   Section of Medical Ethics, Amsterdam University Medical Centre, University of Amsterdam, Amsterdam, The Netherlands

Sue Ziebland   Primary Care Health Sciences, University of Oxford, UK

Sociology of Health & Illness Vol. 41 No. S1 2019 ISSN 0141-9889, pp. 1–15
doi: 10.1111/1467-9566.12898

Understanding digital health: Productive tensions at the intersection of sociology of health and science and technology studies

Flis Henwood ⓘⅅ and Benjamin Marent ⓘⅅ

School of Applied Social Science, University of Brighton, Brighton, UK

Abstract   In this editorial introduction, we explore how digital health is being explored at the intersection of sociology of health and science and technology studies (STS). We suggest that socio-material approaches and practice theories provide a shared space within which productive tensions between sociology of health and STS can continue. These tensions emerge around the long-standing challenges of avoiding technological determinism while maintaining a clear focus on the materiality and agency of technologies and recognising enduring sets of relations that emerge in new digital health practices while avoiding social determinism. The papers in this Special Issue explore diverse fields of healthcare (e.g. reproductive health, primary care, diabetes management, mental health) within which heterogenous technologies (e.g. health apps, mobile platforms, smart textiles, time-lapse imaging) are becoming increasingly embedded. By synthesising the main arguments and contributions in each paper, we elaborate on four key dimensions within which digital technologies create ambivalence and (re)configure health practices. First, *promissory digital health* highlights contradictory virtues within discourses that configure digital health. Second, *(re)configuring knowledge* outlines ambivalences of navigating new information environments and handling quantified data. Third, *(re)configuring connectivity* explores the relationships that evolve through digital networks. Fourth, *(re)configuring control* explores how new forms of power are inscribed and handled within algorithmic decision-making in health. We argue that these dimensions offer fruitful perspectives along which digital health can be explored across a range of technologies and health practices. We conclude by highlighting applications, methods and dimensions of digital health that require further research.

Keywords: Digital health, digital sociology, sociotechnical practices, socio-materiality, care, e-health, telemedicine, science and technology studies (STS)

Introduction

'Digital health' is both easy and hard to define, not least because of its close relationship to other broad terms such as 'e-health' or more specific terms that might be seen as sub-sets of digital health, such as 'telehealth', 'telemedicine' or 'mobile health', which imply more mobile forms of care. Several definitions have been put forward by sociologists seeking to make sense of digital health (Lupton 2018a, Petersen 2019). Lupton, for example, has described digital health as

> 'a wide range of technologies directed at delivering healthcare, providing information to lay people and helping them share their experiences of health and illness, training and educating healthcare professionals, helping people with chronic illnesses to engage in self-care and encouraging others to engage in activities to promote their health and well-being and avoid illness'
>
> (Lupton 2018a, p. 1).

She and others have also identified the range of technologies and/or the various theoretical approaches that have contributed to our understanding of digital health in attempts to map the field (see, e.g., Lupton 2016b, 2017, 2018a, Petersen 2019). These contributions serve as important reminders of the depth and breadth of the digital health field and its constitution in different disciplines and have provided clear insights into the ways in which digital devices are becoming increasingly embedded in healthcare organisations and care delivery. These include attention to the mutually constitutive relationship between digital technologies and healthcare practices. Despite this, there remains a tendency in many digital health studies to 'read off' from the functionalities or capacities of specific digital devices to assess their likely implications for healthcare or to attribute transformations in healthcare delivery to devices without any clear analysis of *how* digital technologies are implicated in the (re)configuration of healthcare practices. One of the main motivations for us in putting together this collection was to examine this question more directly.

At this point, we must locate ourselves more fully. As sociologists working at the boundary of sociology of health and science and technology studies (STS), our main interest is with exploring understandings of digital health at the intersection of these two fields. We do this by reflecting, briefly, on how technology has been understood in both sociology of health and STS and suggest that socio-material approaches and practice theories provide a shared space within which productive tensions between sociology of health and STS continue to be addressed. We then introduce the papers in this collection to illustrate these points.

Health sociology and STS: Overlaps and productive tensions

A central focus of much sociology of health has always been a critique of individualised, behaviour change models (derived from health psychology) where human agency is foregrounded, where individuals are the unit of analysis and where change comes as result of rational decision-making and informed choice. Sociology of health has typically countered this understanding by drawing attention to the structural determinants of health, where social structures are foregrounded, where health outcomes are determined by structural factors (e.g. class, gender, ethnicity etc.) and where positive change comes as result of improving conditions in which people live and work. In both these approaches, technology is often understood, rather uncritically, as a *tool*. In behaviour change models, it is understood as a tool to achieve goals, either for individuals (e.g. health benefits through use on Internet to inform oneself) or for organisations (e.g. to deliver more effective and efficient healthcare by application of new technologies). In a structural determinants approach, technology is also often seen as a *tool* – here, used by dominant groups to rationalise work (de-skilling argument) or to further oppress marginalised groups (e.g. women in the case of reproductive technologies type arguments). Even in some post-structuralist/Foucauldian approaches, especially in critiques of neo-liberalism and 'responsibilisation', technology is often presented as a tool – in this case, for disciplining patients and citizens and leading to negative outcomes for health. Such formulations might be understood as enacting a soft technological determinism, which is surprising given the close link between Foucauldian approaches and practice theories which challenge all forms of determinism. The challenge of avoiding technological determinism while maintaining a clear focus on the materiality and agency of technologies has been best addressed through practice theory, especially in its post-humanist forms.

While humanist practice theories (Bourdieu 1984, Giddens 1984) might be seen as overlooking the agency of technologies, post-human practice theories, associated with the 'material turn' in social theory, understand materials as active agents and participants in practice (Reckwitz 2002, Schatzki 1996). Here, while the human subject is still understood as having agency, s/he is de-centred. Working in sociology, but at the intersection with STS, Shove et al.'s (2012) practice theory defines practices to include three key elements – meanings, *materials* and skills/competences, with materials being further defined as objects, tools and infrastructures. In this version of practice theory, people are understood as carriers of practice, with practices understood as performance. This approach has been particularly well developed in relation to public health (Harries and Rettie 2018, Keane et al. 2017, Supski et al. 2017, Williams et al. 2018).

There is a close overlap here with practice theories that have emerged within STS, from actor network theory (ANT) onwards (Latour 2005). From an STS point of view, science (including medical science) and technologies have always been a specific focus of analysis and part of the *raison d'être* of this field has been to critique all forms of technological determinism and instrumentalism in social theory. Thus, social shaping theory (MacKenzie and Wajcman 1999) drew attention to the social, political and economic forces that shape technology's funding, design and innovation processes. Social constructivism (Bijker et al. 1987) pointed to the mutually constitutive relationship between technology and the social, so that technologies have 'interpretive flexibility' as they develop (albeit achieving 'temporary closure' at specific points, understood as allowing the 'black boxing' of technologies). Following ANT, more recent accounts of the relationship between technology and the social in STS derive from, and in different ways enact, a post-humanist understanding. Here, the unit of analysis is heterogeneous practices which carry and produce relations and both humans and technologies are effects or 'achievements' of these practices. In socio-materialist accounts of practice, both material and discursive relations are addressed – hence Haraway's (1991) term 'material-semiotics'. Again, there are different versions, but all emphasise 'relational networks' or 'assemblages' of human and non-human actors and materiality is understood in a relational, emergent sense, with an emphasis on performativity – on 'becoming rather than being' (Barad 2007, Braidotti 2006, Knorr-Cetina 1997, Latour 2005, Mol 2002). For example, adopting a material-semiotic approach to the study of telecare, Pols demonstrates the value of analysing what people and devices 'do' as the achievement of practices rather than as points of departure (Pols 2012). She shows that while different devices may support different forms of care or help them emerge, they do not lead inevitably to those places (Pols 2012). In her study, webcams, introduced to encourage patient peer support, worked best when patients already knew each other, showing that, while webcams could not create intimacy, they could help maintain it.

While it is interesting to note how socio-materialism offers a point of overlap between sociology of health and STS and creates a space within which to examine the heterogeneous practices of digital health, it is equally important to note on-going tensions between sociology of health and STS. As Law (2008, p. 632) has pointed out in his discussion of sociology's relationship to STS, theories and approaches that rely on systems or network logics (as socio-material practice theories do) tend to 'undo social foundations as an explanatory resource'.

This is because, 'since systems have their own relational logic, the latter is likely to reshape the social as much as the technical' and thus the social is 'just as much in need to explanation as the technical' (ibid.). This can be problematic for sociologists working on health and illness, especially those working in a more critical tradition, who seek to explain enduring social orders such as health inequalities. A second, linked, tension arises because STS systems/network approaches tend to focus on *how* things happen, not *why* they do, so that questions focus on: '*How* they arrange themselves. *How* the materials of the world (social, technical, documentary, natural, human, animal) get themselves done in particular locations for a moment in all their heterogeneity' and how these interactions between elements enact realities and knowledges (Law 2008, p. 632, italics in the original), again raising concerns for those working with more foundational and more critical sociologies that develop and rely on more explanatory theories to address 'why?' questions. In summing up the value of the concept of practice for the sociology of health, Cohn (2014, p. 160) makes a similar point when he notes that, in addition to having the potential to resist both the psychological and the individualising features that have come to define the term health behaviour, the concept of practice 'also potentially resists the search for causal explanations, in the form of identifying determinants, and instead embraces the idea that practices are contingent on a whole variety of social and material factors'.

The papers in this collection all illustrate, to different degrees, this resistance to the search for overall causal explanations. However, there are important differences in emphases across the papers in terms of how they discuss the relationship between the social and the technological and how far and how explicitly they engage with deterministic and/or relational thinking. Thus, while it is probably fair to say that all papers share the assumption that digital health comprises sociotechnical practices and not simply technologies that impact upon health, they differ in the extent to which they engage with the materiality *in a relational sense*. Some papers give more emphasis to human than to non-human agency and give little insight into the specificities of the material devices and systems that help constitute the practices as they emerge. Others engage more directly with socio-materialism to show how the practices observed come into being and are sustained.

As a collection, the papers illustrate well the point that no, one, definition or theory of digital health will be sufficient to capture the diversity of sociotechnical practices involved. The collection is offered as a set of individual cases of digital health and a contribution to what we see as an on-going and productive debate between sociology of health and STS that addresses long-standing challenges of avoiding technological determinism while maintaining a clear focus on the materiality and agency of technologies and recognising enduring sets of relations that emerge in new digital health practices while avoiding social determinism.

In the next section, we introduce the papers in this collection. They cover diverse fields of healthcare (reproductive health, primary care, mental health, diabetes care) and diverse technologies (health apps, mobile platforms, smart textiles, time-lapse imaging) and are therefore able to demonstrate clearly the heterogeneity of digital health practices. However, as we suggest below, they can nevertheless be grouped to highlight key aspects of healthcare being (re)-configured in response to the contradictions arising within new practices of digital health.

Key dimensions for approaching ambivalence of digital health

The papers in this collection explore the ambivalence at play when digital technologies become embedded within health practices. The notion of ambivalence has been developed to elaborate contradictory values that are experienced while engaging with quantified data, new forms of connectivity and algorithmic decision-making (Marent *et al.* 2018). By synthesising the main arguments and contributions in each paper of this collection we elaborate on four key dimensions within which digital technologies create ambivalence and (re)configure health practices.

First, *promissory digital health* outlines the configuration of discourses that enact contradictory virtues and imaginaries by which digital technologies and practices gain momentum within the provision of health. Second, *(re)configuring knowledge* highlights how ambivalence is experienced when digital information and data is generated, negotiated and shared within practices of care. Third, *(re)configuring connectivity* elaborates new digital networks and their often contradictory implications for relationships and collaboration between different actors in healthcare. Fourth, *(re)configuring control* investigates how algorithms may produce new forms of authority within decision-making, diagnosis and treatment. In the following, we illustrate how these dimensions are helpful in exploring the ambivalence of digital health across the range of technological devices and fields of practices that are investigated in the papers of this collection.

Promissory digital health

The first important dimension of digital health we highlight concerns the question of how digital health is talked into being through promissory discourses and practices. Law and Singleton (2014, p. 381) have shown that policies can be seen as sets of heterogenous practices (done across various locations) that have potential to 'enact (phenomena) into being'. The first two papers in this collection show how digital health is discursively configured within policy documents including those of professional associations, governments and funding bodies.

Analysing policy documents through the lens of sociology of expectations (Brown and Michael 2003), Martyn Pickersgill (in this collection) reconstructs the dynamics and momentum by which biomedical virtues generate legitimating tropes for new ventures in technology development. Pickersgill develops the notion of 'performative nominalism' in order to draw attention to the strategies of field-building by which professional associations, governments and funding bodies use their own neologisms to talk new therapeutic interventions into being. While Pickersgill's engagement with promissory digital health focuses on the specific case of digital psychiatry, his argument that 'purportedly novel fields have been constituted in part through practices of 'performative nominalism' (whereby articulations of a neologism in relation to established and recent developments participate in producing the referent of the new term)' (Pickersgill, in this collection) could apply to digital health as a whole. Therefore, it is important to recognise how digital health becomes part of 'professional projects' (Abbott 1988) and works as a means to gain status and expand territories. This is highlighted by other papers in this collection, for example, by demonstrating how online information is symbolically transformed in doctor-patient consultation to underscore professional competence (Stevenson *et al.*) or by reconstructing how global actors (such as the World Health Organisation) have built specific types of professional expertise into an algorithm that influences diagnosis of mental disorders on a global scale (Mills and Hilberg).

Another paper concerned explicitly with promissory discourse is by Emma Rich and colleagues (in this collection) who focus on digital health policy and undertake a critical discourse analysis of how inequality is performed within significant UK policy documents to reconstruct the *imaginary* that underpins digital health. Building on critical sociological approaches to public health and health promotion (Baum and Fisher 2014, Petersen and Lupton 1996), they draw attention to the narrow framings of inequalities in digital health policy. They argue that while digital inclusion and inclusion in healthcare remain priorities for government, equality is being reassembled in ways that reflect broader discourses of neo-liberalism, empowerment and the turn to the market for technological solutions which may have the effect of exacerbating inequalities. Thus, digital health policy reflects and reinforces such wider health policy in trying to tackle health inequalities via downstream solutions (reflected in the notion of 'lifestyle drift' (Willams and Fullagar 2019). Rich *et al.*'s examination of the promissory discourse of digital health policy leads them to argue that the discourse enacts specific conditions of actions and types of selfhood, with citizens being positioned as objects of policy interventions in ways that assume particular agential capacities while, at the same time, obscuring the many social, political, cultural and economic inequalities that impede engagement with digital health.

While only these two papers deal explicitly with promissory digital health, we suggest that promissory discourse is more or less explicit within and across all further dimensions of digital health we discuss below and, as we introduce the rest of the papers, we point to the workings of such promises in both their positive and negative forms.

(Re)configuring knowledge
Under the topic '(Re)configuring knowledge', the contributions to this collection address the question of how health information and data is generated, interpreted and shared by digital means in ways that might (re)configure knowledges about medicine, the body and health. Since the early days of the Internet, the sociology of health has contributed useful insights in how this new digital landscape might be contributing to the reconfiguration of knowledge and provide a challenge to traditional doctor-patient relationships (Hardey 1999, Henwood *et al.* 2003). Nettleton's (2004) paper on 'e-scaped medicine' provided a particularly useful provocation for further studies to address the ways in which medical knowledge is being transformed into 'informational knowledge' (Lash 2002) and thereby seen as potentially more accessible by, and shared between, patients and citizens. Many of these studies examined where and how such processes lead to challenges to medical authority and in what circumstances such challenges might result in the recalibration of doctor-patient asymmetries (Kivits 2004, 2009, Mager 2009, Ziebland and Wyke 2012). Even these early studies showed clearly how becoming *informed* about one's health is not a simple matter of having access to information but requires complex processes of navigating, evaluating and negotiating different sources and types of knowledges, especially when their roots are obscured through these very processes of 'informatisation' (Henwood *et al.* 2008) and how challenges to medical authority can lead to re-entrenched, as well as reconfigured, relationships. The continuing growth and diversification of the Internet, especially the development of social media, the increasing use of mobile devices and the extension of consumer-facing developments such as 'direct-to-consumer' marketing, are all associated with a new set of tensions in digital health. The papers in this section seek to explore how the widespread availability of different types and forms of health information, discussion and debate across a range of platforms and enacted across a range of practices, complicates questions of credibility and trust, reconfigures notions of expertise and of citizen reflexivity and, in the context of quantified data, in particular, contributes the emergence of new and diverse patient and citizen subjectivities.

The paper by Alan Petersen and colleagues (in this collection) provides a particularly good example of the complexities and challenges of e-scaped medicine. They explore the criteria employed by Australian patients and carers to establish the credibility of information on controversial and unproven stem cell treatments, increasingly marketed directly to potential consumers. Seeking to find trustworthy information upon which to base their decisions about whether or not to travel abroad for such treatments, Petersen *et al.*'s patients attempt to enact the promissory 'informed patient' but are faced with the challenges of e-scaped medicine and competing claims about stem cell treatments from clinics, patient groups and other sources. The authors develop the concept of 'cartographies of trust' to describe the complex, often tortuous and emotionally fraught, paths by which individuals navigate various online and offline resources in order to decide for or against travelling abroad to receive treatments that are not provided in Australia. The authors show how, in the case of stem cells, where the scientific justification for many treatments offered was nascent, or in some cases non-existent, matters of opinion and belief are liable to be interpreted as matters of fact.

In contrast, Stevenson and her colleagues (in this collection) examine how General Practitioners (GPs) handle online resources in consultations to validate and explain knowledge to patients and offer them self-help outside the clinic. Using conversational analysis of videoed consultations, Stevenson *et al.* demonstrate the 'interactional delicacy' with which such resources are introduced and they discuss and develop Nettleton's (2004) idea of e-scaped medicine explicitly to argue that, in this case, Internet resources are 'recaptured' by GPs with information 'transformed and translated' (following Berg 1992) into a medical offering that works to maintain the asymmetry between patients and practitioners necessary for successful functioning of medical practice.

In the work of Numerato and colleagues (in this collection), concerning how the vaccination debate unfolds on social media, promissory digital health is visible again – here, in the notion that the range of health resources available online can support the emergence of reflexive patients and citizens. The authors argue that the current information environment, dominated by digital communication platforms such as social network sites, requires further developments of our sociological imaginations of the 'reflexive' patient or citizen. Analysing vaccination debates on Facebook, the authors show how proponents and opponents of vaccination actively manage contradictory information about vaccination (content-related reflexivity) in specific economic, political and informational environments (form-related reflexivity). They develop the notion of 'multi-layered reflexivity' to acknowledge social media sites as vehicles as well as objects of reflexivity and to problematise the epistemological capacities of agents to engage and validate public debates on health matters in the post-truth era, joining a broader debate about how 'informational knowledge' changes ways of thinking and reasoning about health and medicine (Lash 2002, Nettleton 2004).

Relatively new literature on self-tracking has highlighted the ways in which digital technologies produce numerical data to provide novel opportunities to track health and monitor bodily conditions, which may produce new 'quantified selves' (Lupton 2016a, Ruckenstein and Schüll 2017, Schüll 2016, Sharon 2017). Pols and colleagues (in this collection) make the case for an 'empirical ethics' approach to this debate as an alternative to 'certain strands of critical sociology of technology', particularly that which focuses on the disciplining character of self-tracking devices, often linked to the responsibilisation thesis. The authors argue that this construction imagines a 'too uniform neo-liberal subject' that relies on a determinist understanding of technology as well as too broad a concept of reflexive modernisation. Through a re-interpretation of key texts on self-tracking (Schüll 2016, Sharon 2017, Sharon and Zandbergen 2017), and new empirical data on everyday self-trackers, they seek to explore how people 'make sense with numbers' and how numbers 'make sense of people' in ways that show the interplay between freedom and power, determining and being determined, acting and being acted upon. They argue that it is precisely within these tensions that exist in different sets of relations that different 'selves' emerge. For example, only some subjects of self-quantification were found to present the 'objectivist-changer style' that is envisaged by health technology developers and problematised by health sociologists. The authors also identify 'aesthetic-semiotic subjects' that use quantified data, alongside sensing and feeling, to better know themselves and/or criticise existing norms and medical expertise. Therefore, the authors argue for more research that uncovers the various types of 'ethico-psychological subjects' of self-quantification to counter the assumed correlation between the use of health apps and behaviour change, so often emphasised within the promissory discourse of digital health.

(Re)configuring connectivity

Under the topic '(Re)configuring connectivity', we have grouped contributions that address the question of how new modes of connectivity affect relationships and collaboration between different actors in healthcare. The papers assembled under this topic are interested in how intimacy and mobility are produced and experienced within new forms of digital connection and how these can support remote forms of clinical follow-up, peer-support or bring forth a new kind of subtle medicalisation. Here, practice theories offer ways to move beyond dichotomous notions of 'cold technologies' and 'warm care' to explore the specific circumstances within which telemonitoring and telecare practices can be central to achieving good care (Pols 2012).

Enrico Piras and Francesco Miele follow an explicitly practice theoretical approach (Gherardi 2010) to investigate computer-mediated communication through a remote monitoring platform connecting diabetes patients and healthcare professionals. The platform has an in-built, messaging system that works as a secure email service between patients and the ward, supporting asynchronous communication between healthcare professionals and patients between clinical visits. The authors argue that their case shows that digital care infrastructures can generate new forms of *digital intimacy* through the continuity of care (in-between clinic visits) and by complementing abstract medical knowledge ('knowing the patient') with exchange in personal messages that allowed clinicians to imagine themselves 'knowing about the patient' (Fairhurst and May 2001). Thus, the affordances of platforms do not necessarily lead to more structured and impersonal interactions but can generate deliberative exchanges that complement medical data with patients' lifeworld experiences, contributing to feelings of being on 'the same page' and leading to more collaborative partnerships. Such in-depth empirical analyses challenge both optimistic and pessimistic readings of promissory discourses of digital health and bring forth understandings of how digital technologies can complement, or even enhance, traditional forms of care within specific embedding environments.

Ian Tucker and Anna Lavis (in this collection) explore digital connectivity within an online peer-support community where users may experience acute mental distress. Making the point that, in digital research, one cannot separate the digital device (e.g. an online platform) from the social phenomenon being studied there, they examine the experiences of mental health crisis as shaped by the online platform. Specifically, they examine how crises are 'constituted or disrupted in and through the complexities of fluctuating digital temporalities' (Tucker and Lavis, in this collection). The authors outline how online connections are often understood as transforming the spatial and temporal arrangements of healthcare by allowing support to be 'always on' and 'always there'. Online support can create a digital immediacy that shapes what comes to be seen as a mental health crises, and is set against the punctuated temporality of formal health services (in terms of access) even for people undergoing acute mental distress. However, their study showes that, once part of an online support group, new temporalities are established via new obligations to reciprocate support in a timely manner, via the re-living of difficult pasts and through decisions not to post for fear of triggering others. Their study suggests further areas for health sociology and STS to explore the temporalities of technologically-mediated interactions of mental health within both synchronous and asynchronous platforms.

Another form of connectivity – combining patients, monitoring machines and health professionals – is analysed by Kelly Joyce (in this collection). The focus in this paper is smart textile medical devices – clothing that uses sensors and fabrics to monitor bodily processes and communicates with data systems in formal hospital or clinical settings through wireless transmission. The cases analysed are the 'bellyband' that replaces the tocodynamotor and foetal heart rate monitor during labour and birth in hospitals, and 'babyband' that replaces the cardiopulmonary monitor in neonatal intensive care units. The study examined these devices 'in the making', at the research and development stage. The paper analyses potential users' views of such smart textiles and explores contemporary contours of medicalisation (Conrad 2007) and surveillance medicine (Armstrong 1995). The study suggests that the soft fabrics of the bellyband contributed to feelings of being 'comfortable' with the device and the lack of wires was seen as having the potential to reduce labouring women's experiences of being 'tethered'. These feeling of comfort and potential for greater mobility contributed to its acceptability to intended users. Similarly, with the babyband, intended users were positive as the baby seemed to be wrapped in (babyband) pajamas, not hooked up to wires and machines. In particular, touch (important for parent-baby bonding) was seen as easier with babyband. Joyce argues that her case study suggests that smart textiles blur the boundary between hospital/medicine and home/daily life and, although patients and devices are fully integrated into data systems, in these particular cases of blurring, medicalisation becomes 'cozy' and surveillance takes on a comfortable form. There were even suggestions that smart textiles could, perhaps paradoxically, support more 'natural' birth. Joyce argues that it is the invisibility and intimacy of the smart textiles that is crucial for this achievement. It is interesting to note that intended users were much less positive about the idea of expanding this monitoring into the home, especially in cases of routine pregnancy and infancy, a development that could easily follow the introduction of over-the-counter systems. Thus, their support was limited to cases where such monitoring was prescribed by clinicians in cases where there was a particular cause for concern and monitoring would otherwise take place in the hospital. While this was not a study of the technologies-in-use, users' anticipations about use suggests there is room for further research concerning the circumstances within which smart textiles produce cozy or less cozy forms of medicalisation.

(Re)configuring control

Under the topic '(Re)configuring control', we have grouped papers that examine how digital algorithms might constitute new forms of authority that penetrate and transform practices of diagnosis and treatment. In different ways, these papers draw attention both to the ways in which authority is inscribed into systems at the design and development stage, and the ways in which algorithmic authority is disrupted, negotiated and reconfigured in different practices of use. The three papers in this section can be understood as engaging with promissory digital health as they investigate algorithmic healthcare in the context of conflicting virtues and values surrounding datafication and algorithmic reasoning. Both optimistic and pessimistic accounts circulate (albeit implicitly) within the practices examined, with the former emphasising algorithms' ability to provide more rational forms of diagnosis and prognosis, and the latter emphasising the ways in which algorithms embed new forms of control that threaten to displace human judgement, decision-making and even care.

China Mills and Eva Hilberg (in this collection) analyse the 'social life' of the WHO's mhGAP-IG algorithm (Mental Health Gap Action Programme Intervention Guide) that was created for non-specialists to diagnose mental health disorders globally. Conducting an ethnographic study, the authors observed how numbers and statistics were presented at WHO mhGAP forums and formed narrative tropes that emphasised treatment gaps and priority conditions around mental health. Following epistemic strategies associated with evidence-based medicine, the algorithm is reconstructed as an 'inscription device' (Latour and Woolgar 1979) that reifies mental health in a particular way and thus also constitutes the condition it aims to diagnose. Through their post-colonial analysis of the algorithm's production, the authors reconstruct the power relationships built into this diagnostic tool and illustrate how this tool (already used in 80 countries) powerfully amplifies a narrow view of mental health that, when used on a global scale, risks displacing other forms of knowledge about mental distress. However, as Mills and Hilberg acknowledge, further research could investigate the performance and 'doing' of the mhGAP-IG beyond the development context and thereby contribute to the wider debate about how technologies are being 'tamed' and 'tinkered' with within situated practices, whereby algorithmic authority may become redefined or reduced (Hout *et al.* 2015, Mol *et al.* 2015).

This issue is the focus of Nete Schwennesen's paper (in this collection) which investigates the 'liveliness' (Lupton 2018b) of an algorithm-based 'virtual trainer' that replaces the physical therapist and allows patients to undertake physical rehabilitation after hip replacement in their homes. Re-stating promissory discourse, she notes both optimistic and pessimistic accounts that see algorithms as either 'revolutionising healthcare' for the better through more rational forms of diagnosis and prognosis or as 'new forms of control' that will 'invade our lives' and displace humans. In both scenarios, algorithms are understood as if they are capable of acting alone. Her analysis challenges these perspectives by exploring the 'socio-material entanglements' by which the algorithmic system is made and enabled to work in practice. Through an ethnographic study across different sites, Schwennesen underscores the *liveliness of algorithms* and draws on Jasanoff and Kim (2015) to demonstrate how design 'imaginaries' differ from practices of use. While the system was designed to take on professional tasks in clinical practice (predictive diagnosis and treatment regimes in particular), Schwennesen charts the ways in which this 'algorithmic authority' is, in fact, negotiated and sometimes broken down in use, arguing that agency and authority do not adhere to the algorithm itself but are produced through associations made between social and material agencies including algorithmic imaginaries, policies, sensors, smartphones, IT workers, private companies, municipalities, physiotherapists and patients. In this way, Schwennesen builds successfully on the work of Pink *et al.* (2018) to draw attention to the 'fragility' and 'incompleteness' of data and algorithms – how the algorithmic system needs to be adjusted and creatively 'repaired' to build and maintain meaningful connections that enable a productive (mutually constitutive) relationship between system and bodies undergoing rehabilitation. An important insight from Schwennesen's work concerns how we think about accountability in digital health. Her study demonstrates the need for a new mode of accountability focusing on how algorithmic systems come to work in medical practice. This differs both from a 'transparency' approach (disclosure of factors that influence algorithmic decision-making) and an approach based on identifying 'bias' (embedded norms and values that may have discriminatory effects) and calls for an approach to accountability that takes into account the actual and concrete encounters between algorithms, health professionals and patients and the various forms of repair work that are needed to make algorithms work in practice.

Finally, Lucy van de Wiel (in this collection) focuses on algorithms in the context of datafication of reproduction and how time-lapse embryo imaging enables a new 'algorithmic way of seeing' – *in silico* vision'. Time-lapse embryo imaging is designed to displace the embryologist's manual appraisal of embryos by filming them in the incubator, quantifying the visual information and predicting their viability through algorithmic analysis. Van de Wiel's paper focuses on new forms of knowledge production emerging within this data-driven time-lapse method of embryo selection and sets them in the techo-economic dynamics of an emerging global data infrastructure. She argues that this new method of embryo selection may not just result in more in vitro fertilisation (IVF) success but also affects the conceptualisation and commercialisation of the assisted reproduction process and the coming into being of prenatal life. Although there is not much evidence to support the introduction of this new technology, van de Wiel points out that the market is growing rapidly and people using IVF increasingly have to decide whether to pay for this additional aspect of the IVF process. Unlike Schwennesen, van de Wiel does not examine clinicians and/or patient's engagement with the new technology. Rather, like Mills and Hilberg, she presents a rich and detailed account of the development of the new technology in its global context, tracing the 'genealogy' (following Vertommen 2017) of data-driven embryo selection in the contemporary global fertility sector. As with Mills and Hilberg's paper, then, in addition to offering rich insight into ways in which new forms of algorithmic agency and authority are constituted, van de Wiel's work opens up further interesting avenues for research concerning how such agency and authority may be redistributed in different use practices.

Conclusion

The papers in this collection show how sociology of health and STS can work together, particularly in the space offered by socio-materialism, to develop more nuanced accounts of how digital health emerges in practice. By synthesising the main arguments and contributions in each paper of this collection, we have suggested that they point to four key dimensions within which digital technologies create ambivalence and (re)configure health practices in relation to promises, knowledge, connectivity and control. As suggested earlier, there are important differences in emphasis across papers – particularly in terms of levels of engagement with socio-materialism and on questions of politics and power. Thus, while all papers acknowledge both continuities and changes associated with the uptake of digital technologies, some are more likely to emphasise the disturbances and disruptions to long-established traditions and vested interests in healthcare that arise when new technologies are introduced, drawing attention to power and hierarchy in care work (e.g. Pickergill; Stevenson *et al.*; Joyce) whereas others focus on continuity, understanding practices of care as always changing and therefore focus their attention on the kinds of adjustments made to achieve good fit between new digital technologies and relations of care (e.g. Schwennesen; Piras and Miele). Furthermore, while some papers make little mention of the wider political-economic landscape within which digital health is developing, others show how such developments are located clearly within the global systems of capital and governance (Mills and Hilberg; van de Wiel; Pickersgill) providing a useful prompt for more research into strategies of 'field-building' in digital health, exploring how professional bodies, governments and funders can all play a part in its consolidation. Rather than seeing these differences in emphases as options to choose between, we prefer to see them as examples of the productive tension between sociology of health and STS that encourages on-going debate and resists the closure of controversy that would result from the imposition of a universal perspective on digital health.

As with all collections, there are necessarily absences. The papers in this collection do not focus specifically on artificial intelligence, big data or robotics, although these areas are implicit in papers on algorithms (van de Wiel; Mills and Hilberg) and self-tracking (Pols). These are emerging technologies that will almost certainly dominate research on digital health produced over the next few years. Furthermore, we have not pulled out the spatiotemporal dimension of digital health although this is clearly important. While the papers in this collection arguably touched on spatiality by focusing on situated practices, cartographies of trust, new mobilities and the recapturing of e-scaped medical knowledge, the temporal has not been explicitly explored (Tucker and Lavis, notwithstanding) and a discussion of its relationship with the spatial is also lacking. However, it is clear that digital technologies are implicated in the enactment of new spatiotemporalities in healthcare, such as instant constructions of patient histories and projections about people's health. Future research may explore how lay people and professionals work with these new spatiotemporalities, as Lomborg *et al.* (2018) have done in relation to self-tracking and Marent *et al.* (2018) have done in relation to HIV care. Other emerging areas of digital health that have clear implications for spatiotemporalities include projections of pandemics (Opitz 2017), embryonic evolution (van de Wiel, this collection) or genetic predictions for future health (Prainsack 2017, Saukko 2018).

Digital methods are also largely implicit in our collection, although current digital health technologies challenge researchers to re-think data sources and methods (Hine 2015, Marres 2017, Pink *et al.* 2016, Roberts *et al.* 2016). A key aspect of the digital today is the ongoing capture of vast amounts of data about social life. Whether searching the web, engaging in an online discussion board or carrying the smartphone on us while cycling or running, the digital captures our transactions and movements continuously and in real-time. This creates a new source of, so-called 'natural data' that has not been produced for scientific purposes but, nevertheless, is often used for research or commercial exploitation. Only a few papers in this collection are based upon data sources produced within digitised environments – Facebook posts in a debate about vaccination (Numerato *et al.*), online messaging/posts in a mental health peer support network (Tucker and Lavis) and messages exchanged between health professionals and patients through a mobile health platform for diabetes care (Piras and Miele). These papers raise important questions about how established research methods such as observations or qualitative analysis need to be further developed. It will be important for further research to reflect explicitly on the challenges, opportunities and implications of applying digital methods within health research.

Address for correspondence: Flis Henwood, School of Applied Social Science, University of Brighton, Watson Building, Falmer, Brighton, BN1 9PH, UK.
E-mail: F.Henwood@brighton.ac.uk

Acknowledgements

We are very grateful to the Brocher Foundation (Geneva) for supporting us as Visiting Researchers during February 2019 to complete the final editorial work for this collection. We also wish to thank Dr Catherine Will for her valuable feedback on the first draft of this editorial. Finally, we want to thank all the reviewers for providing constructive and insightful comments on the papers in this collection.

References

Abbott, A. (1988) *The System of Professions: An Essay on the Division of Expert Labor.* Chicago: University of Chicago Press.
Armstrong, D. (1995) The rise of surveillance medicine, *Sociology of Health & Illness*, 17, 3, 393–404.
Barad, K. (2007) *Meeting the Universe Halfway: Quantum Physics and the Entanglement of Matter and Meaning.* Durham, NC: Duke University Press.
Baum, F. and Fisher, M. (2014) Why behavioural health promotion endures despite its failure to reduce health inequities, *Sociology of Health & Illness*, 36, 2, 213–25.
Berg, M. (1992) The construction of medical disposals Medical sociology and medical problem solving in clinical practice, *Sociology of Health & Illness*, 14, 2, 151–80.
Bijker, W.E., Hughes, T.P., Pinch, T. and Douglas, D.G. (1987) *The Social Construction of Technological Systems: New Directions in the Sociology and History of Technology.* Cambridge, MA: MIT press.
Bourdieu, P. (1984) *Distinction: A Social Critique of the Judgement of Taste.* Abingdon: Routledge.

Braidotti, R. (2006) Posthuman, all too human: towards a new process ontology, *Theory, Culture & Society*, 23, 7–8, 197–208.

Brown, N. and Michael, M. (2003) A sociology of expectations: retrospecting prospects and prospecting retrospects, *Technology Analysis & Strategic Management*, 15, 3–18.

Cohn, S. (2014) From health behaviours to health practices: an introduction, *Sociology of Health & Illness*, 36, 2, 157–62.

Conrad, P. (2007) *The Medicalisation of Society*. Baltimore: John Hopkins University Press.

Fairhurst, K. and May, C. (2001) Knowing patients and knowledge about patients: evidence of modes of reasoning in the consultation?, *Family Practice*, 18, 5, 501–5.

Gherardi, S. (2010) Telemedicine: a practice-based approach to technology, *Human Relations*, 63, 4, 501–24.

Giddens, A. (1984) *The Constitution of Society: Outline of the Theory of Structuration*. Berkeley: University of California Press.

Haraway, D. (1991) *Simians, Cyborgs and Women: The Reinvention of Nature*. London: Free Association.

Hardey, M. (1999) Doctor in the house: the Internet as a source of lay health knowledge and the challenge to expertise, *Sociology of Health & Illness*, 21, 6, 820–35.

Harries, T. and Rettie, R. (2018) Walking as a social practice: dispersed walking and the organisation of everyday practices, *Sociology of Health & Illness*, 38, 6, 874–83.

Henwood, F., Wyatt, S., Hart, A. and Smith, J. (2003) 'Ignorance is bliss sometimes' constraints on the emergence of the 'informed patient' in the changing landscape of health information, *Sociology of Health & Illness*, 25, 6, 589–607.

Henwood, F., Harris, R., Burdett, S. and Marshall, A. (2008) Health intermediaries? Positioning the public library in e-health discourse. In Wathen, C.N., Wyatt, S. and Harris, R. (eds) *Mediating Health Information: The Go-Betweens in a Changing Socio-Technical Landscape*, pp 38–55. Basingstoke: Springer.

Hine, C. (2015) *Ethnography for the Internet: Embedded, Embodied and Everyday*. London, UK: Bloomsbury Publishing.

Hout, A., Pols, J. and Willems, D. (2015) Shining trinkets and unkempt gardens: on the materiality of care, *Sociology of Health & Illness*, 37, 8, 1206–17.

Jasanoff, S. and Kim, S.-H. (2015) *Dreamscapes of Modernity: Sociotechnical Imaginaries and the Fabrication of Power*. Chicago: University of Chicago Press.

Keane, H., Weier, M., Fraser, D. and Gartner, C. (2017) Anytime, anywhere': vaping as social practice, *Critical Public Health*, 27, 465–76.

Kivits, J. (2004) Researching the 'Informed Patient', *Information, Communication & Society*, 7, 4, 510–30.

Kivits, J. (2009) Everyday health and the internet: a mediated health perspective on health information seeking, *Sociology of Health & Illness*, 31, 5, 673–87.

Knorr-Cetina, K. (1997) Sociality with objects: social relations in postsocial knowledge societies, *Theory, Culture & Society*, 14, 4, 1–30.

Lash, S. (2002) *Critique of Information*. London: Sage.

Latour, B. (2005) *Reassembling the Social: An Introduction to Actor-Network-Theory*. Oxford: Oxford University Press.

Latour, B. and Woolgar, S. (1979) *Laboratory Life: The Construction of Scientific Facts*. Princeton, New Jersey: Princeton University Press.

Law, J. (2008) On sociology and STS, *The Sociological Review*, 56, 4, 623–49.

Law, J. and Singleton, V. (2014) ANT, multiplicity and policy, *Critical Policy Studies*, 8, 4, 379–96.

Lomborg, S., Thylstrup, N.B. and Schwartz, J. (2018) The temporal flows of self-tracking: checking in, moving on, staying hooked, *New Media & Society*, 20, 12, 4590–607.

Lupton, D. (2016a) *The Quantified Self*. Cambridge: John Wiley & Sons.

Lupton, D. (2016b) Towards critical digital health studies: reflections on two decades of research in health and the way forward, *Health*, 20, 1, 49–61.

Lupton, D. (ed) (2017) *Self-Tracking, Health and Medicine: Sociological Perspectives*. Abingdon: Routledge.

Lupton, D. (2018a) *Digital Health: Critical and Cross-Disciplinary Perspectives*. New York: Routledge.

Lupton, D. (2018b) *How do Data Come to Matter?* Living and becoming with personal data: Big Data & Society.

MacKenzie, D. and Wajcman, J. (1999) *The Social Shaping of Technology*. Maidenhead: Open University Press.

Mager, A. (2009) Mediated Health. Sociotechnical practices of providing and using online health information, *New Media & Society*, 11, 7, 1123–42.

Marent, B., Henwood, F., Darking, M. and EmERGE Consortium. (2018) Ambivalence in digital health. Co-designing an mHealth platform for HIV care, *Social Science & Medicine*, 215, 133–41.

Marres, N. (2017) *Digital Sociology. The Reinvention of Social Research*. Cambridge: Polity Press.

Mol, A. (2002) *The Body Multiple: Ontology in Medical Practice*. Durham, NC: Duke University Press.

Mol, A., Moser, I. and Pols, J. (eds). (2015) *Care in Practice: On Tinkering in Clinics, Homes and Farms*. Bielefeld: Transcript.

Nettleton, S. (2004) The emergence of E-scaped medicine?, *Sociology*, 38, 4, 661–79.

Opitz, S. (2017) Simulating the world The digital enactment of pandemics as a mode of global self-observation, *European Journal of Social Theory*, 20, 3, 392–416.

Petersen, A. (2019) *Digital Health and Technological Promise: A Sociological Inquiry*. Abingdon: Routledge.

Petersen, A. and Lupton, D. (1996) *The new Public Health: Health and Self in the age of Risk*. Thousand Oaks, CA: Sage Publications, Inc.

Pink, S., Heather, H., Postill, J., Hjorth, L., *et al.* (2016) *Digital Ethnography*. Principles and practices: Sage.

Pink, S., Ruckenstein, M., Willim, R. and Duque, M. (2018) Broken data: conceptualising data in an emerging world, *Big Data & Society*, 5, 1, 2053951717753228.

Pols, J. (2012) *Care at a Distance: On the Closeness of Technology*. Amsterdam: Amsterdam University Press.

Prainsack, B. (2017) *Personalized Medicine: Empowered Patients in the 21st Century?* New York: NYU Press.

Reckwitz, A. (2002) Toward a theory of social practices a development in culturalist theorizing, *European Journal of Social Theory*, 5, 2, 243–63.

Roberts, S., Snee, H., Hine, C., Morey, Y., *et al.* (eds) (2016) *Digital Methods for Social Science: An Interdisciplinary Guide to Research Innovation*. Basingstoke: Palgrave Macmillan.

Ruckenstein, M. and Schüll, N.D. (2017) The datafication of health, *Annual Review of Anthropology*, 46, 261–78.

Saukko, P. (2018) Digital health–a new medical cosmology? The case of 23andMe online genetic testing platform, *Sociology of Health & Illness*, 40, 8, 1312–26.

Schatzki, T. (1996) *Social Practices. A Wittgensteinian Approach to Human Activity and the Social*. Cambridge: Cambridge University Press.

Schüll, N.D. (2016) Data for life: wearable technology and the design of self-care, *Biosocieties*, 11, 3, 317–33.

Sharon, T. (2017) Self-tracking for health and the quantified self: re-articulating autonomy, solidarity, and authenticity in an age of personalized healthcare, *Philosophy & Technology*, 30, 1, 93–121.

Sharon, T. and Zandbergen, D. (2017) From data fetishism to quantifying selves: self-tracking practices and the other values of data, *New Media & Society*, 19, 11, 1695–709.

Shove, E., Pantzar, M. and Watson, M. (2012) *The Dynamics of Social Practice: Everyday Life and how it Changes*. Thousand Oaks, UK: Sage Publications.

Supski, S., Lindsay, J. and Tanner, C. (2017) University students' drinking as a social practice and the challenge for public health, *Critical Public Health*, 27, 2, 228–37.

Vertommen, S. (2017) From the pergonal project to Kadimastem: a genealogy of Israel's reproductive-industrial complex, *Biosocieties*, 12, 2, 282–306.

Willams, O. and Fullagar, S. (2019) Lifestyle drift and the phenomenon of 'citizen shift'in contemporary UK health policy, *Sociology of Health & Illness*, 41, 1, 20–35.

Williams, R., Weiner, K., Henwood, F. and Will, C. (2018) Constituting practices, shaping markets: remaking healthy living through commercial promotion of blood pressure monitors and scales, *Critical Public Health*, 1–13. https://doi.org/10.1080/09581596.2018.1497144

Ziebland, S. and Wyke, S. (2012) Health and illness in a connected world: how might sharing experiences on the internet affect people's health?, *Milbank Quarterly*, 90, 2, 219–49.

Sociology of Health & Illness Vol. 41 No. S1 2019 ISSN 0141-9889, pp. 16–30
doi: 10.1111/1467-9566.12811

Digitising psychiatry? Sociotechnical expectations, performative nominalism and biomedical virtue in (digital) psychiatric praxis

Martyn Pickersgill ⓘ

Centre for Biomedicine, Self and Society, Edinburgh Medical School, University of Edinburgh, Edinburgh, UK

Abstract   Digital artefacts and infrastructures have been presented as ever more urgent and necessary for mental health research and practice. Telepsychiatry, mHealth, and now digital psychiatry have been promoted in this regard, among other endeavours. Smartphone apps have formed a particular focus of promissory statements regarding the improvement of epistemic and clinical work in psychiatry. This article contextualises and historicises some of these developments. In doing so, I show how purportedly novel fields have been constituted in part through practices of 'performative nominalism' (whereby articulations of a neologism in relation to established and recent developments participate in producing the referent of the new term). Central to this has been implicit and explicit extolment of what I term biomedical virtues in public-facing and professionally orientated discourse. I document how emphases on various virtues have shifted with the attention of psychiatry to different digital modalities, culminating with knowledge-production in mental health as one significant focus.

Keywords: E-health, health technology/technology assessment, mental health and illness, psychiatry/psychiatric care, STS (science and technology studies)

Introduction

Within psychiatry and psychology, digital artefacts and infrastructures have been presented as urgent and necessary. In the UK, for instance, Prime Minister Theresa May promised 'a £67.7 million digital mental health package' (HM Government, 2017). Various articles ostensibly focused on the digital within mental health in general or psychiatry specifically attend to heterogeneous (and often mundane) information and communication technologies (ICT) such as text messaging, web sites, blogs, social media and apps (Harding *et al.* 2015, Mohr *et al.* 2017, Torous 2014). Mobile digital technologies have been employed not only as interventions for mental ill-health, but are on occasion positioned as a means of generating new kinds of information for psychiatrists about patients and pathologies.

Technologies currently in regular operation include therapeutic interactions enabled by videoconferencing (i.e. telepsychiatry), and computer-based interventions like online cognitive behaviour therapy (CBT) platforms that are advocated by programs such as NHS England's Improving Access to Psychological Therapies (IAPT) initiative. Furthermore, commonly and sometimes enthusiastically used mobile phone applications have proliferated. These often promise to help individuals live with or recover from feelings and experiences associated with psychiatric disorders. Such apps have been argued to widen the 'possibilities of therapeutic engagement' (ibid: 262) and 'recast the spatiality and temporality of healthcare' (Trnka 2016: 248, see also Fullager *et al.* 2017).

In this article, I contextualise and historicise some of these developments, charting innovation and discussion about telepsychiatry, mHealth and what has more recently been called digital psychiatry. I argue that these purportedly novel fields have been constituted in part through the implicit and explicit extolment of biomedical virtues in promissory statements about them. I demonstrate how emphases on various virtues have shifted with the attention of psychiatry to different digital modalities, culminating with knowledge-production in mental health as one significant focus.

Conceptual Background

In this article, I employ the concept of 'biomedical virtue' to characterise some of the positive impulses and practices of psychiatry (as understood by practitioners) that are variously framed as being enhanced through, or deactivated by, digital developments. By this term, I do not quite mean 'medical ethics' – in either a straightforwardly moralistic way, or in Osborne's (1994) more capacious definition – nor what Freidson (1988[1970]: 160) called the 'operative norms of performance' within medicine. Instead, biomedical virtue refers to the (profession-defined) praxis of goodness within the laboratory and the clinic. Through widespread instantiation across a range of registers (e.g. public-facing documents and intra-professional conversations), I suggest that articulations of virtue might exert disciplining effects on actual practices. Consequently, biomedical virtue can have an ambiguous existence as both aspiration and actuality.

The rhetoric of biomedical virtue can be strategically and more spontaneously deployed in support of various professional projects and goals. This is particularly evident when what is perhaps the canonical biomedical virtue, the prevention of death, is used to justify continued symbolic and material investment in technological processes that are yet to demonstrate clinical worth. Martin *et al.* (2008) provide a striking example of this through a case study of private umbilical cord blood stem cell banking. They demonstrate how a market has emerged, underpinned by visions of cord blood as having *potential* therapeutic application for assorted life-limiting or threatening disorders that a new-born baby might one day experience. Accordingly, the biomedical virtue of preventing death (or at least, severe suffering) has played a key role in powering a promissory bioeconomy (ibid). More generally, diverse forms of therapeutic promise (Rubin 2008: 13) have been constituted with and through various kinds of biomaterials, configuring these as promissory matter (Brown *et al.* 2006: 330) to which hopes and capital are associated. In effect, articulating virtue can generate value.

Professional projects that might involve the strategic deployment of biomedical virtues to justify their necessity include practices of what I call 'performative nominalism'. Intellectual debts are owed here to Ian Hacking, whose concept of dynamic nominalism captures how, sometimes, 'our classifications and our cases emerge hand in hand, each egging the other one' (Hacking 2002: 106). My adaptation of Hacking's term underscores the role of agency: co-emergence can be deliberately and actively fostered by agents who reflexively reconfigure their (e.g. professional) identities in the process. Practices reminiscent of performative nominalism come from a variety of fields; sociologists of biomedical ethics, for instance, have demonstrated how ethical commentary shapes technoscientific development and thus the need and role of bioethicists (Hedgecoe and Martin 2003). Closer both to psychiatry and to my specific framing of performative nominalism, scholars like Brosnan (2011) and Conrad and De Vries (2011) have detailed how the deployment of the neologism 'neuroethics' has contributed to the organisation of a field and to consolidating its authority.

Such insights emerge from wider work on the sociology of expectations, and form a more general backdrop to the analysis presented here. As Brown and Michael (2003: 3) argue, expectations 'are crucial to providing the dynamism and momentum upon which so many ventures in science and technology depend' (see also Borup et al. 2006, Brown 2003). In the case of biomedicine, the promise of new health technologies involves the mobilisation of 'a range of claims about their future therapeutic impact' (Webster 2002: 443). This includes psychiatry, where investments in neuroscience, for instance, are predicated in part upon the promise that these will enhance clinical practice (Pickersgill 2011). In what follows, I regard performative nominalism as one mechanism within the sociology of expectations, and biomedical virtues as legitimising tropes for promises made. As we will see, promissory discourse has been a key feature of commentary upon and pronouncements regarding the role and impact of digital technologies in and on psychiatry.

Methodological Approach

This article follows a similar methodological approach to Williams et al.'s (2015) analysis of trends and transformations in the area of digital interventions for monitoring and managing sleep. Specifically, I interrogated various (online) documents to ascertain how 'problems, prospects and possibilities' (Williams et al. 2015, : 1041) relating to the use of mobile digital technologies psychiatry were expressed. I was particularly attentive to what had come to count as 'digital psychiatry', how this discourse was being propelled, and what its antecedents were. In so doing, I was alert to 'uncertainty statements' (Webster 2002: 443); that is, comments suggestive of an organised ambivalence (cf. Benjamin 2011) within psychiatry that simultaneously embraces hope for innovation while recognising the potential for disappointment.

Some of the texts discussed in this article were initially collected and examined as part of three Wellcome Trust projects on the sociology of mental health. The first, which took place over 2011–2015, considered how the need for enhancing access to mental healthcare had emerged as a political and clinical concern in the UK, how it was being addressed, and what the ramifications of change were for clinicians and patients. The second study, begun in 2015 and ongoing, analyses how ideas about the nature of diagnosis in US and UK psychiatric research and practice are moving in response to various challenges within and beyond the mental health disciplines. Initiated in 2017, the third project forms part of a wider programme of work on 'Biomedicine, Self and Society'. Through this, I am exploring shifting logics of neuroscience and mental health that migrate away from an exclusive focus on psychopathology and extend into the study of 'normal' subjective experience.

As part of the continuing documentary analysis, interviewing, focus groups and observation at clinical symposia that comprises these projects, I realised I was encountering seemingly increasing – and increasingly high profile – references to digital mental health technologies. Discussions of apps, for instance, were found within government agenda-setting documents, research funder roadmaps and commentaries in high-impact psychiatry journals. The data corpus for this article thus developed from these materials, and was augmented through additional targeted searches in key journals and websites such as that of the UK Department of Health and the American Psychiatric Association (as well as through examining links between the aforementioned documents and other relevant commentaries and position statements). My broadly abductive (Timmermans and Tavory 2012) analysis accordingly entailed both a close reading of isolated texts referring to digital mental health, and a consideration of these in relation to the data collected within the aforementioned studies, and the larger problematic they address: that is, in what ways is mental health praxis changing, and what is powering those shifts?

Psychiatry and Technology

> What greater scourge could befall psychiatry than becoming impersonal – which means losing sight of the persona of the patient? The great technological advances that have taken place in medicine within the last three-quarter century raise this threat – the loss of the personal relationship with the patient. The whole tradition is based on healing and caring for the sick as persons, through constant personal contact between the doctor and the patient
>
> (Bartemeier 1952: 1)

The comments above come from Leo H. Bartemeier's 1952 Presidential Address to the American Psychiatric Association (APA). He used this to sound caution at the rise of techn(olog)ical approaches to clinical practice, and to underscore the therapeutic import of interpersonal relationships. Bartemeier's anxieties orientate us to the great degree to which psychiatrists have long engaged with a wide range of technologies. These often emerged from within allied disciplines such as neurology (e.g. EEG; Schirmann 2014), physiology (e.g. PET; Dumit 2004) and nuclear medicine (e.g. MRI; Joyce 2008). In the mid-20th-century US, psychiatrists like Bartemeier were often highly psychoanalytically orientated, (Hale 1995); yet, interventions into neurological structure and function to treat mental ill-health were widely employed. Most controversially, these included ECT and lobotomy. Sadowsky (2006: 22) has illuminated how receptive many psychoanalysts were to ECT, underscoring 'the extent of eclecticism in American psychiatry'. For lobotomy, Raz (2008: 387) demonstrated that 'psychosurgical discourse adopted key concepts from psychoanalytical discourse' and vice versa. Hence, technical apparatuses within psychiatry can be understood to help direct practitioner attention, while also becoming enfolded within existing theoretical and operational regimes (Pickersgill 2010).

'Telepsychiatry' is a more contemporary instantiation of a (partial) psychiatric embracement of an external technological innovation; namely, telemedicine (APA, 2017b). Now a heterogeneous discipline encompassing an array of technologies and applications (Lupton and Maslen 2017), this was defined in the first editorial of the Telemedicine Journal as: 'the delivery of care to patients anywhere in the world by combining communications technology with medical expertise' (Goldberg 1995: 1). For almost 30 years, clinicians and policymakers have advocated telemedicine as a means of containing healthcare costs and enhancing access (Lehous et al. 2002). In the UK, for instance, early policy announcements emphasised 'the novelty and potential of telemedicine systems in a rhetoric that stresses the technology's place in a paradigm shift in the conceptualization and organization of British health care' (May et al. 2001: 1890). It was in part through such discourse, and via journals, research groups, professional associations and conferences that bore the name 'telemedicine', that the field was constituted (ibid: 1981). This can be regarded as a form of performative nominalism: the coining of 'telemedicine' and the badging of activities as such contributed to galvanising hopes and resources in ways that facilitated its consolidation.

Telepsychiatry is defined straightforwardly by organisations like the APA as an operation whereby 'psychiatric services [are] provided remotely via a video link' (APA, 2017b), and the

Royal Australian & New Zealand College of Psychiatrists (RANZCP) as 'a consultation between a patient and a psychiatrist conducted via video-conference' (RANZCP, undated). These professional bodies suggest that specific uses of telepsychiatry include 'psychiatric evaluations, therapy (individual therapy, group therapy, family therapy), patient education and medication management' (APA, 2017b; see, similarly, RANZCP, 2013: 5). Telepsychiatry apparently 'offers many advantages and is becoming more available' (APA, 2017b); as current APA President Anita Everett stated, one such advantage includes the use of telepsychiatry to 'help increase access' to care (APA, 2017a; see also Bender 2008). Similarly, the RANZCP website poses the question, 'Why use telepsychiatry?', and goes on to answer that it 'can greatly improve access to psychiatric services for people in rural and remote areas, and in other situations where face-to-face consultations are impracticable' (RANZCP, undated).

More generally, research and practice initiatives around telepsychiatry in a range of nations have been inscribed (Akrich 1992) with this logic of access; intervention trials, for instance, commonly note the utility of the technology in terms of enhancing admission into therapy for those who might otherwise be excluded from care (e.g. Kessler *et al.* 2009, Nelson *et al.* 2003, O'Reilly *et al.* 2007).[1] Clinicians, though, have often been presented as resistant to the introduction of telepsychiatry due to assumed deleterious effects on the relationship between doctor and patient deemed central to therapeutic engagement and success. As May *et al.* (2001) and (Wagnild *et al.* 2006) have shown, such matters have inflected the reception of telepsychiatry – and telemedicine more generally (May *et al.* 2003) – for two decades now, with the technological shaping of inter-subjective action constitutive of telepsychiatric practice considered an object of clinical concern.

Telepsychiatry, then, has been constructed as simultaneously enabling and curtailing different kinds of biomedical virtue in psychiatry. On the one hand, and most importantly within promissory discourse, telepsychiatry might increase access to therapy. Even half a century ago, access had been – in the words of APA Medical Director Walter Barton – 'a concern of the APA for a long time' (Barton 1971: 522). Today, the enhancement of access continues to be a virtue (co-)constituted through a range of (inter)national policy and clinical debates. These are underpinned by a form of humanitarian reason (Fassin 2011) in which access is configured as an unproblematic social good. On the other hand, telepsychiatry – as May *et al.* (2001) and Wagnild *et al.* (2006) have documented, and as I have sometimes encountered in my wider fieldwork – is judged to have the potential to undercut a positive doctor–patient relationship. The degree to which the development, maintenance and promotion of this dynamic is felt by many to be virtuous is apparent through recurrent celebrations of the doctor–patient relationship as (for instance) 'a keystone of care' (Goold and Lipkin 1999: S26). The import of this virtue is also illuminated by a wide-ranging literature describing various purported challenges to it, including industrial, economic and political impacts on healthcare systems. Perhaps, especially significant in psychiatry, given the role of inter-subjectivity *as* therapy, the doctor-patient relationship is recurrently underscored as of 'central importance' (as Allan Tasman put it during an APA Presidential Address) (Tasman 2000: 1762). In the case of psychiatry, then, discourse upon the use of communicative technologies within the broad field of telepsychiatry directs attention to two different modes of biomedical virtue, one of which may interfere (Pols 2003) with the other.

'Mobilising' Psychiatry

In the previous section, I introduced some of the ways psychiatry has negotiated new biomedical technologies, focussing in particular on telepsychiatry. This has been a major focus for psychiatric thought about how to interweave information and communications technologies into clinical practice, as well as a striking example of how particular biomedical virtues configure field-building and the reception of innovation. It is not, of course, the only illustration that could be advanced. Online psychological therapy, in particular CBT, has likewise been advocated and debated, with a range of articles appearing in widely read periodicals (e.g. Psychiatric News and the American Journal of Psychiatry). In the UK, online therapy portals like Beating the Blues have been rolled out across the NHS, and are endorsed by bodies such as the National Institute of Health and Care Excellence (NICE) in England and the Scottish Intercollegiate Guidelines Network (SIGN). Online therapies, where users navigate through pre-set text and exercises, tend to be associated with the treatment of so-called 'mild to moderate' instantiations of common conditions like depression, and are deployed through psychological and primary care services. As well as pre-set content, newer tools using chatbots are more interactive – like 'woebot', a 'fully automated conversational agent' (Fitzpatrick *et al.* 2017). Considerations of telepsychiatric approaches as avenues for treatment vary more widely across a range of conditions, including those for which psychiatrists often take clinical responsibility (e.g. schizophrenia). In recent years, telepsychiatry has become frequently operationalised through mobile phones, and online therapies – once accessed largely through desktop PCs – have been 'mobilised' as smartphone applications (i.e. apps).

In this section, I explore how apps are being promoted through the diverse field of 'mHealth' (or 'm-health'; i.e. 'mobile health'). As sociologists Williams, Coveney and Meadows have discussed, through mobile digital technologies 'patients, proto-patients and the wider public may now track their bodies, share their data, participate in online discussion and support groups, and use the information they gather to improve or optimise their health' (Williams *et al.* 2015: 1045). mHealth is a key facet of this matrix of illness, optimisation and technology. In one public-facing article, the UK Medical Research Council (MRC) defined mHealth as 'the name for medicine and public health supported by mobile phones; now a burgeoning field' (MRC, 2015). According to the APA (undated), the 'expanding use of mobile health (mHealth) technologies is unprecedented in the history of medicine' – and there has been 'growing patient, clinical, government, and payer interest in the potential of mHealth technologies for psychiatric clinical care'. To this end, the APA convened a working group to interrogate mobile phone apps which assert that they promote wellbeing and treat mental ill-health. The group went on to develop an evaluation model for psychiatrists to use when ascertaining whether an app might afford a patient therapeutic benefit.

One key difference between the deployment of telepsychiatry and mental health apps is the responsibilisation of the user. In the former case, the onus lies with the clinician to learn and implement new skills and care practices; in the latter, the responsibility lies primarily (though as we will later see, not exclusively) with the purportedly empowered patient. For instance, the World Health Organization recommended in their Mental Health Action Plan that 'the promotion of self-care' for mental ill-health could be encouraged through 'the use of electronic and mobile health technologies' (WHO 2013: 14). In the UK, the MRC (2015) has argued that mHealth 'offers a simple and low cost way to empower patients to take responsibility for their own health – something that's particularly effective in mental health'.

The innovation and implementation of mHealth within the UK has been supported by a strong policy push towards innovation (HM Government, 2017; Mental Health Taskforce, 2016: 38; National Information Board, 2014). Investment has come, for instance, from the NHS National Institute for Health Research, such as in the MindTech Healthcare Technology Co-operative: 'a national centre focussing on the development, adoption and evaluation of new technologies for mental healthcare and dementia'.[2] Indeed, the NHS hosts an online library of apps where patients are invited to 'Find digital tools to help you manage and improve your health' (NHS, 2018). In August 2018, 19 apps featured under the 'Mental Health' section of the site, three of which were badged as 'Being Tested in the NHS'. One of these, Chill Panda, carries the strapline, 'Learn to relax, manage your worries and improve your wellbeing with Chill Panda'. Nevertheless, a disclaimer notes that apps in the Library 'are not intended to be a substitute for a consultation with a healthcare professional. It is up to you to contact a healthcare professional if you are concerned about your health' (NHS, 2018). Clinical expertise thus remains salient, even as (potential) patients are encouraged to contribute to their care.

In the US, the National Institute of Mental Health (NIMH) has, like other sponsors internationally, actively fostered research into mHealth in part through promissory statements articulating tropes of biomedical virtue. It was, for instance, explicitly flagged within the agency's Strategic Plan for Research. This 60-page document described four Strategic Objectives for the NIMH, each of which included two 'Highlights' which contextualised the Objectives through details of existing and anticipated research. The final Highlight – 'A Therapist in One's Pocket: mHealth to Improve Access to Mental Health Care' – posited digital technologies 'such as smartphones, wearable sensors, and video games' as having the capacity to address ongoing problems around access to healthcare. (NIMH, 2015: 51). Like telepsychiatry before it, then, mHealth was thus presented as a technological fix to an issue of healthcare policy, planning and delivery. Nevertheless, the biomedical virtue of direct clinical care was inscribed into the Highlight, with the NIMH making clear that digital tools will 'extend rather than replace the therapist' – at least for 'those with the most disabling illnesses' (ibid). As for specific uses, mobile technologies were described as being employed currently 'for improving adherence to treatment or for collecting passive data about activity or sleep, but the additional possibilities of these technologies are just emerging' (NIMH, 2015: 51). Such entangling of the actual and the anticipatory lends credibility to the promise underpinning the forward-looking statements threading through the Highlight.

More recently, a NIH-wide Funding Opportunity Announcement (FOA; posted 30 November 2017) encouraged applications that 'develop or adapt innovative mobile health (mHealth) technology specifically suited for low- and middle-income countries (LMICs) and determine the health-related outcomes associated with implementation of the technology' (NIH, 2017). The specifically NIMH component of the FOA called for the 'development or innovative application of cost-effective, sustainable, and scalable technologies to improve the accessibility, effectiveness, or delivery of mental health care in LMICs'. Similarly, the MRC (2015) has noted that 'the popularity of mobile phones isn't confined to developed countries. Their widespread use, even in the most remote locations, could help people get faster and easier access to healthcare'. Such calls and statements from funders like the NIMH and the MRC underscore how mHealth, including for psychiatric intervention, is being folded into highly financed regimes of what has been termed 'global health' (as intimated by Williams *et al.* 2015: 1051).[3]

One means of tracking the evolution and increasing visibility of mHealth is through the statements made about it by the psychiatrist and former NIMH Director Thomas Insel (in post 2002–2015). Once cautious about the use of technological interventions in mental health (Shoham and Insel 2011), Insel has become an ever more vocal advocate of (mobile) digital techniques in psychiatric settings. When, during a 2013 *Boston Globe* interview, he was queried about the future of psychotherapy, Insel described how it 'might be that what we call "psychotherapy" is a mobile app that you download and is crafted for your specific cognitive domain' (Koven 2013). A year later, *Psychology Today* asked Insel 'What's a clinical innovation you're excited about?'; he responded: 'Web-based and mobile CBT' (Nemko 2014). The following March, Insel was quoted in *Counseling Today* describing how the 'advent of new devices, mHealth (mobile health), cognitive training and social media will likely change the landscape of mental health care' (Burnett 2015). In 2015, Insel left the NIMH to work for Alphabet on device-orientated approaches to mental health. In a discussion with *Fortune* magazine, he accounted for this interest in technology as relating to wider shifts in understandings of psychopathology: where once disorders like depression were seen as 'just a chemical imbalance', now they are considered to be 'problems with how neural circuits are communicating' – an issues that 'we may be able to modulate with devices' (Sukel 2015).

Despite a widespread lauding of mHealth, concerns have also been raised about the security and commodification of the data that apps might harness, given their commonly commercial origins (Lupton 2014). This includes mental health apps (Nicholas *et al.* 2015), with one news piece for instance addressing the problem explicitly and bluntly: 'Many app developers may be selling patient data for profit' (Torous *et al.* 2016). In a review of opportunities and challenges associated with apps, psychiatrists Marley and Farooq (2015) also highlighted concerns about the clinical accuracy of information presented, and the (lack of a) role of medical expertise in the development of some software – as well as overt risk to patients using apps partly as a consequence of errors and omissions (see also Zhang *et al.* 2015). In an analysis of the challenges associated with digital technologies and mental health, Ben-Zeev (2017: 108) argued that the 'client-clinician therapeutic alliance will be affected by the introduction of telecommunication and telemonitoring technology'. The discussions about the hazards of mHealth proliferating within psychiatric discourse underscore the increasingly everyday nature of mobile digital technologies for mental health, as well as the responsibility many clinicians feel regarding the need to better understand the risks and benefits associated with them when negotiating patients' own questions and concerns.

Through disseminating and defining the concept of mHealth, and generating ethical discourse around its instantiations, professional associations like the APA and funders like the MRC and NIMH contribute to processes of performative nominalism, helping to reify mHealth as an object of (cautious) fascination. Within (for instance) the concerns of physicians, the disclaimers of NHS websites, and the tacit and overt endorsement of mental health apps by health-related organisation, we can see at least two biomedical virtues (beyond the enhancement of access) as playing a role in this performative nominalism. For one, there is – as explicitly stated by the WHO (2013: 14) – the virtue of encouraging self-care. As Rose (2001), among others, has pointed out, public health in a range of countries commonly emphasises care of the self in order to stave off pathology and optimise present health. Self-care is increasingly presented as a virtue, with clinical professionals and societies framing it as a means of empowering patients and cutting healthcare costs (see Rimmer (2014) for a striking example).

Second, we can see the virtue of clinical responsibility. When the NIMH (2015: 51) advances statements that mHealth should 'extend rather than replace the therapist', and when the apps recommended by the NHS carry with them a disclaimer that they are not a substitute for a medical consultation, we can see how the ultimate responsibility for defining and treating mental ill-health is apportioned to a clinician. While articulations of clinical responsibility are necessarily demarcations of power and expertise, they are also configured as virtuous in legalistic healthcare contexts where responsibility is inscribed in hard and soft law. Hence, the formal holding of clinical responsibility, and the performance of being a *responsible* clinician (in a broader sense), are mutually reinforcing and blur the lines between descriptive and normative dimensions of responsibility. Through reminders to patients and professionals within writings on mHealth that mobile technologies should not be substituted for clinical responsibility, the virtue of responsibility comes to legitimise endeavours to innovate the development and implementation of digital devices.

Consolidating 'Digital Psychiatry'?

The year 2017 saw the publication of The World Psychiatric Association-Lancet Psychiatry Commission on the Future of Psychiatry: a report 'intended to stimulate thought, debate, and the change necessary for psychiatry to fulfil its potential as an innovative, effective, and inclusive medical specialty in the 21st century' (Bhugra *et al.* 2017: 776). An accompanying editorial highlighted 'the apparently relentless progress of digital technology', which has 'the potential to render physical distance irrelevant to some areas of psychiatric practice' (Anon, 2017: 733). This creates a new 'challenge' to psychiatry 'to use such innovations to enhance, rather than replace, the humane and humanistic aspects of practice' (ibid). Similar comments about progress and risks were made in the report Executive Summary:

> Digital technology might offer psychiatry the potential for radical change in terms of service delivery and the development of new treatments. However, it also carries the risk of commercialised, unproven treatments entering the medical marketplace with detrimental effect. Novel research methods, transparency standards, clinical evidence, and care delivery models must be created in collaboration with a wide range of stakeholders. Psychiatrists need to remain up to date and educated in the evolving digital world. (Bhugra *et al.* 2017: 775)

The Commission comprised six key sections, one of which was a segment specifically on 'digital psychiatry'. This level of attention to the role of digital technology within mental health research and practice is indicative of a wider growth in prominence that, as we have seen, has been constituted through political position statements, funding policy and outcomes, and research articles and commentaries. What comprises 'digital psychiatry' in the Commission, as elsewhere, is wide-ranging: smartphones, virtual reality and machine learning are all included. Smartphones, as in many writings on mHealth, are given primary prominence; in the Commission, discussion of apps is juxtaposed with more futuristic possibilities such as augmented reality glasses which are 'entering the mental health space' (Bhugra *et al.* 2017: 799), albeit in somewhat undefined ways. Through talk of apps, and of more advanced technologies that 'are already projected to change health care' (Bhugra *et al.* 2017: 799), digital psychiatry can be presented as moving 'beyond traditional telepsychiatry' (ibid: 798) – and hence requiring new and focused attention and debate.

As Hedgecoe (2010: 172) has demonstrated in pharmacogenetics, 'scientific review papers bolster expectations' that new technologies 'will come into everyday clinical use'. The Commission and other writings reviewing the state of digital psychiatry likewise point to the apparent inevitability of innovation and implementation. One recurrent figure within contemporary writings on technology and mental health is US psychiatrist John Torous. Digital Psychiatry Editor for the Psychiatric Times, Chair of the APA Smartphone App Evaluation Task Force and a co-author of the WPA-Lancet Psychiatry Commission, Torous can be regarded as actively constituting a dedicated field of digital psychiatry through documenting its possibilities. This includes articles examining the ethical hurdles associated with the use of digital technologies in mental health, and providing provisional roadmaps for navigating these (e.g. Torous *et al.* 2014, Torous and Nebeker 2017). Through raising (and sometimes resolving) ethical issues, Torous and others contribute to performing the novelty and import of digital innovation in psychiatric praxis. 'Digital psychiatry', then, and 'digital mental health' more generally, appears not so much as a relatively bounded site of sociotechnical practice, but rather manifests through often promissory discourse about the rise of information and communication technologies and their ramifications for research and therapeutic interventions (cf. Brown 2003, Hedgecoe and Martin 2003).

According to the WPA-Lancet Psychiatry Commission report, the 'digital psychiatry revolution has arrived' (Bhugra *et al.* 2017: 798). As indicated above, this includes smartphone apps to treat mental disorders – but also highlighted in the report, and elsewhere, is the possibility of enrolling these as sources of data for research into the nature of psychopathology. As Dror Ben-Zeev (2017: 107) wrote in the first column of his new series in Psychiatric Services on technology and mental health: 'Advancements in Web, mobile, sensor, and informatics technology can do more than serve as tools to enhance existing models of care. Novel technologies can help us better understand the very nature of mental illness'. With similar optimism, the NIMH noted on one of their public-facing pages how receiving 'information from a large number of individuals at the same time can increase researchers' understanding of mental health and help them develop better interventions' (NIMH, 2017).

The direct data that people themselves enter into apps is described in the Commission report as one example of this. Other writing discussing the use of mobile technologies to enhance knowledge-production in psychiatry has emphasised, for instance, the collection of 'data on health behaviours and symptoms in real time and outside of the clinic setting, using text messages' (Vahia and Depp in Jeste 2013). With regards to self-inputted data, new industry-academic partnerships are emerging: for example, between the mental health social networking app TalkLife, Microsoft Research, MIT and Harvard University, which are using machine learning to 'better understand and predict self harm' (TalkLife, 2018). The Commission also noted the importance of passive data obtained via some of the additional features of smartphones (like GPS) (Bhugra *et al.* 2017: 799). Other articles and commentaries have similarly flagged this, with sleep- and activity-tracking highlighted as means of generating new temporally fine-grained insights into psychopathology as experienced in everyday life (e.g. Marzano *et al.* 2015). According to former NIMH Director Thomas Insel, such 'digital phenotyping' is already 'revealing new aspects of behaviour that appear clinically relevant' (Insel 2017: 1217). Threading through all these commentaries is the biomedical virtue of the enhancement of clinical wisdom: digital technologies might impart new means of comprehending mental ill-health, and hence of understanding individual patients.[4]

Conclusion

Innovations in digital mental health promotion and treatment have generated particular excitement internationally (e.g. Hollis *et al.* 2015, Miner *et al.* 2017, Torous 2016) – with one corollary of this being concern and disquiet (Ennis *et al.* 2012, Hayes *et al.* 2016). Through interrogating telepsychiatry, m-health, and digital psychiatry, I have sought to historicise and enrich contextual understandings of digital developments in mental health. We have seen how, in each of these cases, current uses and future possibilities are connected in ways that imply the inevitability and desirability of innovation.

Through discussions of probable and potential sociotechnical scenarios emerging from commentaries on digital psychiatry and the like, some organisations and individuals adopt roles as 'mediators of hope' (Martin *et al.* 2008: 127) regarding new technologies. Of these, agencies like the NIMH have the economic capacity to materialise a selection of the innovations they anticipate and the discourses they promote. Strategies of field-building are consequently occurring with and through concrete investment and change and seem likely to be playing out with a view to propelling such expenditure and innovation. Some of these strategies can be characterised as practices of what I have termed performative nominalism (following Hacking (2002)). In this respect, purported members of ostensibly new fields act, in effect, to talk these into existence. Through mirroring such rhetoric (e.g. about mHealth), funders and governments themselves contribute to this consolidation.

Within the promissory statements that are so important to the constitution of new endeavours, the implicit and explicit extolment of what I call biomedical virtues plays an important legitimising function. Emphases on various virtues have shifted over time, as the attention of psychiatry has ranged around different digital modalities. To date, the promotion of access to treatment has been a key virtue propelling technological innovation in mental health (as, more recently, has the encouragement of self-care). Today, mobile technologies are also now being folded into new regimes of psychiatric data collection, constituted through the virtue of the enhancement of clinical wisdom. In particular, service-orientated research is being conducted and urged, to ascertain the potential for information gleaned from mobile phones (including via apps, but also through activity-monitoring functions) to assist with clinical decision-making. This work has been argued to have the potential to reshape therapeutic encounters, whereby the epistemic salience of patient testimony regarding their subjective experience is dissipated as clinically relevant objectivity is delegated to devices. Investigations are also emerging into how digital technologies might provide new insights into the nature (especially, the temporalities) of symptoms like low-mood. Research in this vein resonates with wider epistemological shifts in psychiatry into the analysis of symptoms and mechanisms of psychopathology (Pickersgill 2014, Rose, 2016), which have (again) rendered problematic the existence of established nosological categories like schizophrenia.

Interfering (Pols 2003) in all this is another biomedical virtue: the maintenance of a positive doctor–patient relationship. As one commentary recently asserted, this relationship is of 'singular importance' in psychiatry (Steingard 2018: 1). It is striking how much the editorial accompanying the WPA-Lancet Psychiatry Commission report, which advanced concerns about the 'challenge' of innovation for 'humane and humanistic aspects of practice' (Anon, 2017: 733), echoes the worries of psychiatrists in decades past. In particular, Leo Bartemeier's anxieties about the 'threat' of technology to the psychiatrists' 'personal relationship with the patient', set out 65 years ago in his APA Presidential Address, seem to be little changed. It thus remains unclear how straightforwardly psychiatrists will accommodate much-vaunted digital developments in their practice. Nevertheless, based on the eclecticism and pragmatism of psychiatry that I illustrated earlier in this analysis, we might reasonably expect more accommodations than the aforementioned concerns might suggest. Regardless, the normative dimensions of (any) new digital instantiations within psychiatric praxis will certainly continue to bear sociological scrutiny.

Address for correspondence: Martyn Pickersgill, Centre for Biomedicine, Self and Society, Edinburgh Medical School, University of Edinburgh. E-mail: martyn.pickersgill@ed.ac.uk

Acknowledgements

I am very grateful to the Wellcome Trust for supporting this research [209519/Z/17/Z; 106612/Z/14/Z; 094205/Z/10/Z]. My analysis has also benefited from my role as a collaborator on a Wellcome Trust Seed Award [201652/Z/16/Z] ('Patienthood and Participation in the Digital Era'). I have appreciated the conversations with Sarah Chan (PI) and Sonja Erikainen that this award has enabled, and which have shaped my thinking around digital health. Finally, I want to thank the Sociology of Health & Illness Special Issue editors and peer-reviewers for constructive and insightful comments on this article during its preparation.

Notes

1   See also Hubley *et al.* (2016) for a review of trials which foregrounds the import of access.
2   See: http://www.mindtech.org.uk.
3   A field that itself could be regarded as consolidated in large part through its naming.
4   One corollary of this is a potential intensification of medicalisation. As Insel's comments imply, prac-
    tices engaged in by individuals categorised with a psychiatric disorder could be (increasingly) associ-
    ated with that psychopathology by virtue of the correlational data collected by digital devices.

References

Akrich, M. (1992) The description of technical objects. In Bijker, W.E. and Law, J. (eds) *Shaping Tech-
    nology/Building Society: Studies in Sociotechnical Change.* Cambridge: MIT Press.
Anon. (2017) New wave, *Lancet Psychiatry*, 4, 733.
APA. (2017a) 'Anita Everett Takes Office as APA President', Available at https://www.psychiatry.org/
    newsroom/news-releases/anita-everett-takes-office-as-apa-president (Last accessed 30 Aug 2018).
APA. (2017b) 'Telepsychiatry: Advances and Challenges'. Available at https://www.psychiatry.org/news-
    room/apa-blogs/apa-blog/2017/09/telepsychiatry-advances-and-challenges (Last accessed 30 Aug 2018).
APA. (undated) 'Mental Health Apps'. Available at https://www.psychiatry.org/psychiatrists/practice/me
    ntal-health-apps (Last accessed 30 August 2018).
Bartemeier, L.H. (1952) Presidential address, *American Journal of Psychiatry*, 109, 1–7.
Barton, W.E. (1971) Report of the Medical Director, *American Journal of Psychiatry*, 128, 522–4.
Bender, E. (2008) 'New APA resource addresses psychiatry in underserved areas', Psychiatric News, 7th
    March 2008. Available at https://psychnews.psychiatryonline.org/doi/full/10.1176/pn.43.5.0017 (Last
    accessed 30 August 2018).
Benjamin, R. (2011) Organized ambivalence: when sickle cell disease and stem cell research converge,
    Ethnicity and Health, 16, 447–63.
Ben-Zeev, D. (2017) Technology in mental health: creating new knowledge and inventing the future of
    services, *Psychiatric Services*, 68, 107–8.
Bhugra, D., Tasman, A., Pathare, S., Priebe, S., *et al.* (2017) The WPA-lancet psychiatry commission on
    the future of psychiatry, *Lancet Psychiatry*, 4, 775–818.
Borup, M., Brown, N., Konrad, K. and Van Lente, H. (2006) The sociology of expectations in science
    and technology, *Technology Analysis & Strategic Management*, 18, 285–98.
Brosnan, C. (2011) The sociology of neuroethics: expectational discourses and the rise of a new disci-
    pline, *Sociology Compass*, 5, 287–97.
Brown, N. (2003) Hope against hype: accountability in biopasts, presents and futures, *Science Studies*,
    16, 3–21.
Brown, N. and Michael, M. (2003) A sociology of expectations: retrospecting prospects and prospecting
    retrospects, *Technology Analysis & Strategic Management*, 15, 3–18.
Brown, N., Kraft, A. and Martin, P. (2006) The promissory pasts of blood stem cells, *BioSocieties*, 1,
    329–48.
Burnett, F. (2015) 'Four questions for NIMH Director Thomas R. Insel', Counseling Today. Available
    at http://ct.counseling.org/2015/03/four-questions-for-nimh-director-thomas-r-insel/ (Last accessed 30
    Aug 2018).
Conrad, E.C. and De Vries, R. (2011) Field of dreams: a social history of neuroethics. In Pickersgill, M.
    and Van Keulen, I. (eds) *Sociological Reflections on the Neurosciences.* Emerald: Bingley.
Dumit, J. (2004) *Picturing Personhood: Brain Scans and Biomedical Identity.* Princeton: Princeton
    University Press.
Ennis, L., Rose, D., Denis, M., Pandit, N., *et al.* (2012) Can't surf, won't surf: the digital divide in men-
    tal health, *Journal of Mental Health*, 21, 395–403.

Fassin, D. (2011) *Humanitarian Reason: A Moral History of the Present*. Berkeley: University of California Press.

Fitzpatrick, K.K., Darcy, A. and Vierhale, M. (2017) Delivering cognitive behavior therapy to young adults with symptoms of depression and anxiety using a fully automated conversational agent (Woebot): a randomized controlled trial, *Journal of Medical Internet Resarch*, 4, e19.

Freidson, E. (1988[1970]) *Profession of Medicine: A Study of the Sociology of Applied Knowledge*. Chicago: University of Chicago Press.

Fullager, S., Rich, E., Francombe-Webb, J. and Maturo, A. (2017) Digital ecologies of youth mental health: apps, therapeutic publics and pedagogy as affective arrangements, *Social Sciences*, 6, 135.

Goldberg, M.A. (1995) Telemedicine journal: a new journal for a new age, *Telemedince Journal*, 1, 1–2.

Goold, S.D. and Lipkin, M. Jr. (1999) The doctor-patient relationship: challenges, opportunities, and strategies, *Journal of General and Internal Medicine*, 14, Suppl, S26–33.

Hacking, I. (2002) *Historical Ontology*. Cambridge, MA: Harvard University Press.

Hale, N.G. (1995) *The Rise and Crisis of Psychoanalysis in the United States: Freud and the Americans, 1917–1985*. Oxford: Oxford University Press.

Harding, C., Ilves, P. and Wilson, S. (2015) Digital mental health services in general practice, *British Journal of General Practice*, 65, 58–9.

Hayes, J.F., Maughan, D.L. and Grant-Peterkin, H. (2016) Interconnected or disconnected? Promotion of mental health and prevention of mental disorder in the digital age, *British Journal of Psychiatry*, 208, 205–7.

Hedgecoe, A. (2010) Bioethics and the reinforcement of socio-technical expectations, *Social Studies of Science*, 40, 163–86.

Hedgecoe, A. and Martin, P. (2003) The drugs don't work: expectations and the future of pharmacogenetics, *Social Studies of Science*, 33, 327–64.

HM Government. (2017) 'Press release: Prime Minister unveils plans to transform mental health support'. Available at https://www.gov.uk/government/news/prime-minister-unveils-plans-to-transform-mental-health-support (Last accessed 30 Aug 2018).

Hollis, C., Morriss, R., Martin, J., Amani, S., *et al.* (2015) Technological innovations in mental healthcare: harnessing the digital revolution, *British Journal of Psychiatry*, 206, 263–5.

Hubley, S., Lynch, S.B., Schneck, C., Thomas, M., *et al.* (2016) Review of key telepsychiatry outcomes, *World Journal of Psychiatry*, 6, 269–82.

Insel, T. (2017) Digital phenotyping: technology of a new science of behaviour, *JAMA*, 318, 1215–6.

Jeste, D. (2013) 'Psychiatry joins the digital revolution', Psychiatric News. Available at https://psychnews.psychiatryonline.org/doi/full/10.1176/appi.pn.2013.3b7. (Last accessed 30 August 2018).

Joyce, K.A. (2008) *Magnetic Appeal: MRI and the Myth of Transparency*. Ithaca: Cornell University Press.

Kessler, D., Lewis, G., Kaur, S., Wiles, N., *et al.* (2009) Therapist-delivered internet psychotherapy for depression in primary care: a randomised controlled trial, *Lancet*, 374, 628–34.

Koven, S. (2013) 'Taking a new approach to psychiatric research', Boston Globe. Available at https://www.bostonglobe.com/lifestyle/health-wellness/2013/12/16/with-thomas-insel-director-national-institute-mental-health/nZ9Qjw88QmJtXWNQft1CFN/story.html. (Last accessed 30 Aug 2018).

Lehous, P., Sicotte, C., Denis, J.-L., Berg, M., *et al.* (2002) The theory of use behind telemedicine: how compatible with physicians' clinical routines?, *Social Science & Medicine*, 54, 889–904.

Lupton, D. (2014) Critical perspectives on digital health technologies, *Sociology Compass*, 8, 1344–59.

Lupton, D. and Maslen, S. (2017) Telemedicine and the senses: a review, *Sociology of Health & Illness*, 39, 1557–71.

Marley, J. and Farooq, S. (2015) Mobile telephone apps in mental health practice: uses, opportunities and challenges, *British Journal of Psychiatry Bulletin*, 39, 288–90.

Martin, P., Brown, N. and Turner, A. (2008) Capitalizing hope: the commercial development of umbilical cord blood stem cell banking, *New Genetics & Society*, 27, 127–43.

Marzano, L., Bardill, A., Fields, B., Herd, K., *et al.* (2015) The application of mHealth to mental health: opportunities and challenges, *Lancet Psychiatry*, 2, 942–8.

May, C., Gask, L., Atkinson, T., Ellis, N., *et al.* (2001) Resisting and promoting new technologies in clinical practice: the case of telepsychiatry, *Social Science & Medicine*, 52, 1889–901.

May, C., Harrison, R., Finch, T., MacFarlane, A., *et al.* (2003) Understanding the normalization of telemedicine services through qualitative evaluation, *Journal of the American Medical Informatics Association*, 10, 596–604.

Mental Health Taskforce. (2016) The Five Year Forward View for Mental Health: A Report from the Independent Mental Health Taskforce to the NHS in England. Available at https://www.england.nhs.uk/wp-content/uploads/2016/02/Mental-Health-Taskforce-FYFV-final.pdf (Last accessed 30 August 2018).

Miner, A.S., Milstein, A. and Hancock, J.T. (2017) Talking to machines about personal mental health problems, *JAMA*, 318, 1217–8.

Mohr, D.C., Weingardt, K.R., Reddy, M. and Schueller, S.M. (2017) Three problems with current digital mental health research and three things we can do about them, *Psychiatric Services*, 68, 427–9.

MRC. (2015) 'Mobile medicine: using phones to improve health'. Available at https://mrc.ukri.org/news/browse/mobile-medicine/ (Last accessed 30 August 2018).

National Information Board. (2014) Personalised Health and Care 2020: Using Data and Technology to Transform Outcomes for Patients and Citizens. A Framework for Action. Hm Government/NHS. Available at https://www.gov.uk/government/uploads/system/uploads/attachment_data/file/384650/NIB_Report.pdf (Last accessed 30 August 2018).

Nelson, E.L., Barnard, M. and Cain, C. (2003) Treating childhood depression over videoconferencing, *Telemedicine Journal and E-Health*, 9, 49–55.

Nemko, M. (2014) The Present and Future of Treatments for Depression, Psychology Today. Available at https://www.psychologytoday.com/blog/how-do-life/201409/the-present-and-future-treatment-depression. (Last accessed 30 Aug 2018).

NHS. (2018) Digital Apps Library – Mental Health. Available at https://apps.beta.nhs.uk/?category=Mental%20Health. (Last accessed 30 August 2018).

Nicholas, J., Lerson, M.E., Proudfoot, J. and Christensen, H. (2015) Mobile apps for bipolar disorder: a systematic review of features and content quality, *Journal of Medical Internet Research*, 17, e198.

NIH. (2017) Mobile Health: Technology and Outcomes in Low and Middle Income Countries (R21 Clinical Trial Optional). Funding Opportunity Announcement. Available at https://grants.nih.gov/grants/guide/pa-files/PAR-18-242.html. (Last accessed 30 August 2018).

NIMH. (2015) Strategic Plan for Research. Available at https://www.nimh.nih.gov/about/strategic-planning-reports/nimh_strategicplanforresearch_508compliant_corrected_final_149979.pdf (Last accessed 30 August 2018).

NIMH. (2017) Technology and the Future of Mental Health Treatment. Available at https://www.nimh.nih.gov/health/topics/technology-and-the-future-of-mental-health-treatment/index.shtml. (Last accessed 30 Aug 2018).

O'Reilly, R., Bishop, J., Maddox, K., Hutchinson, L., *et al.* (2007) 'Is telepsychiatry equivalent to face-to-face psychiatry? Results from a randomized controlled equivalence trial, *Psychiatric Services*, 58, 836–43.

Osborne, T. (1994) Power and persons: on ethical stylisation and person-centred medicine, *Sociology of Health & Illness*, 16, 515–35.

Pickersgill, M. (2010) From psyche to soma? Changing accounts of antisocial personality disorders in the American Journal of Psychiatry, *History of Psychiatry*, 21, 294–311.

Pickersgill, M. (2011) 'Promising' therapies: neuroscience, clinical practice, and the treatment of psychopathy, *Sociology of Health & Illness*, 33, 3, 448–64.

Pickersgill, M. (2014) Debating DSM-5: diagnosis and the sociology of critique, *Journal of Medical Ethics*, 40, 521–5.

Pols, J. (2003) Enforcing patient rights or improving care? The interference of two modes of doing good in mental health care, *Sociology of Health and Illness*, 25, 320–47.

RANZCP. (2013) Professional Practice Standards and Guides for Telepsychiatry. Available at https://www.ranzcp.org/Files/Resources/RANZCP-Professional-Practice-Standards-and-Guides.aspx (Last accessed 30 August 2018).

RANZCP. (undated) Telehealth in psychiatry. Available at https://www.ranzcp.org/Publications/Telehealth-in-psychiatry.aspx (Last accessed 30 August 2018).

Raz, M. (2008) Between the ego and the icepick: psychosurgery, psychoanalysis, and psychiatric discourse, *Bulletin of the History of Medicine*, 82, 387–420.

Rimmer, A. (2014) GPs urge government to create a national self care strategy, *BMJ*, 348, g3533.

Rose, N. (2001) The politics of life itself, *Theory, Culture & Society*, 18, 1–30.

Rose, N. (2016) Neuroscience and the future for mental health?, *Epidemiology and Psychiatric Sciences*, 25, 2, 95–100.

Rubin, B. (2008) Therapeutic promise in the discourse of human embryonic stem cell research, *Science as Culture*, 17, 13–27.

Sadowsky, J. (2006) Beyond the metaphor of the pendulum: electroconvulsive therapy, psychoanalysis, and the styles of American psychiatry, *Journal of the History of Medicine*, 61, 1–25.

Schirmann, F. (2014) "The wondrous eyes of a new technology"—a history of the early electroencephalography (EEG) of psychopathy, delinquency, and immorality, *Frontiers in Human Neuroscience*, 8, 1–10.

Shoham, V. and Insel, T.R. (2011) Rebooting for whom? Portfolios, technology, and personalized intervention, *Perspectives on Psychological Sciences*, 6, 478–82.

Steingard, S. (2018) Therapeutic alliance: implications for practice and policy, *Psychiatric Services*, 69, 1.

Sukel, K. (2015) 'Google's NIH health hire: Smartphones can detect mental health breakdowns', Fortune. Available at http://fortune.com/2015/09/17/googles-nih-health-hire-smartphones-can-detect-mental-health-breakdowns/ (Last accessed 30 Aug 2018).

TalkLife. (2018) Research. Available at https://talklife.co/research/ (Last accessed 30 August 2018).

Tasman, A. (2000) Presidential address: the doctor-patient relationship, *American Journal of Psychiatry*, 157, 1762–8.

Timmermans, S. and Tavory, I. (2012) Theory construction in qualitative research: from grounded theory to abductive analysis, *Sociological Theory*, 30, 167–86.

Torous, J. (2014) Digital psychiatry in Asia, *Asian Journal of Psychiatry*, 10, 1–2.

Torous, J. (2016) Digital psychiatry: the year ahead, Psychiatric Times. Available at http://www.psychiatrictimes.com/telepsychiatry/digital-psychiatry-year-ahead (Last accessed 30 Aug 2018).

Torous, J. and Nebeker, C. (2017) Navigating ethics in the digital age: introducing connected and open research ethics (CORE), a tool for researchers and institutional review boards, *Journal of Medical Internet Research*, 19, e38. https://doi.org/10.2196/jmir.6793.

Torous, J., Keshavan, M. and Gutheil, T. (2014) Promise and perils of digital psychiatry, *Asian Journal of Psychiatry*, 10, 120–2.

Torous, J., Chan, S. and Luo, J. (2016) 'Are your patients using 'digital supplements'?'. Psychiatric Times. Available at https://psychnews.psychiatryonline.org/doi/full/10.1176/appi.pn.2016.11b16 (Last accessed 30 Aug 2018).

Trnka, S. (2016) Digital care: agency and temporality in young people's use of health apps, *Engaging Science, Technology and Society*, 2, 248–65.

Wagnild, G., Leenknecht, C. and Sauher, J. (2006) Psychiatrists' satisfaction with telepsychiatry, *Telemedicine and e-Health*, 12, 546–51.

Webster, A. (2002) Innovative health technologies and the social: redefining health, medicine and the body, *Current Sociology*, 50, 443–57.

WHO. (2013) Mental Health Action Plan: 2013-2020. Available at http://apps.who.int/iris/bitstream/10665/89966/1/9789241506021_eng.pdf?ua=1 (Last accessed 30 August 2018).

Williams, S.J., Coveney, C. and Meadows, R. (2015) 'M-apping' sleep? Trends and transformations in the digital age, *Sociology of Health & Illness*, 37, 1039–54.

Zhang, M.W.B., Ho, C.S.H., Cheok, C.C.S. and Ho, R.C.M. (2015) Smartphone apps in mental healthcare: the state of the art and potential developments, *British Journal of Psychiatry Advances*, 21, 354–8.

© 2018 The Author
Sociology of Health & Illness published by John Wiley & Sons Ltd on behalf of Foundation for SHIL.

Sociology of Health & Illness Vol. 41 No. S1 2019 ISSN 0141-9889, pp. 31–49
doi: 10.1111/1467-9566.12980

Is digital health care more equitable? The framing of health inequalities within England's digital health policy 2010–2017

Emma Rich[1] [iD], Andy Miah[2] and Sarah Lewis[1]

[1]*Department for Health, University of Bath, Bath, UK*
[2]*School of Environment and Life Sciences, University of Salford, Salford, UK*

Abstract Informed by a discourse analysis, this article examines the framing of equity within the UK's digital health policies between 2010 and 2017, focusing on England's development of NHS Digital and its situation within the UK Government's wider digital strategy. Analysis of significant policy documents reveals three interrelated discourses that are engaged within England's digital health policies: equity as a neoliberal imaginary of digital efficiency and empowerment; digital health as a pathway towards democratising health care through data-sharing, co-creation and collaboration; and finally, digital health as a route towards extending citizen autonomy through their access to data systems. It advances knowledge of the relationship between digital health policy and health inequalities. Revealing that while inclusion remains a priority area for policymakers, equity is being constituted in ways that reflect broader discourses of neoliberalism, empowerment and the turn to the market for technological solutionism, which may potentially exacerbate health inequalities.

Keywords: E-health, Health Policy, Healthism, Internet, Social determinants of health, Youth

Introduction

Health inequalities and the social determinants of illness and disease have received growing attention within public health research, which has focused attention on policymaking as a route towards making meaningful changes to the fair distribution of healthcare services. This is crucial, as it has been found widely that social inequalities have deleterious consequences for population health (Marmot and Wilkinson 2001, Peacock *et al.* 2014, Scambler 2012). Indeed, even in countries where the reduction of health inequalities has been a stated policy priority (Smith and Kandlik Eltanani 2015), disparities persist. Numerous authors note that this is partly due to the 'lifestyle drift' (Popay *et al.* 2010) in which policies begin by recognising the need for upstream action to address wider social and economic determinants of health, only to be reduced to a focus on individual behaviour (Baum and Fisher 2014, Williams and Fullagar 2018).

  In this context, digital health technologies have been positioned by governments around the world as central to the delivery of a fair healthcare system and 'promise to transform healthcare systems including strategies of personal risk management, modes of treatment and

Digital Health: Sociological Perspectives, First Edition.
Edited by Flis Henwood and Benjamin Marent.

practices of care' (Petersen 2019: 22). Yet, the presumption that conversion to digital health services from an analogue world will deliver on such ambitions needs careful analysis and verification, not least there is great variation in the way in which digital health is experienced by citizens/patients. Thus, digital health encompasses web-based solutions, mobile phone and tablet applications, the integration of artificially intelligent platforms, the utilisation of wearable devices that track biometric information and the proliferation of social media environments, each of which may have varying impacts on health care equity.

Our starting point is to argue for the need to clarify the impact of digital health on fostering health equality across different settings. To do so, we argue that there is a need to examine the policy discourse that surrounds the drive towards digital health care and focus, here, on the recent work of the UK Government, notably through its ambitions for care provision within England.[1] Since the inception of the United Nations E-Government survey, the United Kingdom has appeared in the Top 10 countries and has been in the Top 5 in its 2 most recent iterations (2016 and 2018), making it a country valuable to analyse. The UK has also been a primary international influence in matters of diversity and inclusion, as articulated in its various Acts of Parliament, including recently the Health and Social Care Act (2012) and the Care Act (2014). The UK has also sought to position itself as a global leader in digital health, evidenced through the implementation of various programmes since the early 2000s (Cabinet Office 2013, Department for International Trade, 2018; Department of Health and Social Care. 2014) and early digital adoption in the 1980s (National Advisory Group on Health Information Technology in England, 2016). Finally, in 2014, the UK Government also published its 'Digital Inclusion Strategy' (Cabinet Office, 2014a) and a Digital Inclusion Charter (Cabinet Office 2014b), which reiterate the ambition to improve equality within health and care provision, made apparent in the strategy of its Department of Health and Social Care's Executive Agency, Public Health England (Public Health England (2017). Yet, despite these initiatives, there remain key inequalities within public provision.

As such, this article considers how discourses of equity are framed in public policy on digital health within England, so as to ascertain where there are gaps and need for further development or investigations. Informed by Rizvi and Lingard (2011: 6), we examine how these policies are linked to 'a broader set of conditions in which its meaning and significance are articulated'. In so doing, we critically analyse a decisive period in the development of the UK Government's digital health trajectory, encompassing a period of two government cycles (2010–2018), during which time a remarkable amount of investment in and discussion about digital health has taken place. Notably, since 2013, a new English body named 'NHS Digital' has emerged, as the 'trading name of the Health and Social Care Information Centre (HSCIC), which was established in April 2013 by the Health and Social Care Act 2012'. In large part, telling the story of England's digital health strategy is well articulated by the story of NHS Digital, the work of which is now the focal point for all other plans (Health and Social Care Information Centre, 2015).

By analysing influential digital health policy documents specifically in England over this period, this article develops our understanding of how health inequalities emerge and persist, which we assert as a crucial complement to other methods of assessing inequalities, such as patient/citizen experience surveys. Indeed, presently, there is no adequate data to assess the impact of many digital health services, but the principles by which such services are designed through policy can reveal insights into how such concerns are understood. Thus, we foreground the contribution of policy analyses to our understanding of these digital health inequalities and present the findings of an analysis of UK and English governmental and policy documents as discourse.

Throughout our analysis, we highlight concerns about how digital access and equality are constituted through and absent within these discourses, questioning how this reifies or challenges the above dominant 'policy paradigm' (Scott-Samuel and Smith 2015: 418) within neoliberalism which 'restricts the ability of policy actors to image alternative, more equitable scenarios'. In this regard, while digital health is often described as a solution to various health crises, including those of widening health inequalities, such policies are being introduced within a policy climate that is persistently focused on tackling health inequalities via downstream solutions (Baum and Fisher 2014, Popay *et al.* 2010, Smith and Kandlik Eltanani 2015, Williams and Fullagar 2018). As such, our analysis examines how digital health is being positioned by and constituting these broader discourses of health inequalities. Furthermore, we examine how these policy texts establish conditions of actions and types of selfhood and subjectivities, specifically in terms of how citizens are positioned as objects of policy interventions. This article describes these current policy directions in resolving health inequalities more broadly before making the case for critical analyses of the positioning of digital health within these public health responses. Following this, we present three key discourses that emerge from our analyses, concluding with suggestions for future policy research and theorisations of digital health inequalities.

Current limitations in public health responses to health inequalities

In recent times, ample evidence from non-governmental and research organisations has revealed the marked and persistent health disparities among and across different social groups, which specifies the extent to which social inequalities have deleterious consequences for population health (Marmot and Bell 2012, Marmot and Wilkinson 2001, Peacock *et al.* 2014, Scambler 2012; WHO, 2008). These circumstances have led to increasing pressure on governments to respond and develop public health policies to address these gaps in provision. For example, in the UK, there was a period of focused policies intended to reduce health inequalities between 1997 and 2010, which led the UK to be 'recognised as a global leader in health inequalities research and policy' (Garthwaite *et al.* 2016: 459). Despite such efforts, inequalities persist and, in some cases, have widened (Bambra 2012; Mackenbach 2011). Indeed, Mackenbach (2011) notes that, although England was the first European country to pursue a systematic policy to reduce socioeconomic inequalities in health, it has failed to reach its own target of a 10% reduction in inequalities in life expectancy and infant mortality.

Although government strategies and systematic policy responses will vary, attempts to addressing population health and accompanying disparities are usually 'characterised by a chasm between two central views of how population health may be improved through action to prevent ill health and promote health' (Baum and Fisher 2014: 214). On the one hand, as certain chronic diseases or conditions (such as obesity) have ostensibly increased, governments have targeted individual behaviours such as physical activity, diet and smoking to address the risks associated with these conditions. However, targeting individual lifestyle and behaviour within new public health approaches (Petersen and Lupton 1996) has been heavily critiqued, not least because of its narrow focus on individual empowerment and on nudging people to change their behaviours. Conversely, perspectives which focus on broader social, cultural and economic factors, which influence and determine health outcomes, highlight the need for health policy and interventions that direct collective action.

As Baum and Fisher (2014) argue, despite the increasing evidence about social determinants of health, many governments continue to draw from behavioural explanations in developing policy responses. This common (re)framing of structural forces as matters of individual will is a tendency that is anticipated under conditions of neoliberalisation and 'healthism' (Crawford 1980) and is now well documented within the sociological literature as a lifestyle drift in health policy which involves a 'tendency for policy to start off recognising the need for action on upstream social determinants of health inequalities only to drift downstream to focus largely on individual lifestyle factors' (Popay *et al.* 2010: 148). Baum and Fisher (2014: 216) consider this lifestyle drift as 'a by-product of the appeal of behavioural health promotion'. Elsewhere, Williams and Fullagar (2018: 2) examine this drift through an exploration of the complexities of advanced liberal governance that help explain 'discrepancies between policies that address health inequalities and the interventions designed to reduce them'.

The rise and promise of digital health solutions

Alongside the increasing interest in health inequalities, there has been a significant growth in digital health technologies and their integration into health care systems. It has been argued that discourses of 'promise' play a crucial role in the development of such digital health policies (Petersen 2019) whereby digitality is positioned as a necessary component of all healthcare solutions. Digital health technologies are increasingly viewed by health organisations, governments and health professionals as crucial components in the advancement of preventative medicine/health care and are rationalised 'against the backdrop of contemporary public health challenges that include increasing costs, worsening outcomes, "diabesity" epidemics, and anticipated physician shortages' (Swan 2012: 93). Indeed, there has been a great deal of excitement among healthcare providers and governments about the potential of these technologies to develop a more effective healthcare system (European Commission, 2014) and to foster the 'digitally engaged patient' (Lupton 2013). As such, digital health has emerged as a priority focus in a range of UK and European Government and health organisation policies and reports (Department of health (2012a), European Commission, 2014, UK Government Digital Strategy (2013)) and consultations (European Commission public consultation, 2014) and the digital agenda is seen as a flagship initiative for public health as part of the Europe 2020 growth strategy. These policies are also assembled through a range of different bodies and affects, such as the desires of different lobby groups or citizens (e.g. quantified self movement) policymakers, health professionals and other agents.

Within the area of inequalities more broadly, not just health, Robinson *et al.* (2015: 569–570) argue that 'digital inequality deserves a place alongside more traditional forms of inequality in the twenty-first century pantheon of inequality' claiming that 'it has the potential to shape life chances in multiple ways'. Indeed, this connection between digital inequalities and other inequalities is becoming increasingly important given the trend towards digital health interventions and this is made evident in the UK Government's wider strategies on digital inclusion (Cabinet Office, 2014a,b).

As the responsibility for the prevention and management of health shift increasingly onto patients (as consumers) and to technological systems, this raises questions about the potential for digital health to widen or narrow health inequalities. Those who experience high levels of social disadvantage are at risk of experiencing the worse health outcomes, yet may also lack the access, digital skills and knowledge to make sense of digital health systems.

Petersen (2019) argues that digital health is 'a field underpinned by promise and optimism, but accompanied by relatively little critical assessment of its social, economic, political and personal implications'. In this context, we caution against an uncritical widespread adoption digital health solutions and the assumption that digital solutions will always be better (see Rich and Miah 2014). Indeed, there is emerging evidence that some digital health technologies might worsen inequalities. For example, the use of mobile health apps and other mobile technologies to improve women's access to health resources has not shown clearly positive effects (Jennings and Gagliardi 2013). Alternatively, digital solutions might not address the needs of health services in rural areas or even save travel costs. Thus, we must ask critical questions about how digital technologies are negotiated, taken up and managed in the contexts of these broader social inequalities. It is also crucial to consider people's shifting investments in health or anxieties about technologies and surveillance, as many people may find digital solutions to be outside of their abilities to manage. Given the continued investment in digital health, a rapid response is imperative in addressing this knowledge deficit to inform the long-term development of digital health policy and practice.

Much of the discourse around digital health and inequalities has been framed by the established notion of a digital divide, which evidences a sizeable majority who do not have access to the internet. This digital divide 'represents inequalities across income, education and age groups, and between the most and least healthy' (McAuley 2014: 1119). Recent research suggests there may be a lack of access to the Internet amongst populations of those with long-term illness, health problems or disabilities (Dutton *et al.* 2013).

Such concerns are increasingly important, given that it is 'now well understood that digital inequality and exclusion cannot be analysed apart from the offline circumstances of individuals and groups and that specific forms of digital exclusion map onto particular kinds of offline disadvantage' (Robinson *et al.* 2015: 570). Similar approaches need to examine the social inequalities that preclude particular forms of digital health engagement, before they are exacerbated by an unscrutinised drive towards further digital health solutionism. This is especially important as digital health expands into even more complex territories, such as artificial intelligence, for which there is already a burgeoning enthusiasm within the healthcare sector. For example, the UK Health Tsar Sir John Bell advocates investment into artificial intelligence, as a crucial criterion of all future health care, saying how it could 'save the NHS' (Bell cited in Ghosh 2018).

Discourse analysis of digital health policies

This article arises from a wider study on digital health and young people during which an analysis of digital health policy documents was undertaken.[2] Our approach draws on a poststructuralist analysis of policy which foregrounds the concept of discourse. Foucault (1977: 49) describes discourses as 'practices that systematically form the objects of which they speech … Discourses are not about objects; they do not identify objects, they constitute them and in the practice of doing so conceal their own invention. We utilise the concept of discourse to explore the ways in which equity is constructed within recent digital health policies in the UK. This draws attention to the power and privileging or constraining affects of '*policy as discourse*' (Ball 2015). As Maguire and Ball (1994: 6) claim; 'Discourses thus provides for or privileges certain relationships and types of interaction, certain organisational forms and practices, certain forms of self-perception and self-presentation, and at the same moment, excludes others'.

Through this analysis, we address questions such as how is equity articulated and what are the implications of the ways in which this is framed? In other words, through this analysis we aim to identify the main policy positions and the discourses specifically in relation to representations of equity. Foucault (1978) identifies policy as a technology of governmentality, which constitutes and regulates conduct. In considering digital health *policy as discourse* we need consider they ways in which 'subjects and subject positions are formed and re-formed by policy' (Ball 2015: 2) Through the concept of discourse, we ask which values, norms and subjectivities are being constituted through language. From this perspective, digital health policy discourse therefore provide us with ways of thinking about digital health, but also about ourselves and others; constituting subject positions through which we might come to understand ourselves as productive, healthy or informed citizens. This requires our analysis goes beyond analysing the content of a text. Instead, we draw attention to how particular articulations of equity and digital health are made possible. As Ball (2015: 6) argues 'discourse is the conditions under which certain statements are considered to be the truth'. Our analysis thus explores the discourses which come to constrain, enable, frame and make possible ways of speaking about equity and digital health within the selected policy texts. The analysis we present below therefore focuses on how expressions of equity are articulated and justified through particular discourses. To do so, we undertook a Discourse Analysis of a selection of policy documents as detailed below.

Document selection
The articulation of national strategic ambitions within any sector context is inherently complex, as many different organisations work towards adoption and delivery of policy. As such, to assist in the identification of relevant policy directions, documents were selected using keyword searches of policy archives on the following government websites: gov.uk and england.nhs. The search terms used on these websites included; digital health, mhealth, telehealth, health, digital literacy and inequalities. A list of search results by term was created and documents that appeared across these lists were read in more detail. If they were deemed relevant to the broad theme of digital health, then they were placed on a shortlist. Documents on this shortlist were then read, compared and discussed among the authors. In this article, we report on an analysis of the following UK documents, each of which were developed during the critical period of the UK Government's digital health trajectory described above (2010–present):

1 Department of Health (2012a) Digital Strategy: Leading the culture change in health and care (DoH, 2012a)
2 Department of Health (2012b) 'The Power of Information: Putting Us All in Control of the Health and Care Information We Need' (DoH, 2012b)
3 National Information Board (2014, Nov) Personalised Health and Care 2020 Using Data and Technology to Transform Outcomes for Patients and Citizens A Framework for Action
4 NHS England Publications (2016) 'Healthy Children: Transforming Child Health information' (NHS England, 2016).

The analysis of these documents differs from more traditional policy analysis, as it moves beyond single case policy analysis to provide cohesive comparative policy analysis, which has long been called for in the wider policy analysis literature (Taylor 1997, Walt *et al.* 2008). Our analytical approach to examining policy as discourse involved a series of steps similar to those undertaken by Carabine (2001) in her genealogical analysis of how lone motherhood was spoken of in Britain in the early 1990s.

Initially, reports were read in detail for their framing of equity and how this was assembled through broader values and discourses. To aid this process, we undertook a keyword analysis using WordSmith software. These two forms of familiarisation occurred simultaneously and invariably influenced one another. Close reading provided an opportunity to engage with the documents, ask questions of the content, gain an understanding of the social and political context in which they exist, and adjust to the differences in language useful between documents. WordSmith was used as an overviewing tool, which allowed authors to query language use in

.

more detail and get a sense of language in context over such a vast amount of data. Keyword analysis made the qualitative analysis more approachable as a body of data. Some of the keywords analysed were; empower/empowerment, engage/engagement, adolescence/adolescents, access, management, self, individual, potential, responsibility, digital. The analysis then built on this familiarisation, concepts that were flagged as interesting were substantiated through further linguistic inquiry, comparison between documents and critical questioning of what was happening in these texts (and the concepts under analysis) in terms of social practices, actors and structures. Not all concepts could be substantiated and it became apparent that much was *missing* from these discourses. Essential in this analysis was the interplay of discourses thus, from a Foucauldian perspective, understanding how they constrained and enabled what could be said; for example how they conformed to neoliberalism, shaping the ways in which inequality can be perceived, discussed and acted on, in these documents.

The inter-relationships between key discourses were then explored (e.g. equity and neoliberal discourses of empowerment). One of the aims of this study was to understand how subject positions were being (re)formed through these digital health policies; what expectations were being constituted in terms of the roles for citizens or 'users' of these technologies. Subsequently, our reading involved identifying how equity was performed through discursive strategies and how the digital *user* as subject was being imagined in relation to particular values, norms and subjectivities. This analytical process involved comparison of documents, discussion between authors and critical reflection on the analysis as it was being conducted. Our analysis focuses on how these policies impact upon equality, asking how they matter, who they exclude/marginalise and what policies can achieve. Finally, the transcripts were analysed in terms of notable absences or silences (e.g. what was not spoken) in relation to the above literature on inequalities which informed the research. This involved multiple readings but also looking across the policies which reflected a crucial period in the UK government's digital health trajectory. Thus, in addition to what was presented through reading and keyword analysis of the policy texts, we also explore the similarities, silences and anomalies. Following Carabine (2001: 281), this approach can be considered an overlapping and iterative process, taking us back and forth between data, analysis, theory and literature.

Findings

Given the emphasis on downstream policy interventions to tackle inequality described above, we were interested in how individuals were described and positioned in the policy document sample and how these approaches were justified. Our analysis reveals three interrelated discourses drawn upon in the policy orientations towards equity; equity as a neoliberal imaginary of digital efficiency and empowerment; digital health as a pathway towards democratising health care through data-sharing, co-creation and collaboration; and finally, digital health as a route towards extending citizen autonomy through their access to data systems. We organise our discussion of the findings around these three discourses.

Equity as a neoliberal imaginary of digital efficiency and empowerment
As recognised elsewhere, 'a range of governmental processes are involved in defining a policy problem, in diagnosing deficiencies and in making promises of improvement' (Rizvi and Lingard 2011: 8). In the context of digital health policy, given the concerns about austerity and welfare cuts, the UK government and various health organisations foreground the benefits of digital strategies for implementing low-cost policy options to address inequalities.

Indeed, across the documents, policy investments in digital health care are justified on the basis of their ability to deliver greater efficiency of overburdened healthcare systems. Throughout, efficiency is rationalised on the basis of developing systems which also enhance empowerment through a 'digitally engaged patient' (Lupton 2013). The rising appeal of digital health solutions to influence individual behaviours is rationalised 'against the backdrop of contemporary public health challenges that include increasing costs, worsening outcomes, "diabesity" epidemics, and anticipated physician shortages' (Swan 2012: 93)

> The accelerating pace of technological change offers unprecedented opportunities to interact with health and care services in ways that are convenient, cost-effective and reliable. In taking advantage of this transformation – as many of us have already done in so many other areas of our lives – we should be confident that personal support is available when needed. (DoH, 2012b: 19)

As described above, despite the development of focused policy strategies to address public health challenges, inequalities persist within health care. Scott-Samuel and Smith (2015: 419–420) suggest that 'one obvious explanation for this phenomenon of ineffective political action on health inequalities is that politicians are attracted by non-controversial relatively low-cost policy options which can be implemented in a short timeframe'. Reflecting this logic, the policy documents are steeped in the language of cost-effectiveness and its benefits in terms of a more efficient healthcare system. This vision for public health is set out in the DoH (2012a) digital strategy:

> There are many advantages to going digital, both for users and for taxpayers. The most obvious improvement will be making public services easier to use, giving people access to services online, reducing the number of forms they need to fill in, giving people the information they need to help them in their everyday lives. (Dr Dan Poulter, Parliamentary Under-Secretary of State for health)

Thus, one way in which equity is (re)framed is through its connection with a range of other values and neoliberal governmental techniques. Echoing a form of market liberalism, these techniques are strongly associated with the turn towards the operations of the market and its assumed efficiencies, where goods and services are seen as critical in preventing illness, managing risk as way of enhancing *health outcomes for all*:

> Better use of data and technology has the power to improve health, transforming the quality and reducing the cost of health and care services [. . .] Digital technologies are changing the way we do things, improving the accountability of services, reducing their cost, giving us new means of transacting and participating. This is more than an information revolution: it puts people first, giving us more control and more transparency. (NIB, 2014: 3)

Policy recommendations put forward are assumed to enhance opportunities by equipping patients as 'informed consumers' to make better choices to manage and gain control over their own health. This emphasis on prevention is clearly linked to the broader vision of the NHS, set out in its five year forward view plan (2014: 7) positioning 'prevention' as crucial to future health and wellbeing as an issue of 'prevention':

> *The health and wellbeing gap*: If the nation fails to get serious about prevention then recent progress in healthy life expectancies will stall, health inequalities will widen, and our ability

to fund beneficial new treatments will be crowded out by the need to spend billions of pounds on wholly avoidable illness.

To ensure sustainability, health and care needs to move from a model of late disease management to early health. Information technology plays an essential and rapidly expanding role in empowering people to take charge of their own health, by providing information, support and control. (NIB, 2014: 9)

These rationalities drive an intensified focus on self-government, preventative medicine and the increased importance of individual responsibility to access health information. Transformation, quality of care and increased inclusion are all implied with the policy commitments of these texts. Rizvi and Lingard (2011: 10) argue that 'the relationship between the values of equity and efficiency is not a simple one, linked to an instrumental logic'. This instrumental discourse features in the DoH Digital Strategy (DoH, 2012a):

In any sector, advances in technology help people to do things quicker, more efficiently and with better results. And launching a health information revolution that puts patients in control of their health and care information, and makes services convenient, accessible and efficient, is now a major priority for the Department of Health.

Similar to the lifestyle drift (Popay *et al.* 2010) described earlier in this article, within existing economic and political systems of neoliberalism, these digital solutions are being positioned as a tool to enhance downstream interventions focused on individual responsibility. These include the promotion of public-facing digital health services which are deemed to both increase efficiency but also empower people, conveying expectations of the responsibilities of citizens as consumers of particular digital goods and services:

In addition, with the growing popularity and use of smartphones and tablets, the health and care system of the future will direct us, as patients and the public, towards accredited health apps to help us keep ourselves healthy and, as appropriate, manage our conditions. (DoH, 2012b: 64)

Digital health care is therefore framed through a 'logic of choice' (Mol 2008) whereby the concept of the patient as a customer or citizen emerges within an instrumental logic oriented towards the market and its health services and products. Many of these digital interventions transfer responsibility away from the state and onto the individual reflecting a broader neoliberal logic of empowerment as part of a focus on predictive, personalised, preventive health care.

While there may be many benefits to the development of these digital systems, they also invoke a series of critical questions about their ideological framing. Through these discourse, digital health users or patients are constituted as rational 'consumers' having agential capacity through which their individual behaviour is amenable to change through engagement with goods, service and information. Arguably, the articulation of these powerful discourses of empowerment, obscure broader social and economic factors, which inhibit individual's opportunity to act upon this knowledge and undertake health practices (Cohn 2014). Furthermore, it suggests that a particular agential capacity, in line with a behavioural model, where digital tools are used for the delivery of health interventions to manage behavioural change such as smoking cessation, alcohol reduction, increasing physical activity or 'managing' mental ill health (e.g. developing resilience).

Many of the policy documents therefore reflect the increased focus on self-management, predicated on the assumed capacity for digital technologies to help engage people in changing or adopting new health behaviours

> Our ambition is for a health and care system that enables people to make healthier choices, to be more resilient, to deal more effectively with illness and disability when it arises, and to have happier, longer lives in old age; a health and care system where technology can help tackle inequalities and improve access to services for the vulnerable.   (National Information Board, 2014: 4)

Such a framing is utilised in policy discourse to judge the 'success' of health outcomes, whereby individual needs can be met through more tailored, precise and personalised digital One of the suggestions put forward by the Department of Health (2012b) is to 'consider what progress the health and care system has already made and what can be learnt from other industries and the wider economy. We then set out a series of proposals that will: "enable me to make the right health and care choices" – citizens to have full access to their care records and access to an expanding set of NHS- accredited health and care apps and digital information services'. Tracking and monitoring may provide tailored benefits to specific communities or provide the means further support, enhancing health equity:

> Information can bring enormous benefits. It is the lifeblood of good health and wellbeing, and is pivotal to good quality care. It allows us to understand how to improve our own and our family's health, to know what our care and treatment choices are and to assess for ourselves the quality of services and support available. (Department of Health, 2012b: 4).

However, it is presumed that people will make better choices, if given information about their behaviour, thus largely overlooking the structural action or upstream interventions required to provide equity of opportunity: As noted earlier, it is well recognised that a focus on changing behaviours remains a dominant and often appealing approach to developing health policies (Kelly and Barker 2016), most notably with regards to state-funded research on the illness-producing behaviours of people in lower socioeconomic groups (Scambler, 2012). However, Blue *et al.* (2016), Ioannou (2005) and Thompson and Kumar (2011) discuss the extent to which they constitute and are constituted by neoliberal notions of the self. Despite this, discourses of empowerment and rationalities of neoliberalism persist across these UK documents.

Although the documents analysed here vary in their terminology, this discourses present within them both promulgate neoliberal imperatives which can reducing issues of equality to a primary focus on empowering agential capacities of individuals. Particular subject positions oriented around healthy, responsible and informed citizens are thus (re)formed through these policies. These documents write about how citizens and individuals are restrained and responsible for their own health and their families. They are positioned as susceptible to prevention messages and willing to self-manage and track their health. Moreover, patients/carers, citizens and individuals are written into these documents as compliant actors, willing to access (outside of a clinical setting) their own health data and seeking to be accessible to healthcare professionals.

Democratising health? Data sharing, co-creation and collaboration
A second core rationale for digital health rests on the techno-utopian vision that digital health will have transformative effects in creating a 'more democratic future' (Petersen 2019: 17) where citizens have more autonomy over their health and care. Information is central to how agencies collaborate, whereby sharing digital information is considered crucial to better

managing health problems and democratising health. One of the guiding principles invoked through these policies is that access to more health knowledge and data may facilitate collaboration and interaction between patients and health. This is a discourse expressed strongly in *The Power of Information* strategy:

'The ability to share information following assessment between all the agencies involved in a child's care would greatly improve joining up of services around the child, and help parents and children better manage the child's condition and retain as much independence as possible'. (DoH, 2012b: 34)

Chapter 2 covers the information held within our individual care records. It sets out a vision in which being able to access and share our own records can help us take part in decisions about our own care in a genuine partnership with professionals. (DoH, 2012b: 7)

The integration of care through information sharing is central to the perceived value of digitisation within health care. Interoperability and openness are positioned as important features to ensure delivery across services and systems, to both enable patient access, but also enable collaboration and sharing of information.

'This is about ensuring that information reduces, not increases, inequalities and benefits all'. (Department of Health, 2012b: 5)

One of the stated goals in this vision of digital health is to dismantle barriers between patients and healthcare professionals and moves beyond techno-determinism through the call for a cultural shift within health care in the UK. An example given in *Department of Health* (2012b) illustrates how a digital tool can be implemented for mental ill health self-management;

South London and Maudsley (SLaM) foundation trust has launched an online health record that gives service users meaningful access to their records as well as allowing them to contribute to the system directly. The open patient record has been developed as a web portal using Microsoft's HealthVault platform. The aim is to allow clinicians and patients to work collaboratively on care and treatment rather than it being an isolated experience. (Department of Health 2012b: 24)

However, it does not set out a blueprint for a devolution of power from healthcare professional to patient. Instead, it acknowledges the social and cultural contexts in which patient/doctor interactions take place, calling for a shift in how these interactions are conducted. Nevertheless, this document has sound principles underpinning its recommendations, attempting to advance digital health in the UK through access to information.

Reflecting a focus on 'citizenship', there also is recognition of the potential use of digital technologies to create more democratic health care policies. One such is example is the use of digital technology to involve the public in the policy process. In 2014, following the launch of the Government's Digital Strategy (2013), the UK Government pioneered the use of digital media, notably Twitter, to encourage pubic commentary on a draft bill. In a news story published by the government, it notes how this 'was the first time a government department had made a draft Bill available for comment online in this way and at such an early stage in the process. The department is 'closing the circle' by explaining how people's comments are influencing changes to the Bill.' Similarly, the National Information Board (2014: 4) identified one of its aims to move towards 'more detailed work on implementation, it will prioritise co-pro-duction with citizens, and partnership with initiatives like NHS Citizen'.[3]

The digitisation of health care has also resulted in an expanding range of agencies who are able to collate and share data. The shift towards the co-production of health between health services and the public, is foregrounded in the NHS England (2016) *Healthy Children: Transforming Health Information*, which sets out a vision for restructuring health information services and systems for children, young people, parents and families. This outlines changes towards 'transformed child health information services' made up of 'various information services exchanging data in a standardised format via a central hub. Information will flow to where it is needed, improving the experience of care and health outcomes for children, young people and their families and supporting the professionals providing that care' (NHS England, 2016: 6). The vision for this Digital Child Health Hub, therefore brings together existing system with care information provided by others (e.g. parents) through the use of online personal health records. Autonomy is promoted as one the key benefits to this development, ostensibly achieved through young people having an online record of their own health and care issues and families having opportunities to co-produce health.

However, as indicated argued elsewhere (Rich and Miah, 2017), the enhanced capacity for data collection and sharing raises some critical questions about the capacity for governmentality of particular social groups. As such, inequalities might arise through the utilisation of data for decision making about health care or future funding plans, raising critical questions about patient autonomy. As Rich and Miah (2017) suggest, it is necessary to examine how data might be used as 'expert knowledge' which far from addressing disparities, might create new inequalities through discourses of risk. Such considerations are relevant to the expansion of organisations who might be involved in the collection of health related data:

> There will be specific informatics requirements to support the new public health system. These include helping local authorities to collect data that was previously collected by the NHS, for example child height and weight surveillance data to track child obesity and data to monitor delivery of the NHS Health Check programme. There is also an opportunity to improve the effectiveness and efficiency of national screening programmes by enhancing the informatics systems that drive them. Finally, the health of our children is of paramount importance to the future health of our nation. An expansion in the Health Visitor service and a series of other public health policies rely on the Child Health Information System to be effective. This system needs to be developed further to provide the best possible support for national and local child health priorities such as vaccination, commissioning care for disabled children and child safeguarding. (DoH, 2012b: 54)

It is now well established that the production of knowledge about and on people's bodies through quantified norms, can be considered to be part of a 'biopolitics' of populations (Foucault 1990) through which particular subjects are normalised and moralised. Yet, there are key questions about social inequalities which arise in relation to how such data/information is utilised in the development of particular health promotion programmes interventions or funding plans.

Autonomy and access to data systems
In this final section, we examine how discourses which emphasise autonomy are assembled alongside those of democracy and empowerment in these policy texts. In part, this perhaps reflects a broader concern about health disparities that 'people with the least amount of autonomy - the least amount of control over their work conditions or other major life circumstances

- have the poorest health' (Buchanan 2008:17). Digital technologies are justified in terms of being able to enhance autonomy, and thereby address this disparity, partly through providing opportunities for patients to access digital systems and take control of their own health care.

In the UK, efforts have been made to advance systems which enable users to access their health information and patient records, with that aim that 'all patient and care records will be digital, real-time and interoperable by 2020' (National Information Board, 2014: 29).

Across the policy texts we analysed, there is clear evidence of the focus on developing digital literacy to enhance accessibility to health care and improve patient autonomy. One of the guiding principles of this approach is the assumption that this enhanced autonomy would therefore facilitate collaboration and interaction between patients and health care professionals;

> The forward view assigns a central place to personal health records as a means of enfranchising parents, families and young people as equal partners in their care and providing a means of collaborative care. (NHS England, 2016: 19)

> The primary use of information is to support high quality care. The most important source of information is the information held in our own health and care records. The information in our records can help make sure our health and care services join up efficiently and effectively, with us at their centre. Being able to access, add to and share our health and care records electronically can help us take part in decisions about our own care. (DoH, 2012b: 16)

As such, there is evidence of recognition within these documents for the need to enhance some aspects of what Sykes *et al.* (2013: 150) describe as 'critical health literacy'

> a distinct set of characteristics of advanced personal skills, health knowledge, information skills, effective interaction between service providers and users, informed decision making and empowerment including political action as key features of critical health literacy. The potential consequences of critical health literacy identified are in improving health outcomes, creating more effective use of health services and reducing inequalities in health thus demonstrating the relevance of this concept to public health and health promotion

The focus on literacy is further elaborated in the Power of Information strategy, in which it is suggested that initiatives may be needed to support individuals in developing appropriate literacy:

> A partnership bringing together representatives from the voluntary sector, health and care professions and industry will consider how to make the most effective use of its combined skills, experience and resources to engage directly with us as patients and the public, increase our health literacy and support information producers to communicate effectively in ways that are meaningful to us. (DoH, 2012b: 66)

The above policy statements offer important steps towards addressing some aspects of digital inequality, particularly given the evidence that digital skills and levels of prior digital engagement (Hargittai and Shaw 2014) may preclude some people from digital health practices. Given that the digital footprint gap is widening, particularly among children (Robinson *et al.* 2015), it is likely that people's health opportunities will develop differently if such disparities are not addressed in future design of digital health. According to McAuley (2014), those who are most in need are the least likely to access and benefit from digital health interventions. Furthermore, Volandes and Paasche-Orlow (2007) argue that poor health literacy ought to be understood as an injustice of the healthcare system given it is a risk factor for poor health outcomes. Failure to address these complexities of digital health literacy might therefore further exclude those considered most vulnerable according to identified social gradient in health outcomes associated with levels of socioeconomic conditions.

Opportunities to utilise technologies to address a range of factors which contribute to health inequalities could be more fully harnessed in future digital health policy. By this, we are referring to the broader range of material, social and cultural inequalities (Krieger *et al.* 2010, Wilkinson and Pickett 2009) and, more specifically, the opportunities to address those inequalities which are the product of relationalities of power (Bambra *et al.* 2005). For example, political action is defined as a feature of critical health literacy, yet the possibilities for digital innovation to enable such collective response is not fully explicated in these policy documents. However, literacy is reduced to a matter of developing the correct competences in order to manage individual health appropriately within a model of behaviour change. The dominant discourse slips back into a focus on the individual; for example on how digital health literacy could be used to develop functional skills to access and interpret information to support healthy lifestyle choices:

> Good information and advice are only useful to us if we have some understanding of the health or care issues and options open to us, i.e. our health literacy. We know that health literacy levels are not high for many people, so initiatives such as health trainers can provide that additional advice and support required to make healthy living choices and decisions about our own care. (DoH, 2012b: 66)

Boyd (2014) and Livingstone and Helsper (2007) highlight the different ways in which particular populations, such as young people, access, use and engage with the Internet. These approaches highlight more complex understandings of digital engagement and exclusion, situated within relationalities of power and agency. Read this way, we need more nuanced approaches that attend to the experiences of users across, what Livingstone and Helsper (2007) describe as, 'a continuum of digital inclusion' (p 684). Thus, further critical exploration must identify how engagement with digital health technologies is shaped by sociocultural context (geographical, familial, spatial, religious, socioeconomic, cultural) and background (age, gender, digital experience). Elsewhere, NHS England (2016: 73) recommend the need to include young people in the design and development of relevant digital services:

> Use the capability of a new digital platform for children's health information to deliver apps and information which are co-created with children and young people and with Education services and which are suitable for teaching and use in schools as part of an ongoing curriculum of self-care.

Differing stakeholders must take into account how people's prior experiences should collectively shape policy. Moreover, this difference may be exacerbated by the use of digital health technologies by key agents or carers in people's lives (carers, teachers, parents, health professionals). In this sense, rather than always offering solutions to inequalities, digital technology can distribute health through a range of relational, multiple and intersecting factors.

While there is recognition that those with greatest health needs might also be those with least opportunity to engage with digital services, there is a need for more nuanced policy recommendations which address differences in conditions within which health practices and choices are made possible (Mol 2008) There is evidence of some initial explorations of this, notably in the UK's Healthy Children Transforming Child Health (2016: 30–2) document, where young people were asked about their concerns when it comes to accessing data. The issues reported highlighted the complexity and challenges of developing digital literacy, including: questions of security, data access, data sharing, language use and data control. Given these concerns, it raises critical questions about expectations on citizens to engage with personal health records and other online information.

As such, increased literacy may also mediate the benefits of using these technologies, which then makes literacy a condition of entry. Consequently, prioritising an egalitarian form of empowerment and access seen in these documents may be detrimental to patients and their (digital) health literacy, as individuals who do not feel ready for empowerment can be over-whelmed by the responsibility this process requires. This is pertinent, as Coulter *et al.* (2014) question whether it is ethical to ask patients to discuss their lived experience, if there is no possibility of intervention. So understood, the presumed empowerment through information sharing may diminish perceived autonomy about one's health and increase feelings of resigna-tion about the fact that knowledge cannot be acted upon. Newly empowered patients, or even healthy citizens, may have information readily available, but might be unable to proceed appropriately, as they still lack crucial medical knowledge and authority or the opportunity for particular health practices (Cohn 2014). The UK documents analysed do not explicitly caution about the misgivings of empowerment. Rather, the tone is positive and optimistic about patient empowerment and, especially, access to information.

Conclusion

All policy language around health care presently reinforces the centrality of digital solutions but there is only sporadic attention given by authorities to matters of variation in the impact or benefit of digital health technologies for different social groups, including those who are mar-ginalised and underprivileged. Yet, understanding this variance – or not assuming that digital solutions diminish health inequalities – has yet to be fully acknowledged as a key area of con-cern for policymakers (McAuley 2014). Such investigations are important especially as evi-dence suggests that equality is improved *only* in circumstances where participants have high levels of digital literacy (Robinson *et al.* 2015). Where this does not exist, then, the drive towards digital health solutions may exacerbate social inequalities due to the displacement of any other solution by digital solutions.

This article has presented findings from a discourse analysis of a selection of UK and Eng-lish governmental and policy documents on digital health, highlighting concerns about how digital access and equality are constituted through and absent within these discourses. We identify the need to understand them in terms of how they establish conditions of actions and types of selfhood. The analysis has revealed how equity is (re)assembled through discourses of efficiency and empowerment, democracy and autonomy. As such, citizens are positioned as objects of policy interventions in ways that assume particular agential capacities, but which obscure myriad forms of social, political, cultural and economic inequalities which impact engagement with digital health.

We recognise that many of the policies we have analysed are relatively new and it will be nec-essary for subsequent research to track the policy effects across time and space and the conditions of possibility that are created through policy-in-action (Fullagar *et al.* 2015). As expressed else-where, 'public policy formations that appear stable, potentially even complete, are never so settled. A great deal of hard political work is done in drawing heterogeneous elements together, forging connections and sustaining them in the face of tensions' (Rizvi and Lingard 2011: 8). Similarly, Bansel (2015: 5) argues that 'the multiple and often contradictory discourses, narratives, practices and experiences through which the subject of policy is governance, are embodied in ways that exceed the rationalities and ambitions of policy' This means attending to the way in which policy knowledge travels in and around different social sites, such as families, health agencies, schools and is taken up, (re)contextualised, negotiated and resisted.

Extending this line of analysis further, there is a need for policymakers to engage with the social, cultural, geographical, political contexts that mediate, limit and provide opportunity for access and engagement with digital health technologies and the data they generate. As Cohn (2014: 157) observes: 'a great wave of research over the last two decades attempting to develop techniques and evidence of behavioural change has proved to have surprisingly limited success'. To this end, a new trajectory of research must explore how cultures, practices and relations of power, shape access, use and engagement with digital health technologies, or else risk replicating or exacerbating existing inequalities.

In the few years, since England's creation of NHS Digital, a great deal more discussion has taken place. For example, in 2017, NHS Digital launched a wide consultation with digital developers to strategically involve itself within the design of third-party platforms, not as co-owners or co-developers, but as an organisation interested in elevating the efficacy and research underpinning of such applications. As well, pilots are underway to launch a single NHS mobile app for patients to use, through which they can check symptoms, book and manage appointments with GPS, order repeat prescriptions, view their medical record, register as an organ donor, and choose whether and how the NHS uses their data (NHS Digital 2018). While there is a great appeal of a single point of access to digital health care, it will be crucial to monitor behaviours around adoption of mobile health applications, else it risks making a dramatic and detrimental impact on the improvement of health inequalities.

Address for correspondence: Emma Rich, Department of Education, University of Bath, Bath, UK. E-mail: E.Rich@bath.ac.uk

Acknowledgements

This work was supported by a grant from the Wellcome Trust: 'The digital health generation: The impact of 'healthy lifestyle' technologies on young people's learning, identities and health practices' reference number: 203254/Z/16/Z.

Notes

1 The governance of healthcare within the United Kingdom is devolved across England, Northern Ireland, Scotland and Wales. Responsibility for public health care in each of these countries lies with respective governments.
2 The project 'the digital health generation: the impact of healthy lifestyle technologies on young people's learning, identities and health practices' was funded by the Wellcome Trust – 2017–2019.
3 'NHS Citizen aimed to "ensure that people and communities have an increasing say in health policy development; and how NHS services are commissioned, designed and delivered"' https://www.england.nhs.uk/participation/get-involved/how/nhs-citizen/

References

Ball, S.J. (2015) What is policy? 21 years later: Reflections on the possibilities of policy research, *Discourse: Studies in the Cultural Politics of Education*, 36, 3, 306–13.

Bambra, C. (2012) Reducing health inequalities: New data suggests that the English strategy was partially successful, *Journal of Epidemiology and Community Health*, 66, 7, 662.

Bambra, C., Fox, D. and Scott-Samuel, A. (2005) Towards a politics of health, *Health Promotion International*, 20, 2, 187–93.

Bansel, P. (2015) The subject of policy, *Critical Studies in Education*, 56, 1, 5–20.

Baum, F. and Fisher, M. (2014) Why behavioural health promotion endures despite its failure to reduce health inequities, *Sociology of Health & Illness*, 36, 2, 213–25.

Blue, S., Shove, E., Carmona, C. and Kelly, M.P. (2016) Theories of practice and public health: Understanding (un)healthy practices, *Critical Public Health*, 26, 1, 36–50.

Boyd, D. (2014) *It's Complicated*. New Haven, CT: Yale University Press.

Buchanan, D.R. (2008) Autonomy, paternalism and justice: Ethical priorities in public health, *American Journal of Public Health.*, 98, 1, 15–21.

Cabinet Office. (2013) Government Digital Strategy: December 2013. Available at https://www.gov.uk/government/publications/government-digital-strategy/government-digital-strategy

Cabinet Office. (2014a) Digital Inclusion Strategy. Available at https://www.gov.uk/government/publications/government-digital-inclusion-strategy/government-digital-inclusion-strategy

Cabinet Office. (2014b) Digital Inclusion Charter. Available at https://www.gov.uk/government/publications/government-digital-inclusion-strategy

Carabine, J. (2001) Unmarried motherhood 1830–1990: A Genealogical Analysis. In Wetherell, M., Taylor, S. and Yates, S.J. (eds) *Discourse as Data: A Guide for Analysis*. London: SAGE Publications, pp 267–310.

Cohn, S. (2014) From health behaviours to health practices: Critical perspectives, an introduction, *Sociology of Health & Illness Special Issue*, 36, 2, 157–62.

Coulter, A., Locock, L., Ziebland, S. and Calabrese, J. (2014) Collecting data on patient experience is not enough: They must be used to improve care, *British Medical Journal*, 348, 2225.

Crawford, R. (1980) Healthism and the medicalization of everyday life, *International Journal of Health Services*, 10, 365–89.

Department for International Trade. (2018) Guidance: UK Life Sciences Trade Organisations, Membership Associations, Clusters, and Research and Innovation Networks. Available at https://www.gov.uk/government/publications/uk-life-sciences-support/uk-life-sciences-membership-associations.

Department of Health. (2012a) Digital strategy: Leading the Culture Change in Health and Care. Available at https://www.gov.uk/government/publications/digital-strategy-leading-the-culture-change-in-health-and-care

Department of Health. (2012b) The Power of Information: Putting all of Us in Control of the Health and Care Information We Need. Available at https://www.gov.uk/government/publications/giving-people-control-of-the-health-and-care-information-they-need

Department of Health and Social Care. (2014) DH digital strategy update: 2014 to 2015. Available at https://www.gov.uk/government/publications/dh-digital-strategy-update-2014-to-2015/dh-digital-strategy-update-2014-to-2015-2

Dutton, W.H., Blank, G. and Groselj, D. (2013). *Cultures of the Internet: The Internet in Britain. Oxford Internet Survey 2013*. Oxford: Oxford internet Institute, University of Oxford.

European Commission. (2014) Green paper on mobile health ('m-health'). Brussels: European Commission. Available at https://ec.europa.eu/digital-agenda/en/news/green-paper-mobile-health-mhealth

Foucault, M. (1977) *The Archaeology of Knowledge*. London: Tavistock.

Foucault, M. (1978) *The history of sexuality: An introduction*. London: Penguin.

Foucault, M. (1990) *The History of Sexuality: An Introduction*, Vol. I. Translated by R. Hurley. New York: Vintage Books.

Fullagar, S., Rich, E. and Francombe-Webb, J. (2015) Assembling active bodies and places: policy tensions across sport, health and equality agendas in the UK. *International Sociology of Sport Association World Conference*. Paris, 09-12 June 2015.

Garthwaite, K., Smith, K.E., Bambra, C. and Pearce, J. (2016) Desperately seeking reductions in health inequalities: Perspectives of UK researchers on past, present and future directions in health inequalities research, *Sociology of Health & Illness*, 38, 3, 459–78.

Ghosh, P. (2018) AI early diagnosis could save heart and cancer patients, BBC News, Available At: http://www.bbc.co.uk/news/health-42357257

Hargittai, E. and Shaw, A. (2014) Mind the skills gap: The role of Internet know-how and gender in differentiated contributions to Wikipedia, *Information, Communication & Society*, 18, 4, 424–42.

Health and Social Care Information Centre. (2015) Information and technology for better care: Health and Social Care Information Centre Strategy 2015–2020, NHS Digital.

Ioannou, S. (2005) Health logic and health-related behaviours, *Critical Public Health*, 15, 3, 263–73.

Jennings, L. and Gagliardi, L. (2013) Influence of mhealth interventions on gender relations in developing countries: A systematic literature review, *International Journal for Equity in Health*, 12, 85.

Kelly, M.P. and Barker, M. (2016) Why is changing health-related behaviour so difficult?, *Public Health*, 136, 109–16.

Krieger, N., Alegría, M., Almeida-Filho, N., Barbosa da Silva, J., *et al.* (2010) Who, and what, causes health inequities? Reflections on emerging debates from an exploratory Latin American/North American workshop, *Journal of Epidemiology and Community Health*, 64, 9, 747–9.

Livingstone, S. and Helsper, E. (2007) Gradations in digital inclusion: Children, young people and the digital divide, *New Media and Society*, 9, 4, 671–96.

Lupton, D. (2013) The digitally engaged patient: Self-Monitoring and self-care in the digital health era, *Social Theory and Health*, 11, 3, 256–70.

Mackenbach, J.P. (2011) Can we reduce health inequalities? An analysis of the English strategy (1997–2010), *Journal of Epidemiology and Community Health*, 65, 7, 568–75.

Maguire, M. and Ball, S.J. (1994) Discourses of educational reform in the United Kingdom and the USA and the work of teachers, *Journal of In-Service Education*, 20, 1, 5–16.

Marmot, M. and Bell, R. (2012) Fair society, healthy lives, *Public Health*, 126, 1, 4–10.

Marmot, M. and Wilkinson, R. (2001) Psychosocial and material pathways in the relation between income and health: A response to Lynch et al., *BMJ*, 322, 7296, 1233–6.

McAuley, A. (2014) Digital health interventions: Widening access or widening inequalities?, *Public Health*, 128, 12, 1118–20.

Mol, A. (2008) *The Logic of Care: Health and the Problem of Patient Choice*. London: Routledge.

National Advisory Group on Health Information Technology in England. (2016) Making IT Work: Harnessing the Power of Health Information Technology to Improve Care in England. Available at: https://assets.publishing.service.gov.uk/government/uploads/system/uploads/attachment_data/file/550866/Wachter_Review_Accessible.pdf

National Information Board. (2014) Personalised Health and Care 2020 Using Data and Technology to Transform Outcomes for Patients and Citizens A Framework for Action. Available at https://www.gov.uk/government/publications/personalised-health-and-care-2020

NHS Digital. (2018) NHS App. Available at https://digital.nhs.uk/services/nhs-app

NHS England Publications. (2016) Healthy Children: A Forward View for Child Health Information.

Peacock, M., Bissell, P. and Owen, J. (2014) Dependency denied: Health inequalities in the neo-liberal era, *Social Science & Medicine*, 118, C, 173–80.

Petersen, A. (2019) *Digital Health and Technological Promise; A Sociological Inquiry*. London: Routledge.

Petersen, A. and Lupton, D. (1996) *The New Public Health: Health and Self in the Age of Risk*. London: Sage.

Popay, J., Whitehead, M. and Hunter, D. (2010) Injustice is killing people on a large scale – but what is to be done about it?, *Journal of Public Health*, 32, 2, 148–9.

Public Health England. (2017) Digital-First Public health: Public Health England's digital strategy. Available at https://www.gov.uk/government/publications/digital-first-public-health/digital-first-public-health-public-health-englands-digital-strategy

Rich, E. and Miah, A. (2014) Understanding digital health as public pedagogy: A critical framework, *Societies*, 4, 296–315.

Rich, E. and Miah, A. (2017) Mobile, wearable and ingestible health technologies: Towards a critical research agenda, *Health Sociology Review*, 26, 1, 84–97.

Rizvi, F. and Lingard, B. (2011) Social equity and the assemblage of values in Australian higher education, *Cambridge Journal of Education*, 41, 1, 5–22.

Robinson, L., Cotten, S.R., Ono, H., Quan-Haase, A., *et al.* (2015) Digital inequalities and why they
matter, *Information, Communication & Society*, 18, 5, 569–82.

Scambler, G. (2012) Health inequalities, *Sociology of Health & Illness*, 34, 1, 130–46.

Scott-Samuel, A. and Smith, K. (2015) Fantasy Paradigms of Health Inequalities: Utopian thinking?,
Social Theory & Health, 13, 3–4, 418–36.

Smith, K.E. and Kandlik Eltanani, M. (2015) What kinds of policies to reduce health inequalities in the
UK do researchers support?, *Journal of Public Health*, 37, 1, 6–17.

Swan, M. (2012) Health 2050: The realization of personalised medicine through crowdsourcing, the
quantified self and the participatory biocitizen, *Journal of Personalised Medicine*, 2, 93–118.

Sykes, S., Wills, J., Rowlands, G. and Popple, K. (2013) Understanding critical health literacy: A concept
analysis, *BMC Public Health*, 13, 150.

Taylor, S. (1997) Critical policy analysis: Exploring contexts, texts and consequences, *Discourse Studies*,
18, 1, 23–35.

Thompson, L. and Kumar, A. (2011) Responses to health promotion campaigns: Resistance, denial and
othering, *Critical Public Health*, 21, 105–17.

Volandes, A.E. and Paasche-Orlow, M.K. (2007) Health literacy, health inequality and a just healthcare
system, *The American Journal of Bioethics*, 7, 11, 5–10.

Walt, G., Shiffman, J., Schneider, H., Murray, S.F., *et al.* (2008) 'Doing' health policy analysis: Methodological and conceptual reflections and challenges, *Health Policy and Planning*, 23, 5, 308–17.

Wilkinson, R. and Pickett, K. (2009) *The Spirit Level: Why More Equal Societies Almost Always do Better*. London: Penguin.

Williams, O. and Fullagar, S. (2018) Lifestyle drift and the phenomenon of 'citizen shift' in contemporary UK health policy, *Sociology of Health & Illness*, 1–6, https://doi.org/10.1111/1467-9566.12783.

World Health Organization. (2008) *Commission on the Social Determinants of Health. Final Report.
Closing the Gap in a Generation: Health Equity through Action on the Social Determinants of Health*.
Geneva: World Health Organization.

Sociology of Health & Illness Vol. 41 No. S1 2019 ISSN 0141-9889, pp. 50–64
doi: 10.1111/1467-9566.12872

Navigating the cartographies of trust: how patients and carers establish the credibility of online treatment claims

Alan Petersen[1], Claire Tanner[2] and Megan Munsie[2]

[1]*Sociology and Gender Studies, School of Social Sciences, Monash University, Melbourne, Vic, Australia*
[2]*Department of Anatomy and Neuroscience, Centre for Stem Cell Systems, School of Biomedical Sciences, University of Melbourne, Melbourne, Vic, Australia*

Abstract   Digital media offer citizens novel ways of 'enacting' health and illness, and treatment and care. However, while digital media may so 'empower' citizens, those searching for credible information will be confronted with various, often-conflicting claims that may have 'disempowering' effects. This article uses Gieryn's concept of the 'cultural cartography' to explore the criteria that patients and carers employ in establishing the credibility of information on alleged treatments. Drawing on data from interviews with Australian patients and carers who have travelled or considered travelling abroad for unproven commercial stem cell treatments, the article examines how individuals assess rival sources of epistemic authority – science-based and non-science-based – as they search for credible information. As we argue, in a context where conventional treatment options are perceived to be limited or non-existent – which is likely to be the case with those suffering severe, life-limiting conditions – and the credibility of sources uncertain, matters of opinion and belief are prone to being interpreted as matters of fact, with potentially far-reaching implications for citizens' health. Revealing the mechanisms by which individuals ascribe credibility to health information, we conclude, has become crucial as digital media assume a growing role in health and healthcare and governments encourage citizens to become 'digitally literate'.

Keywords: trust, credibility, hope, stem cell tourism, cultural cartography, digital technology

Introduction

For those newly diagnosed with a chronic illness or disability, the Internet offers a panorama of possibilities in regards to information about their condition and options for treatment and care. The Internet may be the primary or sole source of information for people or it may be used to supplement health and medical information initially gained from practitioners or other sources (European Commission 2012: 58). Surveys undertaken in the US, Australia and other economically rich nations with a high level of Internet penetration reveal that a significant proportion of those who seek health information begin at, or at some stage use, a search engine such as Google, Bing or Yahoo (Pew Research Centre 2013, Wong *et al.* 2014). Further,

Digital Health: Sociological Perspectives, First Edition.
Edited by Flis Henwood and Benjamin Marent.

citizens may use social media to produce and share content, such as experiences of health, illness and treatment or care options, and to collectively organise to promote research, gain access to treatments, and raise funds to support these activities (Shim 2014, Sosnowy 2014). They may combine credentialed expertise and lay knowledge to form 'epistemic communities', and thereby become influential policy actors or 'evidence-based activists' (Akrich 2010, Rabeharisoa *et al.* 2013). However, while digital media may 'empower' citizens in these ways, their routine use in health and healthcare raises questions about the credibility and trustworthiness of information that is relied upon for decisions about treatment and care. This is particularly pertinent in a context of direct-to-consumer advertising where commercial providers offer therapies yet to be recognised by the established medical authorities.

This article explores the criteria that individuals employ in establishing the credibility of information on claimed treatments as they encounter different sources, and it considers the implications for conceptions of trust in increasingly digitally mediated healthcare. We focus on the experiences of those who have travelled or considered travelling abroad for advertised stem cell treatments (SCTs). This is an area of medical research with a particularly complex topography ranging from proven treatments for a limited number of specific conditions, to clinical trials where promising interventions for additional conditions are evaluated for safety and efficacy. In addition, there are a growing number of interventions being offered outside clinical trials and marketed directly to the consumer where there is little scientific justification for their use. Here, we ask: how do advertised 'treatments' that have been assessed by conventional medical standards to be clinically unproven come to be perceived as credible therapeutic options? On what basis is information about these options and those that provide them judged to be trustworthy or not? The paper draws on interviews with Australian patients and carers (parents or partners of patients), and uses Gieryn's (1999) concept of the 'cultural cartography', that he employed in his analysis of the credibility contests that characterise science, to reveal the mechanisms by which claims come to be judged as having epistemic authority and thus credible or as lacking such authority and thus not credible.

As we argue, in a context where conventional treatment options are perceived to be limited or non-existent – which is likely to be the case with those suffering severe, life-limiting conditions – and the credibility of sources uncertain, matters of opinion and belief are prone to being interpreted as matters of fact, with trust based on a 'leap of faith' or investment in hope. In the article, we explore these complex dynamics of credibility and trust, including their temporal dimensions, as they manifest in the accounts of those with various chronic and acquired conditions who decide to travel and those who decide not to travel for advertised SCTs. As we conclude, understanding the criteria by which citizens ascribe credibility to health information has become crucial as digital media assume a growing role in medicine and healthcare and governments encourage individuals to take a greater responsibility for their own treatment and care. We begin by briefly charting the rise of the market of alleged SCTs, which relies heavily on promissory discourse and online advertising techniques, before introducing our theoretical perspective and the research data upon which we draw.

The Internet and the advertising of SCTs

The growth of the market of alleged SCTs has paralleled and been enabled by growing access to the Internet and use of social media. This market is one that is buoyed by optimism surrounding the potential of stem cell science and its promise to deliver regenerative therapies for many conditions in the future (Morrison 2012). And, it is here that the Internet has played a considerable role. Since approximately 2006, a burgeoning number of these clinically unproven 'treatments' have been advertised directly to consumers via the Internet for various conditions, including spinal cord injury, multiple sclerosis, macular degeneration and Alzheimer's disease (Petersen *et al.* 2017: 6–7).

This 'direct-to-consumer' advertising has been found to employ various techniques to effect a positive portrayal of products and their providers and lend them legitimacy, involving strong emotional appeals: patient testimonials and blogs to connect directly with audiences; links to 'Frequently Asked Questions' with responses that offer reassurances about the safety and efficacy of treatments; the use of scientific and news sources (e.g. about developments in the field) that lend credibility to claims; images and descriptions of clinics and hospitals and of providers' qualifications that convey professionalism, competence and care for patients; and the omission of information on uncertainties and risks (e.g. longer term treatment outcomes and likely additional costs such as travel and accommodation for patients and carers) that would present a more qualified picture of the state of the field (Petersen and Seear 2011). Notwithstanding years of commentary on the state of stem cell science and the difficulties of clinical translation, advertising strategies that use positive claims and portrayals regarding the safety and effectiveness of products have been found to be reasonably consistent over time (Ogbogu *et al.* 2013).

Commercial clinics have sought to leverage the promise and optimism that surrounds the hundreds of trials currently underway to ascertain the safety and efficacy of the different interventions using stem cells or cells made from them (NIH 2017). In advertising their products and services, providers are capitalising on the strong 'translational ethos' and hopeful discourse that attaches to the field of stem cell science (Maienschein *et al.* 2008). At the same time, the rise of the Internet and social media has facilitated the flourishing of online communities of patients with various conditions and/or their families, who share information and personal stories and sometimes lobby for research or to gain access to these products on 'compassionate' grounds (e.g. Margottini 2014, Spalleta 2015).

While science organisations have long argued that the sale of these alleged treatments poses physical and financial risks to patients and potentially undermines confidence and trust in stem cell science (Daley *et al.* 2016), the SCT market has thrived. According to the standards of science, credibility rests on the claim to provide a reliable body of knowledge about the world (Stemwedel 2011). In the case of stem cell science, credibility is founded on the claim that 'evidence' of the efficacy and safety of treatments should be established through 'gold standard' clinical trials, with findings published in peer-reviewed articles, *before* treatments gain regulatory approval (Timmermans and Berg 2003). Yet SCTs that may not find application in mainstream clinical practice for many years to come, given the lengthy period and considerable financial investment required to undertake fundamental research and conduct trials before treatments gain approval (Dickson and Gagnon 2009).

Missing from idealised portrayals of the science is acknowledgement that stem cell-based interventions may need to be tailored for each type of chronic, congenital or acquired condition, and that for some conditions a cellular replacement strategy remains unlikely due to the complexity of the disease. While clinical successes thus far are limited to the use of blood stem cells for the treatment of many types of cancers and diseases of the blood and immune system, and a small number of other applications that capitalise on the presence of stem cells in skin and the surface of the eye, scientific and public optimism for stem cell science remains high, especially with frequent media reports of 'breakthroughs', leading to 'gaps' between people's expectations and clinical practice (Cossu *et al.* 2017: 1). In Cossu, *et al.*'s view, this context has created the conditions for the flourishing of inadequately regulated clinics that appeal to patients and their families who, in the absence of reliable information from trials, cannot be informed of the benefits and risks of advertised SCTs (2017: 1).

While it is difficult to determine the overall size of the SCT market, since there is no systematic mechanism for recording and verifying patient numbers at the country level, the evidence suggests that it is substantial and growing. A 2016 review of the global distribution of businesses advertising stem cells found an increased activity at the global level, with over four hundred websites advertising stem cell-based therapies for a wide range of conditions, a large and growing proportion of which were in rich countries such as the US, UK, Australia, China and Germany (Berger *et al.* 2016). Regulation of this market has proved difficult for various reasons, including its complex character involving opaque and sometimes highly mobile national and transnational actors, the political and practical difficulty of harmonising and coordinating multiple regulatory agencies, regulatory exemptions regarding autologous SCTs in some jurisdictions, the myriad array of claimed stem cell products for a huge range of conditions, and the multiple sources and means by which information on treatments may be procured (Cossu *et al.* 2017, Sleeboom-Faulkner *et al.* 2016). Insofar as individual countries have enacted regulations, these have in some instances been questioned for being insufficiently rigorous. Japan, for example, introduced legislation in 2014 allowing 'conditional', time-limited approval that some argue has set the bar too low in terms of demonstrating clinical utility and may result in patients being exposed to unscrupulous providers and removing the incentive to participate in stem cell trials (Chan 2017: 841–4, Sipp 2015). Meanwhile, individuals who have exhausted current treatment options are presented with various, often-optimistic claims about SCTs that circulate online and offline.

The cultural cartography of credibility

In exploring the criteria used by individuals in establishing the credibility of information on alleged treatments, it is useful to consider the 'cultural cartography' within which credibility contests occur. According to Thomas Gieryn (1999), the establishment of credibility claims can be envisaged in terms of cultural maps used by individuals to 'find workable truths about nature and (sometimes) suffer the consequences of practical choices they make based on where epistemic authority is located' (1999: 12–3). The mapping metaphor serves heuristically to call attention to the process by which boundaries between rival sources of epistemic authority regarding particular knowledge or practice are drawn and then redrawn. According to Gieryn, in such a process, credibility claims are contested and overturned, as some claims become persuasive and others marginalised and denounced as matters of faith, illusion, ulterior motive and so on. As Gieryn argues, those within science may seek to police the boundary of 'real' science by highlighting posers' failure to conform with expected ethical or methodological practice. Those outside science, on the other hand, may draw different cultural maps, using rival epistemic authorities to curtail the reach of science, by pointing to their inadequacy or liability in regards to certain kinds of issues – subjective, political and ethical (1999: 22).

As Gieryn argues, mapping the boundaries of credibility ('boundary-work') has different consequences for different actors, both for those who draw them and those who rely on them, in terms of authority, fame, influence and employment. People's reliance on cultural maps allows them to distribute responsibility for 'facts of nature', some of which may be regarded as provisionally true for the practical choices people make and some fabricated, false or discrepant and therefore disregarded as a basis for action. Decisions may be grounded in science, which is the generally preferred source of knowledge about nature, or some other authority (e.g. religion, personal experience), as people become more convinced of the accuracy, trustworthiness and effectiveness of truth claims, or they may subsequently justify those decisions by reference to the greater expertise and competence of those who are trusted with the truth (1999: 13).

The boundaries of science are 'perpetually contested terrain' since the issues at stake are often significant, in terms of status, power and access to material rewards (Gieryn 1999: 15). While establishing and maintaining credibility is crucial for all professional areas, this is especially so for new or emergent fields of science, such as stem cell science, where the borders and territories are still being mapped and where legitimacy of practice depends crucially on establishing and maintaining public and policy support. For such fields, at stake is the autonomy over scientists' ability 'to define problems and select procedures for investigating them', which is achieved by 'purifying science' and demarcating it from all political and market concerns (1999: 23). In the case of SCTs, those who profit from the early advertising of clinically unproven interventions are seen to 'pollute truth' and to threaten the boundaries that define the very essence of 'science'. Consequently, scientists have sought to police the boundaries of stem cell science by discrediting SCT providers' claims, pointing to the lack of verifiable evidence of benefit for their products, the health risks associated with the intervention or its administration, and to the exploitative character of their practices.

Gieryn's ideas have found useful application in sociological studies of various professional areas, in revealing how disputes between contending experts are negotiated (e.g. Burri 2008, Cadge 2012, González 2016, Kurath 2015). In such studies, the application of the concept of 'boundary-work', whereby the contours of a field are mapped so as to establish claims in a contested territory of legitimacy, has proved insightful. However, Gieryn's ideas have yet to be applied to analysing the negotiations and deliberations that occur as lay citizens encounter different sources of information during their research on conditions and treatments. As noted, in the age of digital media citizens both produce and consume information, often combining credentialed expertise and lay knowledge to form their own epistemic communities. By exploring how people respond to multiple, including discrepant claims about health, illness and treatment that they encounter in these different communities, one can potentially learn much about the changing bases for credibility claims and notions of trust upon which they rely in a digitally mediated age.

Methods

This article draws upon data arising from a 4-year (2012–2015) Australian Research Council funded project on 'stem cell tourism'. This project aimed to explore the sociocultural dynamics of stem cell tourism, particularly the factors shaping Australian's views and expectations of SCTs offered abroad. It investigated the contributions of various factors, including informal networks and information sources – such as the Internet, print media, treatment providers and other travellers – to the shaping of individuals' expectations and decisions about treatments. We did not set out to explore issues of credibility per se; however, our findings revealed the diverse sources consulted by respondents as they sought to gain credible or trusted sources of information on their conditions and treatment options. As part of the study, interviews were undertaken via the telephone with patients or their carers (generally parents or partners) who had been diagnosed with a range of conditions, including lymphoedema, motor neuron disease, chronic obstructive pulmonary disease, autism, multiple sclerosis, spinal cord injury and Parkinson's disease, and who had either travelled abroad for treatments ('travellers') ($n = 24$) or who had considered travelling but at the time of the interview had not yet done so ('non-travellers') ($n = 27$). While phone interviews have limitations, particularly in not allowing observation of respondents' reactions to questions, they enabled us to include respondents from across Australia, some of whom were remotely located.

The sample was self-selected by two principal means: our project's website and through patient organisations, whose representatives distributed (via newsletters) information about our study and contact details to members. In both cases, respondents were able to contact us if they were willing to be interviewed. As noted above, people who underwent treatment or considered undergoing treatment, as well as carers of people, who were often intimately involved in information gathering, decision-making processes and or treatment journeys, were invited to participate. The final sample of travellers comprised 9 males and 15 females, of which 11 were patients and 13 carers; the non-travellers comprised 14 males and 13 females, of which 16 were patients and 11 carers. In the majority of cases, patients (some children) were suffering serious, life-limiting conditions, where prognoses were poor and treatment options limited. Some were developmental or neurological conditions, such as autism or multiple sclerosis, or physical disabilities that affected movement or posture, such as cerebral palsy or spinal cord injury. Many of these conditions involve combinations of symptoms such as loss of motor control, fatigue, and incontinence. Consequently, our respondents may have been especially open to exploring 'non-traditional' treatments. In interviews, they often claimed (and evidently appeared) to have undertaken extensive research on their conditions and in some cases were well versed in their scientific aspects – which may make them atypical of patients and carers in being especially skilled in their ability to make sense of and discriminate between different sources of information.

Interviews were mostly undertaken with individual patients or carers themselves; however, on three occasions, they were undertaken with both the patient and their carer being present. One individual was interviewed on two different occasions – as a 'non-traveller' then a 'traveller'. By interviewing 'travellers' and 'non-travellers', we aimed to ascertain differences in views on and expectations of SCTs and the factors shaping these. While within Australia there was a growing marketplace for unproven stem cell 'treatments' during the time the interviews were conducted, most local clinics limited their services to musculoskeletal conditions (Munsie and Pera 2014), and were rarely a consideration for our participants.

Questions explored with 'travellers' included how individuals learnt about SCTs offered outside Australia, the factors shaping their decisions about treatments, knowledge about treatments undertaken, responses of family, friends, physicians and others to decisions about treatments, and their experiences of treatments and providers. Questions explored with 'non-travellers' included knowledge and perspectives on SCTs, reasons for not undertaking treatments abroad, the influence of family, friends, physicians and others on decision-making, perceptions of risks, and other factors shaping decisions and sources of information (if any) on SCTs. Interviews, which generally lasted 1 hour, were conducted via phone, and the data were coded and thematically analysed with the assistance of NVivo and Word search. Each member of the research team contributed to the analysis and agreed on the themes, with attention paid to the respondents' accounts of their decisions to travel or not to travel and of the factors affecting these decisions, including the influence of different sources of information, and to pre- and post-travel experiences, including engagements with the providers themselves. In analysing the data, we were particularly interested in determining differences in travellers' and non-travellers' views and expectations and the factors shaping these. Pseudonyms are used to protect individuals' privacy.

The findings

Visiting the Internet
Consistent with earlier studies (e.g. Pew Research Center 2013, Wong *et al.* 2014), our research revealed that, for patients and carers, whether travellers or non-travellers, the Internet,

Facebook and blogs were major sources of information regarding treatment options as well as on the condition itself. They also provided a means for individuals to connect with other patients and providers. For some, the Internet provided their sole source of information. However, in the majority of cases, individuals combined different sources – both online and offline – with their reliance on each varying over time as they sought to clarify their treatment options and to confirm the credibility of sources and information. Offline sources included print media such as newspapers, and third parties, often personally significant others, typically members of one's family and trusted doctors, but also those met as a result of chance encounters or during the course of one's daily activities, such as other patients and tradesmen. Some also recounted face-to-face meetings with the providers themselves, generally after having first researched their details online. While we acknowledge the significance of these offline sources in decisions, our main focus in this article is on patients and carers as seekers of credible online information in the context of the direct-to-consumer advertising of treatments.

Searches were undertaken in a context where many individuals felt that the consulting doctors and other health professionals had effectively abandoned them by failing to offer hope in regards to further treatment. However, a range of responses to doctors were noted, ranging from indifference and equivocation to support. For example, some noted that their doctors said that they had read about SCT and heard that it could be beneficial but were reluctant to pass judgement about its efficacy, choosing instead to adopt a 'non-directive' approach (Petersen *et al.* 2017). Many respondents expressed a sense of injustice in being denied the information, or access to trials or treatments that they felt could and should have been made available to them. However, as some expressed it, 'doing nothing' was not an option, and individuals consequently attempted to source information and advice about treatments, using the Internet and personal contacts, often forged online, to inform themselves.

While some searched for treatments in general and then encountered advertisements or personal stories about SCTs, others sought to find out more about SCTs after having first heard about them from other sources such as friends or news coverage. During interviews, some respondents indicated that they began searching the Internet after discovering that SCTs, clinical trials, or information on treatments were not 'available' in Australia. In telling their stories, respondents presented themselves as being well researched and as seeking to leave 'no stone unturned' in their search for treatments but also in their quest to learn 'the truth' about them. As Alex, who had a spinal cord injury and at the time of interview had not travelled for treatment, said, 'I spent every afternoon for probably 2 or 3 years just reading and ... sourcing the information, and as much as I could, and going to meetings and stuff like that'.

Navigating different information sources
During their searches, individuals often explored different information sources, each offering either only partial perspectives on SCTs or views that conflicted with those obtained elsewhere, which served to raise questions about the basis for their belief and trust in the credibility of sources and prompted further investigation. Dan, who had a spinal cord injury and had considered travelling to Germany for SCT because 'it's in Europe, it's got to ... have some legitimacy and ... it's got to be good', but then decided not to travel after further enquiries, offers insight into the often-tortuous route followed:

> Well there wasn't a great deal of information on the web and what was there, thinking about their site, didn't really ... instil a great deal of confidence in you, when you looked at it. So I then went onto another website which was more of a blog type chat forum operated out of the States, and picked up a couple of threads of information there, and followed those, and found a lot more information through this blog site than anywhere else, which

led into newspaper reports from the UK on people who had travelled there, who'd had prob-
lems, which then also led to another newspaper article, which again I think was out of the
UK, that highlighted the fact that they were operating within Germany under a loophole in
German legislation ... .

As Gieryn notes, when faced with multiple and discrepant accounts of nature, people need
'still other maps to assign authority over the task of mapping' – that is, 'second-order boundary-work' – to locate 'credible cultural cartographers' or sources that can be relied upon to dismiss a rival's map as 'unskilled or misleading or deceptive' (1999: 17–8). While both
travellers and non-travellers recounted broadly similar experiences in their quest to confirm
credibility claims, the latter appeared to stay more within the boundaries of science in that they
expressed concerns about lack of transparency of results and outcomes that would have been
found in published peer-reviewed journals. In the above non-traveller's account, the individual's suspicions of a website led to investigation of other, in their view more credible, sources
such as blogs and news articles that tend to rely less on scientific criteria of evidence than on
personal experiences and popularised depictions of science. The use of various media – in the
above case, a US blog and a UK news article – was common. Such sources, it should be
noted, rely heavily on patients' stories, sometimes recounting heroic quests to gain SCTs.
Patient blogs, for example, involve personal experiences of treatment, and sometimes advocate
for 'compassionate use' of experimental therapies, thereby bypassing strict rules qualifying
patients for participation in clinical trials (Zettler 2015). In contrast to Dan's experience,
above, of finding critical media reports which preceded the closure of the X-Cell Centre in
Germany, the 'articles' cited by participants were mostly those appearing in news media or
online forums that focus on scientific 'breakthroughs' and stories of promise.

On the other hand, only a few respondents mentioned consulting medical or scientific journals or deriving sources of information from articles published therein. Theo, a non-traveller,
in the early stages of motor neurone disease, stated that they read 'mainly the scientific journals' and that they were not 'so interested in individual cases', while another non-traveller,
Len, who had an optic nerve problem following a stroke, indicated that they had 'been through
medical journals which most of which don't make sense to me'. However, as the comments of
the latter suggest, individuals may struggle to interpret what they read. As Len elaborated,
'you need to have some sort of medical background or someone that you can rely on who is
going to give you ... an honest opinion or can sort through what you're reading because
there's so much stuff out there'.

In short, while individuals sought an ultimate source of authority to adjudicate between contending claims about SCTs, they often felt unassisted and had to rely on their own judgement
and resources. While it is hazardous to generalise about differences between travellers and
non-travellers in regards to their use of particular sources, since at the time of the interview
some of the latter had adopted a 'wait and see' approach and continued to explore their
options, the non-travellers' responses suggest that they may inhabit epistemic communities that
are more science-based in that they were more inclined to question non-scientific claims.

Symbolic significance of science
Like citizens in general, many of those considering SCTs looked to 'science' as the preferred
source of knowledge when seeking to establish the legitimacy of claims (Gieryn 1999: 14).
While few respondents consulted medical or science journals or read scientific articles, or
talked to scientists, some mentioned that the providers whom they had identified or contacted
had research published in medical or scientific journals or displayed other attributes of scientific expertise or distinction, which they evidently saw as an indicator of their legitimacy. For

example, when asked whether he talked with his treating doctor about his previous experience, Benjamin, who was in 'the final stage' of scleroderma, an autoimmune rheumatic disease, replied:

> He's got 400 or so peer-reviewed articles or 500 peer-reviewed articles. He got named at one stage as one of the leaders in chemotherapy treatments in all of Europe. So it wasn't like I was going to some back-shop operator.

When asked about how they judged the credibility of the doctors in a Panamanian clinic whom they contacted, Faye, the mother of a child with cerebral palsy, responded:

> ... Mostly just reading their bios and just doing some research online then, just Googling the names, Googling the hospitals they used to work at, that sort of stuff. Just tried to authenticate, to a certain extent their credentials. And they all sort of checked out. A couple of them, one of the doctors that I read about at the clinic in Panama has written an article in a medical journal which made me go, 'Yeah, okay, well they wouldn't just let me write in their medical journal and call myself a doctor'.

Comments such as these suggest that individuals saw these articles as lending credibility to the claimed treatments and in some cases the provider, since it offered evidence of a link to legitimate medical research. As noted, advertisements for SCTs have been found to make considerable reference to scientific articles and other symbols of science (e.g. assurances of 'accreditation', the citing of professional qualifications, images of clinics) as an indicator of their legitimacy, along with testimonials recounting positive experiences and assurances of competence and care, as techniques for establishing credibility for treatment and engendering trust in providers (Lau *et al.* 2008, Ogbogu *et al.* 2013, Petersen and Seear 2011).

That evidence of links to legitimate or reputable science may carry considerable weight in credibility contests is supported by some respondents' references to hospitals or websites being 'university-linked' or 'university-run' and to 'trials' being undertaken, when recounting why they decided to proceed with SCTs or visit particular clinics. Respondents were, in short, drawing on the symbolic resources used by scientists to demarcate the boundary between legitimate and illegitimate knowledge (Gieryn 1999: 17). However, interestingly, while respondents' accounts suggest that these symbols of science may carry considerable weight in the assessment of credibility claims, in framing their accounts individuals relied heavily on subjective, non-scientific points of reference – the 'evidence' referred to being one's own or others' experiences or impressions. References to other patients' (generally positive) experiences, to national stereotypes and to 'gut feeling', for example about the 'sophistication' or otherwise of providers' websites, were common. This reflects a more general tendency for epistemic authority to be decided 'downstream', in the local, episodic and contingent rather than the universal, involving formal criteria and actual practices in the laboratory or clinic (Gieryn 1999: 27).

Subjective, non-scientific criteria
The deployment of such subjective, non-scientific criteria in evaluations of credibility was strongly evident in the story of the following individual, Janet, a carer for their partner, a health professional, who had a genetic condition affecting muscle function. In this case, the role of local, contingent factors in decisions was also apparent. As they said, they had starting looking into SCTs in the previous 2 years as they were 'willing to take a few more risks than they would have before' because 'all [my husband's] cousins have died quite suddenly and [my husband] is actually commenting that he's feeling worse' than he was when he was first diagnosed 16 years earlier.

We Googled stem cell therapy which is probably the usual thing that most people do and then we came up with different sort of websites and a lot of India stuff. And we're sort of, even though my husband is from [Asian country] and we're not anti-Asian medicine, we did feel that India may be pushing boundaries or a bit of a rip-off just because that's how we perceive that country ... . We then found an American website which we felt, seemed a lot more credible, and ... I sent an enquiry thing out and it, I guess my little alerts were they rang me. Why would somebody ring STD or internationally to try and get you to do their treatment? That seemed a little odd.

As this excerpt clearly conveys, subjective impressions of credibility may be established during initial searches of websites. However, the process of establishing credibility or implausibility generally involves a series of interactions and observations over time, sometimes entailing engagements with various media. As this respondent elaborated, they received a telephone call from a woman who said her daughter had been treated with cerebral palsy and had made 'great steps'. Further, the doctor at the clinic selling the treatment whom they interviewed 'had very poor command of English and seemed to be reading from a script, which sent up an alert at me'. Their suspicions were further heightened when the provider said they 'offered a discount to doctors'; however, 'the final piece de resistance was, "On the day of your treatment, we take you across the border to Mexico"', when 'I thought, "Oh okay. You're getting us to go outside of a country for treatment because it's not legal"'.

This case reveals how a variety of criteria and rival sources of epistemic authority may shape credibility assessments. Thus, giving weight to non-scientific criteria did not mean that they were oblivious to physical risks and safety – indeed, as noted, the words 'risk' and 'safety' were used by the above respondents, as well as some other respondents – however, these criteria were often considered alongside other factors, including subjective impressions of providers. References to national stereotypes, clearly evident in the above example, were common.

Confirming credibility
In the effort to confirm 'credible knowers and authentic claims' (Gieryn 1999: 22), respondents generally sought to confirm their online impressions through personal recommendations or by contacting providers directly. The role of other patients' stories communicated via blogs, face-to-face meetings and testimonials linked to clinics' websites were evidently of crucial importance in the hierarchy of credibility claims, since they were seen as untutored and authentic. Thomas, who had a rare acquired immune inflammatory disorder, who travelled to the US for a bone marrow-based SCT, reasoned that it was once difficult for patients with a rare disease to 'talk to another patient about their problems, especially when you got a rare disease' and if they did 'they normally lived quite close anyway and they'd normally have the same doctor or they would be treated in the same sort of circle'. However, 'with the Internet and online forums ... I'm talking to people from all over the world ... from Hong Kong to Europe, to America. And we're all seeing different doctors and we're all being exposed to different methodologies and different things'. As this and other accounts highlighted, obtaining a range of perspectives, including personal contacts with other patients and providers, was seen to offer a more comprehensive picture of both the patient experience and of the likely benefits or otherwise of SCTs than that offered by single sources.

A number of respondents recounted personal contacts with providers before deciding on SCTs, sometimes travelling to their clinics to confirm their impressions, after first learning about them on the Internet. Meeting providers face-to-face in their clinic, they said, gave them confidence about their decision whether or not to proceed with a SCT.

Who or what to trust?
Assessing credibility claims can be time-consuming and frustrating, and may ultimately prove fruitless in the sense of being offered no definitive evidence or advice on who or what to trust. Obtaining disinterested information was a challenge, as Phillipa, a carer for her partner with dementia, who, at the time of interview had not travelled for treatment, explained:

> Our concern is establishing the efficacy of the treatment, the clinics and the practitioners. And that's the stumbling block because the information comes either from the providers who have a barrow to push or from scientists and academics who are ... and the Australian medical profession who are naturally cautious.

While feelings of uncertainty, doubt and suspicion were especially pronounced in the accounts of non-travellers, they were evident to some extent in the accounts of virtually all respondents. Individuals often showed acute awareness of the tricks and traps associated with the advertising of SCTs, some using terms such as 'shonky', 'dodgy' and 'cowboy' to convey their impressions of providers whose credibility was deemed suspect. As Benjamin observed, 'there are very, very shady operators out there that'll cut corners and just collect the money and don't care about the consequences'. Suspicions were heightened when providers seemed overly eager, especially in regards to finalising payments for SCTs.

When commercial considerations were seen to take priority, individuals saw this as providing grounds for doubt. On the other hand, demonstration of professionalism and of concern, for example, in positive replies to enquiries, generally served to instil confidence. As was clear from the accounts, assessing credibility is a far from dispassionate matter. Many expressed that they hoped for at least some improvement in their own or, if carers, their partner's or child's condition, which evidently played a role in the decisions of many of the travellers. Despite the frequent failure to uncover definitive information after extensive research (in the above case over approximately 3 years), and sometimes contrary to the advice of their Australian doctors, family or friends, many decided that the potential benefits outweighed the risks or that the risks were small, and embarked on SCTs. Gabrielle, who travelled to X-Cell Centre in Germany before it was closed in 2011, was at first suspicious of its website ('Oh no, that looks too good to be true; I don't trust it') and was warned by her 'best friend', a nurse, about 'the power of the placebo effect'. However, after talking to other people, including another friend 'who's a doctor', they 'threw caution to the wind, and went'. In this case, as in others, respondents recounted hearing or reading about others making miraculous improvements or recoveries after receiving SCTs, which they found encouraging, if not persuasive. While they themselves may not have expected 'miracles' from SCTs, the power of hope in shaping actions was a pervasive theme in interviews.

Discussion and conclusion

Using Gieryn's (1999) concept of the 'cultural cartography', our analysis highlights the often tortuous, emotionally fraught paths taken by those who are seeking to establish the credibility of claims about SCTs. Drawing on the experiences of patients and carers who travelled or contemplated travelling overseas for SCTs, our study reveals that individuals encountered diverse sources, both online and offline, as they sought to clarify options and to confirm whom and what they should trust, with the Internet and social media being especially significant in regards to information about conditions and treatments. In telling their stories, individuals relied heavily on non-scientific criteria of credibility, with references made to third-party recommendations, other patient stories, and their own personal 'feelings'. Scientific sources were infrequently cited although, for many, science evidently held considerable symbolic value, despite the fact that, for many applications, the scientific justification for the treatments offered was nascent or in some cases non-existent. While we have no way of knowing whether our respondents' actions were consistent with their accounts, these non-science criteria may carry considerable weight in credibility contests. Where such contests are yet to be settled and the stakes in their outcomes are high, as is the case with claims about SCTs, matters of opinion and belief are liable to be interpreted as matters of fact.

Gieryn's ideas offer the basis for a dynamic portrayal of the development of science knowledge, highlighting the 'boundary-work' undertaken and contestations occurring at the margins of science as rival groups seek power and influence using different sources of epistemic authority. Such a dynamic portrayal is highly pertinent in the age of digital media characterised by numerous, rapidly circulating claims about health and treatments. We suggest that in markets for new, clinically unproven treatments, such as SCTs, where the boundaries of the field are highly contested and unstable, those who have exhausted their treatment options may be especially vulnerable to the appeals of those who portray themselves as competent and caring. The suspension of doubt or 'leap of faith' in deciding to embark on treatments was a common response to the context in which individuals found themselves; namely one of limited clinically proven options, often inconsistent or conflicting information about alternatives, and the promise and hope offered by SCTs.

In revealing these dynamics of credibility assessments, our study contributes to a growing body of sociological and other social science literature on citizens' engagements with digital health technologies (e.g. Adams and Niezen 2016, Lupton 2016). It highlights that, contrary to the many optimistic portrayals of such technologies as 'tools of empowerment', the potential impacts of their use on users' subjectivities, including sense of agency, are far from uniform, positive and absolute. By enabling access to a wider range of often-discrepant information that is difficult to reconcile, digital media may actually serve to 'disempower' users by making them vulnerable to certain claims. Understanding how people assess whether information on therapies is credible and trustworthy is of great significance in an age when digital media play a growing role in forging affective relations and political identities (Barassi 2016).

While research reveals that consumers are often aware of the limitations of online health information and may question its credibility (e.g. Sillence et al. 2007, Silver 2015), investigations thus far have focused largely on traditional health websites rather than on social media (Dalmer 2017). As the Pew Research Center observes, in its enquiry into 'The fate of online trust in the next decade': 'the rise of the Internet and social media has enabled entirely new kinds of social relationships and communities in which trust must be negotiated with others whom users do not see, with faraway enterprises, under circumstances that are not wholly familiar, in a world exploding with information of uncertain provenance used by actors employing ever-proliferating strategies to capture users' attention' (Rainie and Anderson 2017: 2). Scientists have increasingly recognised that 'fostering trust' in science is crucial for maintaining public support for promising research, yet scientific debate has focused mostly on how to communicate the value and workings of science to citizens and on 'correcting any misunderstandings' of previous work (e.g. Cossu et al. 2017). This assumes that 'facts' will necessarily carry most authority in credibility contests and provide the foundation for engendering public trust. As our work highlights, in their search for information, citizens are likely to encounter claims that may rest on criteria that are very different from those of credentialed experts and traditional trusted authorities.

Given the growing emphasis on enhancing 'digital literacy' among citizens (e.g. Australian Digital Health Agency 2017, NHS 2017), greater attention should be given to how individuals assess the credibility of the diverse sources of health information that they may encounter and how this may shape their conduct, including in relation to alleged treatments. While the issue of establishing credibility is not unique to digital media, the vast quantity and accessibility of online information in the market of healthcare means that the origins of information, its quality and veracity are less clear than they once were (Metzger and Flanagin 2013). Providers can now use the Internet and social media to advertise directly to consumers using strong emotional appeals and promises of self-transformation, while citizens may employ the same media to share stories, mobilise their networks, raise funds and access treatments. These new market relations unsettle accepted criteria of credibility and trustworthiness. As Salter, *et al.* observe, in their analysis of the global political economy of stem cell therapies, hegemonic biomedical expertise, governance and values have come into collision with the demands of increasingly informed health consumers who are pursuing their own interests (Salter *et al.* 2015). The need to develop forms of 'digital literacy' that will enable citizens to safely navigate this treacherous terrain has never been more urgent.

Address for correspondence: Alan Petersen, Sociology and Gender Studies, School of Social Sciences, Monash University, Wellington Road, Clayton, Victoria 3800, Australia. E-mail: alan.petersen@monash.edu

Acknowledgement

This research was support by an Australian Research Council Discovery Project Grant (DP120100921). We would like to acknowledge the support of the many individuals who made themselves available for interviews or who attended project workshops or assisted in other ways.

References

Adams, S. and Niezen, M. (2016) Digital "solutions" to unhealthy lifestyle "problems": the construction of social and personal risks in the development of eCoaches, *Health, Risk and Society*, 17, 7–8, 530–46.

Akrich, M. (2010) From communities of practice to epistemic communities: health mobilizations on the internet, *Sociological Research Online*, 15, 2, 1–17.

Australian Digital Health Agency (2017) Australia's National Digital Health strategy. Available at https://www.digitalhealth.gov.au/about-the-agency/publications/australias-national-digital-health-strategy (Last accessed 19 November 2017).

Barassi, V. (2016) Digital citizens? data traces and family life, *Contemporary Social Science*, 12, 1–2, 84–95.

Berger, I., Ahmad, A., Bansal, A., Kapoor, T., *et al.* (2016) Global distribution of businesses marketing stem cell-based interventions, *Cell Stem Cell*, 19, 2, 158–62.

Burri, R.V. (2008) Doing distinctions: boundary work and symbolic capital in radiology, *Social Studies of Science*, 38, 1, 37–64.

Cadge, W. (2012) Possibilities and limits of medical science: debates over double-blind clinical trials of intercessory prayer, *Zygon*, 47, 1, 43–64.

Chan, S. (2017) Current and emerging global themes in the bioethics of regenerative medicine: the tangled web of stem cell translation, *Regenerative Medicine*, 12, 7, 839–51.

Cossu, G., Birchall, M., Brown, T., De Coppi, P., *et al.* (2017) Lancet commission: stem cells and regenerative medicine, *The Lancet*, 391, 1–27. Available at www.thelancet.com (Last accessed 9 October 2017).

Daley, G.Q., Hyun, I., Apperley, J.F., Barker, R.A., *et al.* (2016) Setting global standards for stem cell research and clinical translation: the 2016 ISSCR guidelines, *Stem Cell Reports*, 6, 6, 787–97.

Dalmer, N.K. (2017) Questioning reliability assessments of health information on social media, *Journal of the Medical Library Association*, 105, 1, 61–8.

Dickson, M. and Gagnon, J.P. (2009) The cost of new drug discovery and development, *Discovery Medicine*, 4, 22, 172–9.

European Commission (2012) Patient involvement. Aggregate report, May 2012. Eurobarometer qualitative study. Brussels: European Commission, Director-General for Health and Consumers.

Gieryn, T.F. (1999) *Cultural Boundaries of Science: Credibility Contests on the Line*. Chicago and London: The University of Chicago Press.

González, A. (2016) Between certainty and trust: boundary-work and the construction of archaeological epistemic authority, *Cultural Sociology*, 10, 4, 483–501.

Kurath, M. (2015) Architecture as a science: boundary work and the demarcation of design knowledge from research, *Science and Technology Studies*, 28, 3, 81–100.

Lau, D., Ogbogu, U., Taylor, B., Stafinski, T., *et al.* (2008) Stem cell clinics online: the direct-to-consumer portrayal of stem cell medicine, *Cell Stem Cell*, 3, 6, 591–4.

Lupton, D. (2016) The diverse domains of quantified selves: self-tracking modes and dataveillance, *Economy and Society*, 45, 1, 101–22.

Maienschein, J., Sunderland, M., Ankeny, R.A. and Robert, J.S. (2008) The ethos and ethics of translational research, *The American Journal of Bioethics*, 8, 3, 43–51.

Margottini, L. (2014) Final chapter in Italian stem cell controversy?, *Science*. Available at http://www.sciencemag.org/news/2014/10/final-chapter-italian-stem-cell-controversy (Last accessed 4 October 2017).

Metzger, M.J. and Flanagin, A.J. (2013) Credibility and trust of information in online environments: the use of cognitive heuristics, *Journal of Pragmatics*, 59, 210–20.

Morrison, M. (2012) Promissory futures and possible pasts: the dynamics of contemporary expectations in regenerative medicine, *BioSocieties*, 7, 1, 3–22.

Munsie, M. and Pera, M. (2014) Regulatory loophole enables unproven autologous cell therapies to thrive in Australia, *Stem Cells and Development*, 23, Supplement 1, S34–8.

NHS (2017) Digital literacy. NHS. Available at https://hee.nhs.uk/our-work/research-learning-innovation/technology-enhanced-learning/digital-literacy (Last accessed 19 November 2017).

NIH (2017) ClinicalTrials.gov. Available at https://clinicaltrials.gov/ (Last accessed 11 December 2017).

Ogbogu, U., Rachul, C. and Caulfield, T. (2013) Reassessing direct-to-consumer portrayals of unproven stem cell therapies: is it getting better? *Regenerative Medicine*, 8, 3, 361–9.

Petersen, A. and Seear, K. (2011) Technologies of hope: techniques of the online advertising of stem cell treatments, *New Genetics and Society*, 30, 4, 329–46.

Petersen, A., Munsie, M., Tanner, C., MacGregor, C., *et al.* (2017) *Stem Cell Tourism and the Political Economy of Hope*. London: Palgrave Macmillan.

Pew Research Centre (2013) Majority of adults look online for health information. FactTank. Available at http://www.pewresearch.org/fact-tank/2013/02/01/majority-of-adults-look-online-for-health-information/ (Last accessed 7 November 2017).

Rabeharisoa, V., Moreira, T. and Akrich, M. (2013) *Evidence-Based Activism: Patients' Organisations, Users' and Activists' Groups in Knowledge Society*. Paris: Centre de Sociologie de l'innovations Mines Paris Tech.

Rainie, L. and Anderson, J. (2017) The fate of online trust in the next decade. Pew Research Center. Available at http://www.pewinternet.org/2017/08/10/the-fate-of-online-trust-in-the-next-decade/ (Last accessed 9 October 2017).

Salter, B., Zhou, Y. and Datta, S. (2015) Hegemony in the marketplace of biomedical innovation: consumer demand and stem cell science, *Social Science & Medicine*, 131, 156–63.

Shim, K.J. (2014) Impact of social media on power relations of korean health activism, *Media and Communication*, 2, 2, 72–83.

Sillence, E., Briggs, P., Harris, P.R. and Fishwick, L. (2007) How do patients evaluate and make use of online health information?, *Social Science & Medicine*, 64, 9, 1853–62.

Silver, M.P. (2015) Patient perspectives on online health information and communication with doctors: a qualitative study of patients 50 years and older, *Journal of Medical Internet Research*, 17, 1, e19.

Sipp, D. (2015) Conditional approval: Japan lowers the bar for regenerative medicine products, *Cell Stem Cell*, 16, 4, 353–6.

Sleeboom-Faulkner, M., Chekar, C.K., Faulkner, A., Heitmeyer, C., *et al.* (2016) Comparing national home-keeping and the regulation of translational stem cell applications: an international perspective, *Social Science and Medicine*, 153, 240–9.

Sosnowy, C. (2014) Practicing patienthood online: social media, chronic illness, and lay expertise, *Societies*, 4, 316–29.

Spalleta, M. (2015) Medical issues in Italian journalism: the journalistic coverage of 'Stamina, *The International Journal of Communication and Health*, 5, 66–76.

Stemwedel, J.D. (2011) Scientific credibility: is it who you are, or how you do it? Scientific American. Available at https://blogs.scientificamerican.com/doing-good-science/scientific-credibility-is-it-who-you-are-or-how-you-do-it/ (Last accessed 13 October 2017).

Timmermans, S. and Berg, M. (2003) *The Gold Standard: The Challenge of Evidence-Based Medicine and Standardization in Health Care*. Philadelphia: Temple University Press.

Wong, C., Harrison, C., Britt, H. and Henderson, J. (2014) Patient use of the internet for health information, *Australian Family Physician*, 43, 12, 875–7.

Zettler, P.J. (2015) Compassionate use of experimental therapies: who should decide?, *EMBO Molecular Medicine*, 7, 10, 1248–50.

Sociology of Health & Illness Vol. 41 No. S1 2018 ISSN 0141-9889, pp. 65–81
doi: 10.1111/1467-9566.12833

General Practitioner's use of online resources during medical visits: managing the boundary between inside and outside the clinic

Fiona Stevenson[1] ⓘ, Laura Hall[1], Maureen Seguin[1], Helen Atherton[2], Rebecca Barnes[3], Geraldine Leydon[4], Catherine Pope[4], Elizabeth Murray[1] and Sue Ziebland[5]

[1]*Research Department of Primary Care and Population Health, University College London, UK*
[2]*Department of Sociology, University of Warwick, UK*
[3]*Department of Primary Care, University of Bristol, UK*
[4]*Primary Care and Population Science, University of Southampton, UK*
[5]*Primary Care Health Sciences, University of Oxford, UK*

Abstract In an increasingly connected world, information about health can be exchanged at any time, in any location or direction, and is no longer dominated by traditional authoritative sources. We consider the ways information and advice given in consultations by doctors transcends the boundary between the clinic and the home. We explore how information that is widely accessible outside the consultation is transformed by General Practitioners (GPs) into a medical offering. Data comprise 18 consultations identified from 144 consultations between unselected patients and five GPs. We use conversation analytic methods to explore four ways in which GPs used online resources; (i) to check information; (ii) as an explanatory tool; (iii) to provide information for patients for outside the consultation; (iv) to signpost further explanation and self-help. We demonstrate the interactional delicacy with which resources from the Internet are introduced and discussed, developing and extending Nettleton's (2004) idea of 'e-scaped medicine' to argue that Internet resources may be 'recaptured' by GPs, with information transformed and translated into a medical offering so as to maintain the asymmetry between patients and practitioners necessary for the successful functioning of medical practice.

Keywords: doctor-patient communication/interaction, E-health, general practice, Internet, conversation analysis (CA)

We live in an increasingly connected world. The percentage of the population using the Internet between 2006 and 2016 was 82% in high income countries, 55% in upper middle income countries, 29.9% in lower middle income countries and 12.5% in low income countries (World Bank Group 2017). In the UK, 90% of UK households have Internet access, with 53% of people over the age of 16 reporting looking for health-related information (Office for National

Digital Health: Sociological Perspectives, First Edition.
Edited by Flis Henwood and Benjamin Marent.

Statistics 2017). Increasing pressure in terms of demand for health services has led to a growing focus on mobilising self-management, part of which can be seen in the pursuit of a 'digital
first' strategy promoting the use of digital resources to protect and improve health (c.f. Public
Health England 2017).

In 2004, Nettleton argued that medical knowledge has 'escaped' from the medical establishment 'into the networks of contemporary info-scapes where it can be accessed, assessed and
reappropriated' (Nettleton 2004: 674). The Internet enables the exchange of information about
health at any time, and in any location or direction, with people able to access information as
well as upload their own content and comment on posts by others (Tan and Goonawardene
2017, Ziebland and Wyke 2012). A surge in layperson broadcasting of experiential knowledge,
coupled with increased patient access to medically and non-medically sanctioned online information on health and illness, means the medical profession is facing a potential challenge to
its legitimacy (Hardey 1999, Naghieha and Parvizi 2016).

Interest in how patients manage the movement and translation of health information
found on the Internet into consultations is ever-increasing (Seguin and Stevenson In press).
Research indicates that patients do not fully disclose their use of online health information
before consultations (Bowes *et al.* 2012, Hardey 1999, Stevenson *et al.* 2007). The Chair
of the Royal College of General Practitioners, Professor Stokes-Lampard, commented that
'Dr Google' appears in 80% of her consultations, suggesting that most patients use the
Internet before consulting (Pulse Today 2017). Stokes-Lampard has encouraged the public
to self-manage minor illness, for example using online resources and community pharmacists, in a bid to reduce GPs' attendance (Mail Online 2017, The Telegraph 2017). Despite
some research interest in the perspective of General Practitioners (GPs) on patients introducing Internet -derived health information in consultations (Ahluwalia *et al.* 2010), there
has been much less consideration of how GPs manage the presentation of online health
information to patients in the consultation. GPs access much of the information via the
Internet is also readily available to patients, raising the question of how information and/or
resources can be (re)presented by GPs to patients as a medical offering. This paper focuses
on references to, or use of, the Internet by GPs during consultations. Specifically, we are
interested in how GPs negotiate using and directing patients to resources that are widely
accessible via the Internet whilst maintaining the position of provider of expert medical
knowledge. We draw on the idea of transformation (Berg 1992, Harding and Taylor 1997)
to argue that GPs seek to transform widely accessible material into something that is
imbued with expertise through the process of explanation and interpretation during
interactions.

Transformations

In his classic paper on medical disposal, Berg (1992) suggests that a patient's problem is solv-
able when the doctor is able to propose a limited set of actions which are perceived to be a
sufficient answer (at this time and place) to the specific problem. The key to such disposal is
the idea that data derived from the patient's reported symptom and the doctor's examination
(as well as medical criteria and disposal options) are not 'givens' which unidirectionally lead
the doctor towards a specific disposal. Rather, elements presented in the consultation are articulated and then actively reconstructed to fit a certain transformation. The patient's problem is
not simply translated but is remoulded through an active articulation of an array of heterogeneous elements in order to effect the transformation.

Harding and Taylor (1997) draw on this idea of transformation in relation to pharmaceutical expertise. They demonstrate how the provision of advice and selection of aspirin by

pharmacists may invest even medicines regarded as familiar with additional value and status. They argue that:

> When aspirin is selected (from a range of alternative drugs) by an 'expert', sanctioned to interpret its appropriateness for a specific individual, this commonly available drug has the potential to be symbolically transformed into a medicine (Harding and Taylor 1997: 554).

The idea of transformation has also been used in relation to medical prescribing, suggesting that a prescription not only provides access to treatment but also possesses symbolic value which legitimises and transforms the presenting problem into a problem worthy of medical treatment (Pellegrino 1976).

In this paper, we draw on the concept of transformation to consider how GPs transform information that is widely available outside the consultation into a medical offering and how this is received by patients (and/or their companions).

Methods

The data originate from a large qualitative mixed methods study; **H**arnessing **R**esources from the Internet (HaRI), in which use of the Internet in consultations is a central concern (Seguin *et al.* 2018). The data used in this paper came from five GPs working at three practices located in the South East of England. Practices varied in terms of level of deprivation. Four of the GPs were male, and GPs varied in terms of ethnicity. Two GPs were trainees, the others reported being registered for 19, 26 and 34 years respectively at the time of data collection. From 144 consultations, we identified 18 consultations in which GPs used or referred to the Internet.

In these 18 consultations, 12 of the patients were female and six were male. They ranged in age from under one (including babies with their carers) to over 65. Four patients were joined by companions during their consultation. The sample predominantly identified as White English, with a minority identifying as Asian. There was a relatively even split between patients who had attained a vocational qualification or higher and those with secondary level education or lower.

For the purposes of this paper, we draw solely on video recordings of consecutive, (as far as possible subject to written informed consent), unselected consultations between GPs and patients. We viewed 144 video recordings to identify consultations which met at least one of the following criteria: (i) the GP used the Internet during the consultation and the computer screen was clearly visible to the patient; (ii) the GP used the Internet during the consultation and referred to it when discussing a problem with the patient (regardless of whether the patient saw the screen); and/or (iii) the GP recommended that the patient use the Internet in relation to their health issue.

We employed conversation analysis (CA), a micro analytic approach to consider how actions are constructed and produced in interaction (Barnes 2005, Drew *et al.* 2001, Sidnell 2010) to analyse our data. Following identification, consultations were viewed repeatedly with specific sequences of interaction between patients (and companions, if applicable) and GPs, transcribed in detail according to the Jeffersonian transcription system (Jefferson 2004) to facilitate analysis of verbal and embodied interactions. A key to the notation used in the transcribed extracts presented is shown in Figure 1.

:	Extended vocal sound. Multiple colons indicate further extension
(0.2)	Pause in tenths of a second
(.)	micro pause
> <	rapid speech
↑	Upward intonation
°°	quiet speech
,	continuing intonation
.hh	in breath
hh	out breath
=	latched talk
(( ))	text between double brackets gives descriptions of action or clarifications of phonetic meaning
_	Underling text used to denote forms of emphasis
( )	Single brackets used to indicate sections that were hard to hear or not hearable

Figure 1 *Transcription symbols used in the analysis [Colour figure can be viewed at wileyonlinelibrary.com]*

Ethical Approval was obtained from a local UK NHS Research Ethics Committee, with governance approval from the Health Research Authority. The data presented here have been anonymised for names and place names. In the extracts presented, GPs' contributions are marked as 'GP', Patients' as PT and companions as 'CM'.

Findings

The GPs in our sample generally used the website www.patient.co.uk to look up information either for themselves or to share with patients. The site describes itself as:

the web's leading independent health platform, established for 20 years. With more than 18 million visits a month, it is a trusted source of information for both patients and health professionals across the globe. The site contains over 4000 health information leaflets and thousands of discussion forums. It is accredited by The Information Standard, NHS England's quality mark and was listed as 'The top health website you can't live without' by The Times newspaper (Jan 2013). (https://patient.info/about-us)

GPs also made use of the Google search engine which has a visually distinctive interface and is arguably easily recognised by patients (or companions) who use the Internet.

In our sample, there were four ways in which GPs used the Internet; (i) to check information to support their practice; (ii) as a tool to explain to patients the reasoning for advice or diagnosis; (iii) to provide printed information about the presenting problem and/or signpost to further assistance outside the consultation, such as helplines or exercises and; (iv) to signpost further explanations and self-help via a web link.

This paper focuses on instances in which it was evident that patients were aware that the GP was searching for information on the Internet.

The consulting room
Before examining the data, it is important to consider the layout of the rooms used by the GPs to consult and how this impacted on the potential for sharing resources from the Internet. GP4 consulted in a room in which the computer screen could not easily be seen by patients. This limited the patients' awareness of what the GP was looking at, including whether GP accessed the Internet. The physical space and orientation of the furniture in the consulting rooms of the other GPs allowed patients a view of the screen, and in some cases the GP also tilted the screen so patients had a better view.

(i) Internet used to check information to support practice
In the example below the patient presented with rectal bleeding. Following a physical examination, the patient and GP return to their seats and the GP suggests restarting a previously prescribed treatment for diverticulitis and initiating a new prescription for antibiotics. The GP initiated a search on the website patient.co.uk. Although it is clear that the patient is also looking at the screen, neither the GP nor the patient refer to the fact the GP is searching for information, and at no point is there an explanation either about the necessity for the search or the information being sought.

Extract 1

1	GP:	°↑let me just have a ↑quick ↑look,° ((brings up patient.co.uk on
2		the screen and scrolls down)) (6.4) can I ↑check your blood
3		pressure while I look,
4	PT:	((patient shifts gaze to raise her sleeve to have her blood
5		pressure taken))yeah and it ↑also ↑leaves a horrible taste you
6		↑know ↑in ↑my↑mou:th, (0.6) whether that's the:: (1.0) the
7		blood I really don't ↑kno:w, (0.8) ((looks back at the screen))
8		it's not nice
9		(4.8)
10	GP:	°°o::h°° (1.6) are you a↑llergic to any↑thing?
11	PT:	↑no:,
12	GP:	((switches back to patient record)))°okay° (0.6).hhhhh (0.6)
13		kuh kuh ku:h ((doctor moves chair to take the blood pressure))
14	PT:	((patient looks at her arm as the blood pressure cuff is
15		readied))
		GP1 R8

At the beginning of the extract, the GP announces his intention to use the Internet using the words 'just have a quick look' (line 1). The soft delivery and use of the words 'quick' and 'just' works to minimise the act of using the Internet, suggesting clarification as opposed to a critical piece of information. The patient looks at the screen, only shifting her gaze when she readies herself to have her blood pressure taken following a request from the doctor (line 4) and shifting it back once she has pulled up her sleeve (line 7). Neither the doctor nor the patient refer to what the GP is looking at or what he is searching for. The patient's only interjection is to provide another symptom, a horrible taste in her mouth (lines 5-8). This is not taken up by the GP suggesting it is not relevant in that place in the consultation. The GP meanwhile shifts his gaze between the computer and the task of preparing to take the patient's blood pressure. He switches the screen back to the patient's medical record following verbal confirmation she is not allergic to anything. It is not possible to ascertain if the question about being allergic to anything related to what the doctor was looking at on the website.

Neither the GP nor the patient comment on what was viewed. The website has a clear banner saying 'patient', so the patient is likely to be aware the GP is using a website accessible to patients, yet neither the patient nor the GP appear to orientate to the website as anything other than a 'medical' resource.

(ii) Internet as a tool to support the reasoning for advice or diagnosis

Below, we present a number of examples in which GPs harnessed the Internet as a communication tool to support explanations of medical problems and provide advice.

In the following example, the patient attends to ask for a letter for his travel insurance company stating that it is safe for him to travel following a stroke. The GP uses the Google search engine and patient.co.uk to check for guidelines on the safety of travelling, specifically flying, after a stroke. The patient and his companion can clearly see the screen, although the GP does not invite the patient to look at the screen and share in the interpretation of the information.

Extract 2

1	GP	°°Right let's have a look°° ((typing and clicking as he reads
2		information on the Internet – patient.co.uk)) (38.9) right
3		↑what ↑they ↑sa:y is (0.4) ↑↑reasons ↑↑not to be allowed to,
4		trave:l (0.6)include a stroke within three da:ys (0.6↑) so
5		you're obviously clear of tha:t,
6		(4.6)
7	?PT	so it ↑should be all ↑right,((unclear who says this))
8		(3.6)((GP continues to look at the screen))
9	PT	yea:h I feel all right,
		GP1 R1

Similar to extract 1, the GP marks the fact he is going to look up information on the computer by saying 'right let's have a look' (line 1). This is said softly but marks the action, with the use of 'let's', as collaboratively seeking to address the patient's query. The GP makes clear his assessment on the safety of flying is based on the information he finds, reporting to the patient 'what they say is' (line 3). The website is presented by the GP as the source of information that will be used to provide a written medical assessment to a bureaucratic body. In this way the information that is readily available to both the patient and the insurance company is transformed into evidence upon which to base a written medical opinion.

In the next example we see how images from the Internet may be used to support explanations and advice. Images are particularly useful when the patient has a visible disorder such as a skin problem. Such images are readily available but may require medical knowledge to transform them into something understandable. In the following case, the patient who had previously been treated for skin cancer, presents with concerns about some moles which he thought had changed; a known indicator of skin cancer. The doctor examines the patient and explains the moles are harmless. He then shares images on the Internet with the patient to support his assessment.

Extract 3

1	GP	This is (certainly?)not skin cancer I will s͟how you the
2		picture so that you can see::((said as he examines the
3		patient with a magnifying glass which is then returned to a
4		drawer))
5		(22 lines omitted in which GP reassures patient he does not
6		have cancer using technical terms to list types of mole)
7	GP:	[th]at's a ↑typi↑ca:l o:ne (0.6) so ↑but at ↑ti::mes
8		it can become ↑thi:s (0.8) len↑t͟igo:: (2.8) and ↑you will see
9		the:, (.) len↑tigo magn) (.) [which is] =
10	PT:	[ri::ght,]
11	GP:	=a super↑ficia::l, (0.6) <ski:n cancer> a form of superficial
12		skin [cancer] that is not it ((GP shakes his head slightly as
13		he says this, patient leans forward and Dr moves screen
14		towards the patient))
15	PT:	[ri:ght]
		GP2 R53

In lines 1–2, the GP informs the patient that the moles are not skin cancer. The GP then states his intention to show the patient some pictures to visually bolster this diagnosis. When the GP uses the computer, the patient moves forward to see the screen which the doctor angles towards the patient once he has located the images he wishes to share (lines 13–14). Notable in this extract is the GP's use of medical terminology throughout, punctuated by pointing at particular images on the screen. The patient produces continuers, all in overlap with the GP's talk (lines 10, 15), indicating engagement with what is being said and shown; however, this cannot be taken to indicate understanding. The GP provides a translation of images which, although readily available using the Google search engine, here called upon medical expertise in order to respond to the patient's concerns.

In the next example we can see how the Internet may be used to support and bolster a diagnosis. Following a physical examination, the GP suggested a diagnosis of phlebitis and shared the website patient.co.uk with the patient.

Extract 4

1	GP	°so° (0.4) ((turns screen towards patient and points at it)) redness
2		and tenderness along the vein with swe↑lling,
3	PT	hm ↑mm::,
4	GP	.hhhh ↑usually in the ↑greater saphenous ↑vei:n ((gestures towards
5		his thigh)) which is ↑just(0.4) just ↑slightly higher u:p and this
6		is the lower pa:rt of that vein ((returns hand to screen and
7		points))
8	PT	↑ri:ght,
9		(0.8)
10	GP	er I ↑don't think you've got cellu↑litis there's ↑nothing to
11		su↑ggest a deep vein thrombos↑is=
12	PT	=↑mm,
13	GP	or any of tho:se really ((moves hand down the screen as he says
14		this))
15	PT	ri:ght,
		GP1R115

The GP turns the screen towards the patient and points at the relevant material, inviting her to view the screen by gesturing towards it. At the same time, he verbally outlines the description on the site that fits with her symptoms and his physical examination (lines 1–4). He then moves to illustrate the patient's problem on his own body (lines 4–6), but following an acknowledgement from the patient in line 8, he once again points at the screen as he verbally lists and physically gestures towards the diagnoses he has discounted. In this way the Internet is used as a primary resource as the GP translates the information on the webpage in order to provide evidence to bolster his diagnosis of the patient's problem via the exclusion of other possibilities.

In the following example the patient had ongoing health issues and one of her reasons for visiting the GP was to find out whether she should avoid contact with her grandson who had chickenpox. The GP uses the Internet to check if this might be a problem. The patient comments on the information on the screen, uninvited, stating that she had tried looking up information on the same site (patient.co.uk) but couldn't understand it.

Extract 5

1	PT	I've read loa:ds on the:re I couldn't make head nor tail of
2		it in the ↑end, (0.6) does your'ead in dunn↑it ↑ha:::::::h
3		↑ha ↑ha ↑ha ↑ha.hhhh and ↑p'raps ↑does ↑it ↑lead ↑to
4		↑shingle:::s a:::nd,
5	GP	no >the the< the ↑only person who can get ↑shingles from
6		chickenpox (.) is the person who's ↑had the chickenpox
		GP1 R17

This is the clearest example we have of both the GP and patient negotiating the boundary between inside and outside the clinic. The patient navigates the moral dimension of what is deemed appropriate consulting by both patients and doctors (Llanwarne *et al.* 2017), while the GP is faced with a situation in which the patient indicates they have already accessed the information the GP is using to address her query, leaving the GP needing to reassert his medical authority. Unlike the previous extracts, the GP does not announce his intention to use the Internet, or look for further information; he just opens up the site on his computer. Uninvited, the patient indicates her recognition of the site and says she has already looked at the information but did not understand it. In this way the patient presents herself as a 'good' patient who has actively researched her query before 'bothering' the doctor. The patient's uninvited comments make clear she has access to the same, or similar, information to that being viewed by the GP. This presents a potential challenge to the expertise of the GP. The laughter in lines 2–3 may be attributed to the delicacy of raising the fact that the information being used by the GP is generally accessible, as well as orientating to the interactional delicacy of her suggestion of a lack of understanding (Holt 2012). Throughout, the patient carefully presents herself as less expert than the GP by indicating she could not understand the information she had read, while at the same time creating an opportunity to ask a question about whether contact with her grandson who has chickenpox could cause her to develop shingles. This provides an opportunity for the GP to reassert his authority as an expert by demonstrating his knowledge of the link between chicken pox and shingles (lines 5–6). It is important to note here the co-constructed nature of the interaction between the patient and the doctor, in particular that it is the patient's utterances in lines 3–4 about the possibility of shingles, left unfinished, that provides the GP with the opportunity to assert his medical expertise and his position of authority in the consultation.

Having considered how the Internet was used by doctors in consultations to support medical explanations, diagnostic reasoning and treatment advice, we now moves on to consider how resources referred to, or discussed, which originate from the Internet were transformed into medical resources for use outside of the consultation by virtue of being printed and given to patients.

(iii) Provision of printed information to take away and/or signposting of resources outside of the consultation

Here we consider examples in which the GP gave the patient printed versions of material from the Internet.

The following extract is from a consultation in which the patient presented with pain in his wrist. Following a physical examination and diagnosis, the GP offers to find the patient a leaflet about the presenting problem and immediately turns to the computer to execute a search.

Extract 6

1	GP:	um I'll ↑try and see if I can <u>find</u> something for you a ↑leaflet,
2		(0.6) which (kinda) explains a bit <u>more</u> about this ((starts
3		searching on Internet))
		GP4R85

The GP uses the Google search engine to locate a fact sheet which includes anatomical diagrams. Although the GP does not invite the patient to share the screen, after 12 seconds the patient shifts forward in his seat and appears to be looking at the screen. After finishing his searching, rather than pointing to what was on the screen (as we saw in extracts 3 and 4), the GP demonstrates the likely cause of the pain using his own wrist.

The GP subsequently prints out the information and uses the printed version to illustrate his message. In summary, the GP uses the Internet as a source of information similar to the previous examples; however, also transforms the information from something that the patient could find themselves via a web search to a printed version shared in the consultation and endorsed for use outside of the consultation. The action of providing a printout may be seen as comparable to the 'gifting' involved in issuing a prescription for a medicine (Cooper 2011, Pellegrino 1976).

The next example is drawn from the same consultation as extract 4. Here, the GP offers the patient a printout of information, noting the version they had viewed together was the medical article and the version he was printing for her to take away was the patient version.

Extract 7

1	GP:	.hh what I could do: is ↑that that was the ↑medical a:rticle I
2		.↑could [ve you] the, (0.4) this is the=
3	PT:	[o:↑kay]
4	GP:	=patient version,
5	PT:	↑oka:y (4.0)((GP scrolling through page)) ↑thank you:
6		(1.6)
7	GP:	↑°e:::r° (.) ↑usually page fou::r (0.6) yeah ↑that's just their
8		advertis↑ing,
9	PT:	hm ↑mm::,
10	GP:	and their disclaimer so if it's all right with you I won't print
11		th[at bit]
12	PT:	[↑no::] no that's fi:ne
		GP1R115

This is the only reference in our data to two versions of patient.co.uk; the information shared with the patient when discussing diagnostic reasoning (the medical version) and the information the GP offers to printout for the patient for use outside the consultation (the patient version) (lines 1–4). The reference to the page containing the advertising (lines 7–8) and the disclaimer (line 10) not only demonstrates the GP's familiarity with patient.co.uk, but also works to distinguish the offering as a 'lay' resource. In this example, the GP demonstrates his expertise in translating the 'medical' version for the purposes of diagnosis in the consultation but also establishes a demarcation between the information he accessed and used and the version of the information he gives to the patient for her use outside of the consultation. Crucially the GP asserts his authority over information sources across the boundary between home and the clinic.

In the following example, the patient reported pain in his foot on walking and was given printed information as well as exercises to alleviate his symptoms.

Extract 8

1	GP:	((GP takes print-out from printer, staples it and shows it to
2		the patient)) Thi this is (0.2), so although this talks about
3		Achilles tendon as well
4	PT:	Mmm
5	GP:	it is (.) for the plantar fascia
6	PT:	Mhm
7	GP:	erm um because of the link er explained there
8	PT:	Right yeah
9		(0.1)
10	GP:	..hh so, (0.6) have a ↑read ↑throu::gh,
11	PT:	↑yeah [I will]
12	GP:	[have a] go at the exer↑cises and [hopef]ully (.)=
13	PT:	[yeah,]
14	GP:	=it will settle down for [you]
15	PT:	[↑lo]vely (0.4) ↑thank you very
16		mu[ch]
		GP1R14

The printout provides information about the problem and self-help resource in the form of exercises. The exercises are not demonstrated in the consultation; however, the doctor imbues them with the authority of medical treatment (lines 12–14), and the patient responds with an appreciation marking this as unproblematic.

A similar scenario was played out in a different consultation (not shown here) in which the GP alluded to the normality of providing printed information about anxiety, stating the resources were bookmarked on his computer for ease of access. In that consultation, the GP provided a print off outlining self-referral to counselling and/or exercises providing another example of resources from the Internet being transformed into treatment recommendations imbued with medical authority.

The patient in the following extract came to see the GP after suffering a panic attack the previous night and being taken to hospital. On her discharge from Accident and Emergency, it had been suggested she visited her GP for a follow up. The GP, as in the previous examples, provides the patient with a print out of information and breathing exercises to address her anxiety. In contrast, however, the patient (and her companion) resist this recommendation and present Kalms (a herbal remedy for anxiety) as an alternative, attributing the suggestion to an unnamed person at the hospital.

Extract 9

1	GP:	so ↑what ↑what ↑what we'd normally do is give you so:me,
2		(0.4).tch (0.6) some ↑tips (.) ↑to:::: (0.4) ↑teach
3		yourself some calming breathing making muscles relax
4	PT:	yeah,
5	GP:	and then there's ↑also::, (0.6) do ↑either of you u- use
6		comput- the com↑puter?
7	PT:	[no:]
8	CM:	[no:]

(continued)

Extract 9   *(continued)*

1	GP:	so ↑what ↑what ↑what we'd <u>normally</u> do is give you so:me,
2		(0.4).tch (0.6) some ↑<u>tips</u> (.) ↑to:::: (0.4) ↑teach
3		yourself some <u>calming</u> breathing making muscles relax
4	PT:	yeah,
5	GP:	and then there's ↑also::, (0.6) do ↑<u>either</u> of you u- use
6		comput- the com↑puter?
7	PT:	[no:]
8	CM:	[no:]
9	GP:	°okay°.hh (0.4) ↑u:::m, hhhh
10		(0.8)
11		((34 lines omitted where the companion talks about the
		patient's recent health problems and whether it
		is alright to go on a planned holiday))
12	GP:	((prints off documents and goes through it with the patient
13		illustrating what he is saying by pointing to the relevant part
14		on the paper)) right ↑the::se, (0.4) so a <u>lot</u> of this is
15		computer based but there is a <u>phone</u> number as well if you (0.6)
16		this is ↑ou::r (.)en aitch ess (NHS) ↑counselling service
17		↑loca↑lly,
18	PT:	↑yea:h
19	GP:	u::m if you ↑ca::n or ↑have ↑got access >to a< computer
20		these are <u>very</u> ↑good, (0.6) but if not don't ↑worry,
21	PT:	↑yea:h
22	GP:	↑that's ↑↑tha::t ((hands a page to the patient and looks at
23		the next page))(0.4) and then <u>this</u> is some <u>written</u>
24		inform<u>ation</u> about rel<u>ax</u>ation. (0.6) so you can do some
25		↑breathing exercises and you can do some <u>muscle</u> exercises
26	PT:	cises yeah (0.2)yeah
27	GP	((moves away to staple pages))
28	CM:	↑wha- (.) what about the:: (.) th- the <u>kalms</u> would ↑the::y ↑
29		be ↑any ↑↑good ↑o::r (.) just in case she feels (satisfied)
30		with that ↓o:r
		GP1R7

The GP introduces the idea of relaxation techniques to help prevent, or at least control, any further panic attacks. This is met with a minimal response from the patient in line 4. The possibility of using a computer to access resources is then raised by the GP but is immediately closed down by both the patient and her companion who, when asked if they use a computer, produce a definitive 'no' response (lines 7–8) in overlap with each other. The GP pursues the suggestion of relaxation exercises (line 10) and having printed off information from the Internet, goes through it with the patient. This receives relatively minimal acknowledgement from the patient (lines 18, 21, 26). The patient, and her companion, appeared to be seeking a different course of action, namely Kalms tablets. The doctor moving to staple the pages (line 27) provides a slot for the question about the use of Kalms to be raised again. Kalms was raised as an option by the patient after she had presented her problem and prior to examination (not shown here) and received minimal uptake from the GP. The re-introduction of Kalms, as the doctor moves to give the patient the printout of information can be seen as a, (at least partial), rejection of the relaxation techniques and information provided by the GP. Moreover, the fact the printout originated from the Internet, a resource the patient categorically stated neither she nor her companion had access to, and that the GP refers to aspects of the information provided which are compromised through lack of Internet access (lines 14, 19–20), weakens the print out as a viable solution for the patient.

Having discussed the provision of printed information from the Internet we now consider examples in which links to websites were given to patients to access medical resources outside of the consultation.

(iv) Signposting via a web link to further explanation and support.

One of the five GPs did not access the Internet in the consultation, but he did provide patients with web addresses for use outside of the consultation. In the following example, the patient is diagnosed with golfer's elbow. At five and again at eight minutes in to the ten and a half minute consultation the GP offers a web link to more information about the problem. When the GP gives the patient a prescription at the end of the consultation, the patient appears unsure of what to do next.

Extract 10

1	GP:	((GP shows the patient the prescription and points to the
2		information on it with his pen))so ↑that's the anti
3		inflammator↑i.e.::s,
4	PT:	↑yea:h
5	GP:	↑that's the websi:te >it's just< ↑patient dot co dot yew
6		↑ka:y, (0.4) >it's called< ↑golfer's elbo:w,
7	PT:	Yeah
8	GP:	the ↑technical name is medial epicondylitis but, (.) >if
9		you put< golfer's elbow in it will tell you all about it
10		((gives patient the prescription script))
11	PT:	thank ↑you:,
12	GP:	↑all ↑right,
13	PT:	what do I do ↑with ↑↑thi:s?((looking at the script))
14	GP:	↑u:m, ((takes the script and turns it over and points to
15		the drug prescription)) (0.4) take ↑any::, (0.4) take that
16		to ↑any: (.)chem↑i:st,
17	PT:	ye[ah,]
18	GP:	[the]y'll have ↑i:t, ((Turns script over))(.) and
19		just ↑tea:r that bit off and >keep it with you<
20	PT:	thanks a ↑lot
21	GP:	↑all ↑right
22	PT:	thank you
23	GP:	no problem
		GP5R131

Following an appreciation in line 11, the patient looks at the prescription he has been given and asks what he should do with it. We can tell the patient is looking at the website written on the blank side of the prescription script as the GP turns the prescription over and then instructs the patient on how to get the prescription filled. The patient's difficulty appears to arise because the website address and details of what to search for are written on the same piece of paper as the prescription for anti-inflammatories. The patient appears unclear how to collect the prescribed medication without giving away the website address and search details written on the prescription script. The GP tells the patient to detach the side with the website written on it and keep it. This last phrase was delivered rapidly, potentially reducing comprehensibility (line 15). This exchange also makes noticeable that although the GP raises the topic of a website on two occasions before the interaction shown the GP does not make it clear what supplementary information the patient should be looking for from the website. This transfer of explanatory work from the clinic to the home did not involve physically seeing or receiving any resources, and as such it remains unclear what information the patient may access as a consequence of the consultation.

In the following extract we see how a direction to a website to support the GP's assessment of a no problem diagnosis received minimal uptake. The consultation concerns a mother who thought her child was developing a curvature of the spine and wanted a referral to a specialist. On physical examination the GP finds no indication of a problem. The mother does not accept this assessment and the GP suggests the mother accesses information on the Internet as further support for the professional assessment.

Extract 11

1	DR:	they ↑won't do anything with i:t (0.8) there's ↑a: (.)
2		↑websi:te tha:t (.) can >tell you a little bit< a↑bou:t ↑it
3		(0.6) I can ↑give ↑you::
4	CM:	↑hm ↑hm:
5	DR:	patient dot co dot yew ka:y but, (0.4) ↑that's ↑mi[:ld]
6	CM:	[but] ↑even
7		like any ↑exer>↑cise you know< like something she could £↑do:£
8		↑↑huh (0.4)it's ↑ho::w ↑the ↑se::lf (0.4) to he[lp thi:s]
		GP5144

The mother displays resistance to the 'no problem' diagnosis, with minimal uptake to the refusal to refer and suggestion of a website to provide more information (line 4) and continues to seek a more limited medical intervention by asking about exercises (lines 6–8). In this situation, resources on the Internet, especially as they are referred to rather than demonstrated, are easily dismissed.

Discussion

This paper explored 18 consultations in which the GP used or referred to the Internet. We identified four ways in which GPs used the Internet in consultations; (i) to check information (ii) as an explanatory tool (iii) to provide resources for patients to use outside of the consultation and (iv) to signpost explanations and self-help. Using conversation analytic methods, we based our observations on recordings and detailed transcripts of routine consultations allowing us to analyse practice-in-action as opposed to accounts of practice. Using video data meant we were able to consider the physical layout of the consulting room, in particular the positioning of the GPs' computer screen and the extent to which patients had a view of the screen.

Information from the Internet appears to be situated somewhere between medical and 'lay' knowledge and as such invoking the Internet as a medical resource may be seen to transcend the boundary between the clinic and the home. Our detailed analysis of data provided example of how this is achieved in practice.

We argue that the Internet may be co-opted by GPs and employed as a medical resource. For example, the Internet was invoked as a resource upon which to base medically authoritative correspondence in the example of the letter to an insurance company to state a patient was fit to fly. The Internet was also utilised to explain diagnoses and deliver self-help resources, such as exercises, either in printed form or as a web link. Information from the Internet was discussed in consultations, as well as provided for use outside. In this way, we suggest that in addition to 'e-scaped medicine' as described by Nettleton (2004), resources from the Internet are 'recaptured' by GPs to facilitate their work. Information and exercises may be transformed from something that patients could access without medical support into a medically sanctioned resource.

The idea of GPs 'recapturing' resources from the Internet purports that instead of health resources that have 'e-scaped' the control of the medical profession creating a challenge to the legitimacy of the medical profession GPs are using these resources to maintain the legitimacy of their position as experts by reframing resources from the Internet designed as a substitute for medical consultations and imbuing them with medical expertise. Thus an unintended consequence of the development of Internet resources to support health outside of the consultation may be time spent by GPs in consultations referring patients to, and using, these resources.

Transforming resources from the Internet into a medically sanctioned resource is not necessarily straightforward. Heritage and Stivers (1999) distinguished online explanation and online commentary to describe instances in which doctors describe what they are doing and what they are seeing, feeling or hearing during a physical examination of a patient. They argue that the latter may be used to pre-empt patient resistance to a 'no problem' diagnosis. In our data, online explanations and online commentary were used to introduce use of the Internet (extracts 1, 2, 6), explain the reasoning for a decision (extract 2), diagnosis (extracts 3, 4) and treatment (extract 9). We argue that initiating use of the Internet in this way presents this use as medically legitimate, particularly when use is presented as collaborative through the use of phrases such as 'let's have a look' (extract 2) or moves to share the screen (extract 3, 4). Conversely, naming as opposed to showing resources on the Internet, as was the case in extracts 10 and 11, reduces the opportunity for full endorsement enabled through physically viewing a resource together, arguably making it easier to miss or dismiss, particularly given what is already known concerning the difficulty patients have remembering information given in consultations (c.f. Kessels 2003).

Extract 5 makes clear the interactional delicacy of using a resource that patients could, or indeed may have, accessed. In this case, the accountability associated with use of the Internet by both the patient and the GP was demonstrated. Although the GP did not announce his intention to access a website the patient recognised the site (patient.co.uk). In response to use by the GP of a website that is accessible to patients, the patient sought to account for her visit and the 'doctorability' (Heritage and Maynard 2006) of her query by reporting that she had tried to resolve her query but could not understand what she read. She is however left with the dilemma of having identified the information the GP was using as generally accessible, potentially presenting a challenge to his authority as a medical expert. It is resolved here when she presents a further medical query which the doctor is able to answer using his medical knowledge; however, this example clearly demonstrates the risks to the authority of the GP of using the Internet in consultations. Awareness on the part of a GP of the potential challenge to their authority through the use of Internet sites is particularly evident in extract 7 in which the GP notes he has shared the medical version of the website (patient.co.uk) with the patient but will give her the patient version to take home with her.

The arguments above all point to the importance of recognising the necessity of asymmetry in relation to knowledge and that both doctors and patients constitute and enact asymmetry throughout interactions in consultations (Pilnick and Dingwall 2011). Pilnick and Dingwall (2011) argued that asymmetry lies at the heart of the medical enterprise and is embedded within a wider functionality of the institution of medicine in society as it is founded in what doctors are there for; namely to provide medical expertise to those in need.

Having mooted the idea of the successful 'recapturing' of resources previously described as having 'e-scaped' (Nettleton 2004), it is also important to consider what happens when resources from the Internet are used to offer an option that the patient does not appear to want. In extract 9, reference to relaxation techniques accessible from the Internet enabled the patient and her companion to dismiss the GP's offer by responding categorically in the negative about use of a computer. Thus the shift of medical resources on to the Internet can be seen to open up an opportunity for resistance on the part of patients based on access to the Internet. In the case cited here, it made it possible for the patient and her companion to return to their preferred option of Kalms tablets.

In conclusion, patients are increasingly encouraged to seek out information before consulting a GP. Previous work has reported patients' accounts of using information from the Internet in this way (Bowes *et al.* 2012). Here we argue that Internet resources may be 'recaptured' by GPs. We have focused on the ways in which information available via a web search can be transformed and translated by GPs into a medical offering. We have demonstrated the interactional delicacy with which resources from the Internet are both introduced and discussed so as to maintain the asymmetry between patients and practitioners that is seen as necessary for the successful functioning of medical practice.

Address for correspondence: Fiona Stevenson, Reader in Medical Sociology, Co-Director eHealth unit, Research Department of Primary Care and Population Health, UCL, Rowland Hill Street, London NW3 2PF. E-mail: f.stevenson@ucl.ac.uk

Acknowledgements

The authors would like to acknowledge the patients, GPs and practice staff who supported data collection. Professor Trish Greenhalgh who was a co-applicant on the original grant, the patient and public involvement representatives, Jon Benford and Charles Prince, as well as the helpful comments of the reviewers. The Harnessing Resources from the Internet (HaRI) project was funded by the National Institute for Health Research School of Primary Care Research. The views expressed are those of the authors and not necessarily those of the NIHR, the NHS or the Department of Health. NHS costs are covered via the Local Clinical Research Network. CP is part funded by NIHR CLAHRC Wessex.

References

Ahluwalia, S., Murray, E., Stevenson, F.A., Kerr, C., *et al.* (2010) 'A heartbeat moment': qualitative study of GP views of patients bringing health information from the internet to a consultation, *British Journal of General Practice*, 60, 88–94.

Barnes, R.K. (2005) Making sense of qualitative research: conversation analysis: a practical resource in the healthcare setting, *Medical Education*, 39, 113–5.

Berg, M. (1992) The construction of medical disposals, *Medical Sociology and Medical Problem Solving in Clinical Practice, Sociology of Health & Illness*, 14, 151–80.

Bowes, P., Stevenson, F., Ahluwalia, S. and Murray, E. (2012) 'I need her to be a doctor': patients' experiences of presenting health information from the internet in GP consultations, *British Journal of General Practice*, 62, 574–5.

Cooper, R. (2011) In praise of the prescription: the symbolic and boundary object value of the traditional prescription in the electronic age, *Health Sociology Review*, 20, 462–74.

Drew, P., Chatwin, J. and Collins, S. (2001) Conversation analysis: a method for research into interactions between patients and health-care professionals, *Health Expectations*, 4, 58–70.

Hardey, M. (1999) Doctor in the house: the Internet as a source of lay health knowledge and the challenge to expertise, *Sociology of Health & Illness*, 21, 820–35.

Harding, G. and Taylor, K. (1997) Responding to change: the case of community pharmacy in Great Britain, *Sociology of Health and Illness*, 19, 547–60.

Heritage, J. and Maynard, D. (2006) *Communication in Medical Care: Interaction between Primary Care Physicians and Patients*. Cambridge: Cambridge University Press.

Heritage, J. and Stivers, T. (1999) Online commentary in acute medical visits: a method of shaping patient expectations, *Social Science and Medicine*, 49, 1501–17.

Holt, E. (2012) Conversation analysis and laughter. In The Encyclopedia of Applied Linguistics, C. A., Chapelle (ed.) http://doi.org/10.1002/9781405198431.wbeal0207

Jefferson, G. (2004) Glossary of transcript symbols with an Introduction. In Lerner, G.H. (ed.) *Conversation Analysis: Studies from the First Generation*. Philadelphia: John Benjamins.

Kessels, R. (2003) Patients' memory for medical information, *Journal of the Royal Society of Medicine*, 96, 219–22.

Llanwarne, N., Newbould, J., Burt, J., Campbell, J.L., *et al.* (2017) Wasting the doctor's time? A video-elicitation interview study with patients in primary care, *Social Science & Medicine*, 176, 113–22.

Mail Online (2017) DO ask Dr Google before you see your GP! Leading doctor urges patients to follow a three-step plan before setting foot in a surgery - including searching their symptoms online. Available at http://www.dailymail.co.uk/health/article-5219409/Leading-doctor-says-think-going-GP.html (Last accessed January 2018).

Naghieha, A. and Parvizi, M. (2016) Exercising soft closure on lay health knowledge? Harnessing the declining power of the medical profession to improve online health information, *Social Theory and Health*, 14, 332–50.

Nettleton, S. (2004) The Emergence of E-Scaped Medicine?, *Sociology*, 38, 4, 661–79.

Office for National Statistics (2017) Internet access - households and individuals. Available at https://www.ons.gov.uk/peoplepopulationandcommunity/householdcharacteristics/homeinternetandsocialmedia usage/datasets/internetaccesshouseholdsandindividualsreferencetables (Last accessed January 2018).

Pellegrino, E.D. (1976) Prescribing and drug ingestion symbols and substances, *The Annals of Pharmacotherapy*, 10, 624–30.

Pilnick, A. and Dingwall, R. (2011) On the remarkable persistence of asymmetry in doctor/patient interaction: a critical review, *Social Science and Medicine*, 72, 1374–82.

Public Health England (2017) Digital-first public health: Public Health England's digital strategy. Available at https://www.gov.uk/government/publications/digital-first-public-health/digital-first-public-health-public-health-englands-digital-strategy (Last accessed January 2018).

Pulse Today (2017) 'Dr Google enters 80% of my consultations', warns RCGP chair. Available at http://www.pulsetoday.co.uk/your-practice/practice-topics/it/dr-google-enters-80-of-my-consultations-warns-rcgp-chair/20035400.article (Last accessed January 2018).

Seguin, M. and Stevenson, F. (In press) Patient engagement in treatment in an information age. In Hadler, A., Sutton, S. and Osterberg, L. (eds.) *The Wiley Handbook of Treatment Engagement*. Wiley-Blackwell, Oxford.

Seguin, M., Hall, L., Atherton, H., Barnes, R., *et al.* (2018) Protocol paper for the 'Harnessing resources from the internet to maximise outcomes from GP consultations (HaRI)' study: a mixed qualitative methods study, *British Medical Journal Open*, 8, e024188. https://bmjopen.bmj.com/content/8/8/e024188.info

Sidnell, J. (2010) *Conversation analysis: An introduction*. Oxford: Wiley-Blackwell.

Stevenson, F., Kerr, C., Murray, E. and Nazareth, I. (2007) Information from the Internet and the doctor-patient relationship: the patient perspective - a qualitative study, *BMC Family Practice*, 8, 1, 47.

Tan, S.S.L. and Goonawardene, N. (2017) Internet health information seeking and the patient-physician relationship: a systematic review, *Journal of Medical Internet Research*, 19, 1, e9.

The Telegraph (2017) Available at http://www.telegraph.co.uk/news/2017/12/29/royal-college-gps-recommends-dr-google-first-time-bid-ease-pressure/ (Last accessed: January 2018).

World Bank Group (2017) World Development Indictors. Available at http://wdi.worldbank.org/table/5.12 (Last accessed January 2018).

Ziebland, S. and Wyke, S. (2012) Health and illness in a connected world: how might sharing experiences on the internet affect people's health?, *Milbank Quarterly*, 90, 2, 219–49.

Sociology of Health & Illness Vol. 41 No. S1 2019 ISSN 0141-9889, pp. 82–97
doi: 10.1111/1467-9566.12873

The vaccination debate in the "post-truth" era: social media as sites of multi-layered reflexivity

Dino Numerato[1] ⓘ, Lenka Vochocová[1] ⓘ, Václav Štětka[2,1] ⓘ and Alena Macková[1,3] ⓘ

[1]Faculty of Social Sciences, Charles University, Prague, Czech Republic
[2]School of Social Sciences, Loughborough University, Loughborough, UK
[3]Faculty of Social Studies, Masaryk University, Brno, Czech Republic

Abstract This paper analyses the contemporary public debate about vaccination, and
medical knowledge more broadly, in the context of social media. The study is
focused on the massive online debate prompted by the Facebook status of the
digital celebrity Mark Zuckerberg, who posted a picture of his two-month-old
daughter, accompanied by a comment: 'Doctor's visit – time for vaccines!'
Carrying out a qualitative analysis on a sample of 650 comments and replies,
selected through systematic random sampling from an initial pool of over 10,000
user contributions, and utilising open and axial coding, we empirically inform the
theoretical discussion around the concept of the reflexive patient and introduce the
notion of multi-layered reflexivity. We argue that the reflexive debate surrounding
this primarily medical problem is influenced by both biomedical and social
scientific knowledge. Lay actors therefore discuss not only vaccination, but also its
political and economic aspects as well as the post-truth information context of the
debate. We stress that the reflexivity of social actors related to the post-truth era
re-enters and influences the debate more than ever. Furthermore, we suggest that
the interconnection of different layers of reflexivity can either reinforce certainty or
deepen the ambiguity and uncertainty of reflexive agents.

Keywords: conspiracy theory, Facebook, post-truth, reflexivity, social media, vaccine

Introduction

On 8 January 2016, Facebook CEO Mark Zuckerberg posted on his Facebook profile a picture of his two-month-old daughter, accompanied by a comment: "Doctor's visit – time for vaccines!" In only few days, the post attracted more than 83,000 comments. The debate between proponents and opponents of vaccination that followed the statement made by the global celebrity provides a unique insight into the contemporary character of the public debate about vaccination, and medical knowledge more broadly.[1] Furthermore, the analysis of this specific case empirically informs the theoretical debate about patient and citizen reflexivity in late modern societies.

Against this backdrop, the aim of this paper is to analyse the debate about vaccination in the global public space. The following questions are addressed: What topics and arguments were articulated during the Facebook debate about vaccination? What are the theoretical

Digital Health: Sociological Perspectives, First Edition.
Edited by Flis Henwood and Benjamin Marent.
Chapters © 2019 The Authors. Book Compilation © 2019 Foundation for the Sociology of Health & Illness/John Wiley & Sons Ltd.

implications for our understanding of public debates about medical knowledge in the digitalised post-truth era? How does this particular analysis empirically inform the theoretical notion of a reflexive patient? These questions are answered utilising a qualitative thematic analysis of the user comments and replies below the aforementioned Facebook status of Mark Zuckerberg.

This paper provides a contribution to the theoretical debate on reflexivity of patients, exemplified by the highly debated case of vaccination. The study is contextualised within the broader theoretical debate about the changing character of the public sphere in the so-called post-truth era, characterised by the intensified marginalisation of factually-based evidence; increasing diffusion of inaccurate claims; 'fake news' and "alternative facts" spread mainly through social media platforms as well as by the fragmentation and polarisation of media audiences.

The study is organised into the following four parts. First, we outline the debate concerning the changing status of expert systems and evidence-based knowledge as one of the main features of the so-called post-truth era, with a particular focus on vaccination. Second, we discuss the notion of a reflexive patient. After presenting our research methods, we provide an empirically informed debate about different facets of reflexivity emerging in the context of the post-truth global public debate. Finally, we discuss the relationship between the multi-layered nature of reflexivity and the construction of new uncertainties in late modern societies.

Internet, post-truth and the transformation of expertise

The contemporary information environment features an increasing dominance of digital communication technologies and social media platforms, becoming an ever more important source of news and general information for the majority of the population. According to Pew Research Centre (2017), two-thirds (67%) of American adults get their news from social media, and 45 per cent of Facebook users say that they get their news from this platform.

However, while certainly contributing to a greater pluralisation of our information ecosystem, the growing penetration and importance of online and social media raises serious concerns over the quality, accuracy and credibility of circulated information and knowledge. The affordances of social networking sites, stimulating the creation of "echo chambers" that amplify and reinforce existing views rather than support confrontation with dissenting perspectives (see e.g. Sunstein 2017), contribute to a faster and deeper polarisation of opinions, whilst allowing for factually incorrect, misleading or entirely fabricated information to gain the kind of prominence and impact that previous communication technologies could never have provided (Iyengar and Massey 2018, Van Aelst et al. 2017).

The viral diffusion and increasing societal and political influence of online 'fake news' and hoaxes has been frequently portrayed as one of the key symptoms of the 'post-truth age' Western societies have now allegedly entered. While the term – often used synonymously with 'post-truth politics' – has been popularised by the media in response to events such as the 2016 US presidential election campaign or the UK Brexit referendum of the same year, both infamous for spreading false and manipulative statements (see e.g. d'Ancona 2017, Levinson 2017), it has recently become an object of academic reflection in many fields (Boler and Davis 2018, Corner 2017, Ylä-Anttila 2018), and particularly in the field of Science and Technology Studies (Fuller 2018, Hoffman 2018, Lynch 2017, Sismondo 2017).

The studies and essays dealing with post-truth published so far often adopt, as a starting point for discussion, the Oxford Dictionaries definition of this term, according to which it is an adjective 'relating to or denoting circumstances in which objective facts are less influential in shaping public opinion than appeals to emotion and personal belief'.[2] Whilst the existing scholarship has not offered a more comprehensive definition yet, and some scholars are explicitly critical of the interpretation established in the popular discourse (Lynch 2017), most authors agree that the concept of post-truth highlights the changing mechanisms of social construction and legitimisation of knowledge, including the decline of trust in institutions that have traditionally been accepted as its symbolic guardians, such as science, universities, and the mainstream and elite media (Brubaker 2017). Fuller (2018) talks in this respect about the post-truth world as 'the inevitable outcome of greater epistemic democracy', enabled by opening access to instruments of knowledge production to the general public, thereby dismantling the old epistemic hierarchies. In a more critical fashion, Brubaker (2017) utilizes the concept of 'epistemological populism', first coined in Saurette and Gunster's (2011) analysis of Canadian political talk radio, to describe the favouring of 'common people's knowledge' over knowledge that is produced by expert systems.

As various authors have argued, this increasing disdain for 'expert' knowledge has been stimulated by the perceived wisdom of the crowd on the Internet and social media. In his book 'The Death of Expertise', Tom Nichols voiced fears 'a Google-fuelled, Wikipedia-based, blog-sodden collapse of any division between professionals and laypeople, students and teachers, knowers and wonderers – in other words, between those of any achievement in an area and those with none at all' (Nichols 2017: 3). Pointing more specifically to the area of scientific knowledge, Brubaker (2017) observes a deepening of the gaps that "divide the views of scientists from those of the public about subjects such as evolution, the causes of climate change, the safety of vaccines, and the safety of genetically modified foods" (Brubaker 2017).

According to d'Ancona (2017), the modern campaign against vaccination is the most palpable example of 'scientific denialism', 'the growing conviction that scientists, in league with government and pharmaceutical organisations ('Big Pharma'), are at war with nature and the best interests of humanity' (d'Ancona 2017: 70). With claims like these, the anti-vaccination campaign often shares common ground with conspiracy theories, which Ylä-Anttila describes as a 'type of counterknowledge' – alternative knowledge which challenges dominant epistemic authorities – centred around the conviction that "common people are misled in secrecy by an elite" (Ylä-Anttila 2018: 361).[3] Even though the rise of conspiracy theories cannot be associated solely with either the digital age or with the "post-truth" era, as they date far back into history (Van Prooijen and Douglas 2017), some authors claim that they are now part of our "contemporary political zeitgeist" (Einstein and Glick 2015) and that the online environment as well as the anti-expert climate of epistemic populism offer them particularly conducive conditions to flourish, as the anti-vaccination campaign arguably demonstrates (Iyengar and Massey 2018, Lewandowsky *et al.* 2017).

While the anti-vaccination movement has a long history, dating back to mid-19th century (Blume 2006, Song and Abelson 2016), the modern-day wave of the campaign was famously sparked after a study by Dr Andrew Wakefield was published in the Lancet in 1998, which claimed to have found a link between the MMR (measles, mumps and rubella) vaccine and autism. Even though the study was eventually retracted and its findings refuted, numerous opponents of vaccination still reference the study, which could have contributed to a decline in MMR vaccinations in many countries, leading to the outbreak of a measles epidemic in the U.S. and Canada in 2014/15 (Song and Abelson 2016).

It is beyond doubt that the Internet and Web 2.0 platforms have been crucial in the spread of the anti-vaccination campaign, bringing it to a global level and enabling the activists and supporters to better organise and efficiently disseminate information among them. The online anti-vaccination movement has also greatly benefited from the involvement of celebrities endorsing the campaign and bringing their own "expertise" in support of claims about the harmful effects of vaccination. The one that received the most publicity was Jenny McCarthy's appearance on Oprah Winfrey's television talk show in 2007, where she defended her competence to speak against vaccination by claiming that she simply found information on Google, adding that "the University of Google is where I got my degree from" (d'Ancona 2017: 73).

Despite the charismatic power of celebrities and viral potential of online misinformation in the alleged post-truth age, the majority of Americans still agree that the benefits of childhood vaccines outweigh the risks, and overwhelmingly trust medical scientists over any other source of information on that issue (Pew Research Centre 2017). However, there seems to be more widespread scepticism among younger generations, with only 39 per cent of 18–29-year olds agreeing that medial scientists understand the effects of MMR vaccines "very well", as opposed to 48 per cent of 30–60-year olds and 51 per cent of people above the age of 61. Likewise, the majority of young people don't believe the media are doing a good job covering science (Pew Research Centre 2017). According to a recent survey focused on medical conspiracy theories in the United States, 20 per cent of Americans believe that doctors are willing to vaccinate children even though they know vaccines can cause autism and physical disorders. A further 36 per cent neither agree, nor disagree with the statement (Oliver and Wood 2014a).

Reflexive patient

Decisions of contemporary social actors about vaccination are potentially made as part of complex reflexive scrutiny. The capacity of social agents to consider the possible risks associated with vaccination emerges in the broader context of reflexive modernisation. Following the sociological meta-narrative about reflexive modernisation that had acquired a prominent position in social theory beginning in the early nineties, the notion of reflexive (Adams 2011, Lupton 1997, Nettleton and Burrows 2003, Newman and Kuhlmann 2007) or informed patient (Kivits 2004) has been elaborated in the context of health care. The modern division between experts and lay persons has been blurred. Notwithstanding a recognition of the possible limits of lay knowledge (Prior 2003, Ziebland 2004), the notion of a reflexive patient referred to "increasingly reflexive and decreasingly deferential citizens" in the "fundamentally changed late-modern society" (Martin 2008: 41).

The notion of a reflexive patient might be discussed through two interconnected dimensions, depending on the object of reflexivity represented either by one's own health or the health care system. Firstly, reflexivity refers to the general capacity of late modern actors to reflexively consider their own health in light of medical knowledge proliferated in late modern societies. In this vein, patients become proto-professionalised (de Swaan 1988); hand in hand with the medicalisation of everyday life, they embrace expert medical vocabulary and knowledge to reconsider their health conditions. Hence, reflexive patients are actors who are informed about and responsible for their own health (Adams 2011, Lupton 1997). In other words, late modern actors incorporate reflexive reasoning while making decisions about health and well-being (Giddens 1991). The increased reflexive engagement is performed by ill patients in search of health care as well as by healthy people who more and more consider their own health vis-à-vis the new expert evidence,[4] frequently mediated by internet platforms and social media (Miah and Rich 2008). Patients become proto-medical experts who either make their own individual choices or just merely reply to the policy or market pressures on patients to behave as reflexive, and therefore responsible, consumers (Dent and Pahor 2015, Nettleton and Burrows 2002, Newman and Kuhlmann 2007) and digitised health citizens (Lupton 2017).[5]

Secondly, reflexivity refers to the critical capacity of patients to express discontent with health-care institutions and professionals. In other words, late modern patients, in addition to being proto-medical experts who embrace medical knowledge to assess their own health conditions, question traditional medical authority, problematise the position of biomedical knowledge or assess the performance of health care professionals and institutions. Reflexive behaviour not only represents a way of coping with new uncertainties and insecurities arising from the application of expert knowledge. Simultaneously, the increased reflexivity also contributes to the production of new insecurities hand in hand with the problematisation of expert knowledge (Beck *et al.* 2003). More specifically, while seeking certainty, the reflexive patient often manufactures new risks and uncertainties.

The topic of vaccination represents a typical example of a specific health-related issue becoming an object of reflexive reasoning. The reflexive stance of citizens constitutes part of the vaccination debate and was apparently influenced by new information and communication technologies that, in the so-called post-truth era, disseminate knowledge and information of different quality, accuracy and credibility. As suggested by the example of the debate around the MMR vaccination, in the context of reflexive modernisation and also in the context of an increasingly digitalised information environment, vaccination appears under reflexive scrutiny (Nettleton and Burrows 2002).

More generally, the Internet provides a platform where simple monitoring or even dissatisfaction with provided health care is confronted and expressed (e.g. Adams 2011, Kivits 2009, Lupton 2017, Miah and Rich 2008). The intensification of information and communication technologies has apparently contributed to the increased reflexivity of patients and with the afore-mentioned dominance of digital communication technologies and social media platforms, more space for various expression of reflexivity has opened up.

Information and digital technologies are therefore understood primarily as facilitators and vehicles of reflexivity. Nettleton and Burrows (2003: 171) argued that proactively engaging in these 'reflexive resource[s]' may result in a 'strategic advantage in the real world'. These ideas were further developed by Martin (2008) who argued that these resources provide people with knowledge which, together with their experience with the disease, can lead to developing 'a new, positioned perspective on the science or delivery of medicine' (ibid: 39). Ziebland (2004), who connects the development of the Internet as an easy source of information with a changing relationship between doctors and patients, points out the complexity of the situation. The potentially negative consequence of this trend, a decline in trust in expert knowledge, may well be compensated for by the rise of self-confident, mutually supported patients who are able to act as partners in the doctor-patient relationship.

While previous studies suggested that information and digital technologies are mere facilitators and vehicles of reflexive scrutiny, our study aims to go beyond this perspective by suggesting that the contemporary information environment, characterised by an increasing dominance of digital communication platforms, itself represents another object of reflexive scrutiny. In other words, our analysis is based upon the assumption that a patient is not only potentially more cognisant of medicine and health care, but also cognisant of the logic of the mass media and social media. The aim of our analysis is to identify different facets of patient reflexivity, analyse the interconnection of these different facets and explore their links with different perspectives on compulsory vaccination.

Methods

A qualitative thematic analysis of user comments and replies below the aforementioned Mark Zuckerberg Facebook status was carried out with a specific focus on the diverse discursive practices of the users. The case of the debate following Mark Zuckerberg's post represents an empirically unique opportunity to understand the nature of contemporary global debate surrounding compulsory vaccination; it resembles a sociological vignette used to stimulate the debate and reaction of respondents in a real-life situation. Mark Zuckerberg's Facebook profile is a relatively neutral site for the exchange of opinions that does not remain closed in their "echo chambers", which would just amplify and confirm existing opinions. Furthermore, the plurality of standpoints and heterogeneity of reactions in the sample was facilitated by the resonance that Mark Zuckerberg's post acquired in mainstream media.[6]

With an aim to explore the complexity of topics and arguments rather than to provide a representative overview of different positions, our data were selected in two steps. First, 1263 most relevant comments and related 9312 replies to comments and replies to replies were selected. We acknowledge that this selection is highly dependent on the power of Facebook algorithms and is not fully representative of the whole debate beyond the Facebook post. However, we acknowledge that these posts attracted the highest attention and were followed by the most intense interaction of Facebook users. Furthermore, considering our data against the previous research, we are confident that the nature and plurality of themes and arguments reflects the main themes and argumentations spelled out in past debates. The first selection of data was, second, followed by a systematic random sampling method and the data collection continued until empirical and theoretical saturation was achieved. More specifically, in total 650 comments and replies were analysed.

We employed the first two steps of the grounded theory approach, open and axial coding (Strauss and Corbin 1998), to categorise the data and identify patterns in the pro- and anti-vaccination comments of discussants with a specific focus on the two abovementioned layers of reflexivity. During the process of open coding, the main topics and arguments in the vaccination debate and the position of the participants were first identified, leading to a basic set of categories structuring the debate, its proponents, topics, and actors (the content related reflexivity). In the second step, we put a systematic emphasis on comments and replies that did not focus on vaccination itself but on the debate about vaccination. These comments represented a significant aspect of the discussion and revealed the form-related reflexivity, i.e. the means by which vaccination proponents and opponents promoted their position by discussing with public health authorities, the pharmaceutical industry, biomedical knowledge production as well as the media (both mainstream and social) and their alleged role in the vaccination discourse.

During this coding phase, we focused specifically and selectively on the presence and type of information sources as well as the links to them, references to and evaluation of the actors considered important in the vaccination discourse, the argumentation position of the participant (i.e. how and whether the commentators reflect and stress their experience with the topic and position in the debate), the level of rationality of the arguments (i.e. the presence of some kind of supportive reasoning or evidence in the comment – Wright, S., Graham, T., Jackson, D., Unpublished data), and the presence of arguments reflecting power relations in the vaccination debate (including conspiracy contributions). This coding phase resulted in a more detailed picture of the argumentation strategies of the vaccination debate participants and the reflexivity of these discussants in relation to various actors in the vaccination discourse, including information sources and the role of the Internet and social networking sites.

The accessibility of social media data does not necessarily indicate their availability for research purposes (Hine 2011). The study has thus necessarily been related to several ethical concerns, also in light of the changing rules governing the privacy settings of social networking sites. At the same time, the intrinsically contextual way in which Facebook users experience their privacy (Marwick 2014) was considered. In our research, we analysed comments and replies below a single post on Mark Zuckerberg's public page. According to the Facebook privacy policy, such content posted with the privacy settings set to public may be accessed and seen by anyone, and it "can be seen, accessed and reshared or downloaded though third-party services".[7] We suppose that users perceived the page as public space where they intentionally wanted to express their own opinion on vaccination. On the other hand, we also suppose that many users are not completely aware of the privacy setting and its consequences (Williams *et al.* 2017) and we thus considered the risk of harm and the sensitivity of the data (see Townsend and Wallace 2016). In light of this consideration, several potentially illustrative quotations were dropped or trimmed down.

Findings

The debate stimulated by Zuckerberg's post (Figure 1) has apparently mirrored the previous debates on vaccination (see e.g. Blume 2006, Hobson-West 2003, 2007, Kata 2012, Poland and Jacobson 2001, Skea *et al.* 2008). Among the users commenting on Zuckerberg's post not only were there strict proponents or opponents of vaccination but there were also those who provided more neutral and ambivalent comments. By advocating different perspectives, Facebook users supported their view with references to their direct experience, instinct, common sense, as well as with references to biomedical expertise, scientific evidence, the statements of celebrities, and articles in the mass media and on social media platforms. Furthermore,

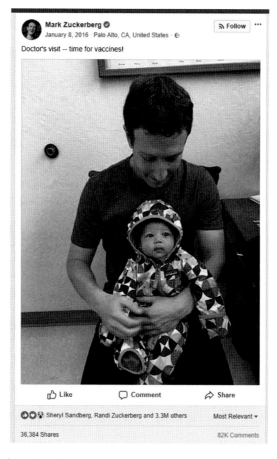

Figure 1 *A printscreen of Mark Zuckerberg's post [Colour figure can be viewed at wileyonlinelibrary.com]*

discussants commented on the risks related to vaccines and their quality, and reminded others of their secondary and adverse effects. Opponents of vaccines juxtaposed their criticism of the unnatural character of vaccines with comments about their toxicity. Based on historical and epidemiological evidence, individual responsibility for collective immunisation was emphasised against the "free riding" behaviour of some parents and "pro-choice" calls, framed by broader arguments such as civic liberties and human rights.

In a more theoretical vein, the richness of arguments and themes in the debate puts the contributors in the position of reflexive agents who are "(. . .) faced with an overwhelming range and chaotic juxtaposition of (re)sources, making time and space for considered reflection virtually impossible" (Nettleton and Burrows 2003: 181). Considering the rich plethora of arguments, the example of discussion below Zuckerberg's post would lead us to a similar theoretical observation. However, considering this quote relates to the early stages of Internet diffusion, we should emphasize that reflexivity of actors in the so-called post-truth era is different, notably thanks to the proliferation of social media platforms. In this context, not only is the diffusion of the variety of arguments intensified, but the nature of the arguments changes as well. More specifically, the content-related reflexivity focused on vaccines is more commonly accompanied with form-related reflexivity, focused on the debate about vaccines. Under these circumstances, the overwhelming range of resources and the questions of their origin not only presented an object of sociological commentary but also increasingly an object of the lay comments of social actors.

The debate about the vaccination debate: multi-layered reflexivity

The data analysis suggests that in addition to the debate about vaccines, increasing attention is paid to the economic, political, and information environments in which this debate takes place. The identification of economic, political and information layers of the vaccination debate leads us to the introduction of the notion of *multi-layered reflexivity*. The concept of multi-layered reflexivity puts a stronger emphasis on the capacity of social actors to reflect upon the processes of production, governance, distribution and, most importantly, a mediated interpretation of the role of vaccines.

Reflexivity and information environment

As part of the vaccination debate, Facebook users, regardless of their standpoint towards vaccination reflected the role played by the information environment, in particular the role of the mainstream media, the Internet and social media platforms. The opponents of vaccination warned against some of the politicoeconomic aspects behind the production of media content. More specifically, they blamed the mainstream media and a political or economic interest group for denying access to alternative voices and those revealing the negative effects of vaccination, as can be illustrated by the following quote: 'Why parents of vaccine injured child are not permitted to talk in mainstream television. Thinks about it.'[8] , or explicitly labelled them as propagandist or manipulative.

Considered a member of the elites, Mark Zuckerberg himself was often blamed by anti-vaccination users for having a financial interest in promoting vaccination. These discussants also frequently claimed they did not believe Mark Zuckerberg was vaccinating his child – an argument stemming from a conviction that elites are informed about the harmful nature of vaccines and protect their children from it (or have access to better-quality vaccines):

> How much were you paid to post this? I know there's no way you'd vaccinate for many reasons the truly informed parents already have stated. Do you not make enough from Facebook or is your back pocket change running low?

Comments criticising Mark Zuckerberg as a personification of digital media's financial interests belong to a wider trend noticeable also among vaccination proponents (see below) who employed reflection on the role of the Internet in current information exchange and approached online media with scepticism. However, the pro-vaccination stance focused mainly on digital media as a possible source of misinformation in the post-truth era, opponents of vaccination stressed the importance of financial interests of both media owners and individual people (labelled as trolls or fake profiles) allegedly using social media to make money by serving the interests of the pharmaceutical lobby.

On the proponents' side, the argumentation concerning the role of the media in the vaccination debate dominantly stemmed from a focus on facts and truth, the responsibility of informed people (responsible parenting, responsibility concerning herd immunity) and 'real science' providing actors with facts. These aspects were presented in strong opposition to what people could get from online information sources, mainly search engines represented by Google and social networking sites such as Facebook or YouTube. The anti-vaccine position was often labelled as 'anti-science' or 'pseudo-science' by proponents of vaccination and was typically connected to the allegedly poor role the Internet and social media platforms played in informing people. In this logic, Zuckerberg was celebrated for 'being a responsible parent [...] listening to the experts and not following an antiscience, trendy, elitist, poorly educated stance' who could, unlike many "antiscience, trendy, elitist" and 'Google-miseducated', tell which information sources were valid, and which were not.

As mentioned above, reflections on the role of the Internet in the distribution of knowledge, and specifically disinformation, were an inherent part of the pro-vaccination discourse. Digital media (specifically Web 2.0) were considered the main source of '*anti-science*' or lay knowledge opposed to expert, well-informed knowledge deriving from scientific research. The voice of the opponents of vaccination was disputed due to low media literacy related to an uncritical approach towards the Internet and social media platforms, ironically referring to 'Google University', 'Facebook scientists' or the truth about vaccination which "is out there", on YouTube.

We identified stress on factual correctness and explicit mention of the difference in relevance of internet sources and scientific information as a crucial part of pro-vaccination argumentation. Together with references to social media platforms and Internet more broadly as a non-reliable source, accompanied by suggestions such as 'Don't ever take advice from someone on the Internet. Or Google. Or Facebook,' or 'Don't ever listen to uninformed crazies on Facebook', vaccination proponents often employ biting humour and sarcasm to laugh at the other side's argumentation:

> Vaccine research laboratory: 200 years of research and development. Anti-vaccine research laboratory: 200 minutes of web browsing.

It is precisely in the comments of pro-vaccination discussants where the penetration of the discourse on the 'post-truth' age and 'fake sources' in the vaccination discourse becomes most obvious. Proponents of vaccination and those relativising the veracity of anti-vaccination claims reveal alleged 'fake profiles' or 'trolls' as unworthy participants of the discussion[9] and name specific websites as well-known sources of unreliable information, referring to *Collective Evolution*, *NaturalNews* or to chat forums such as *The Agenda*, *The Illuminati Revealed* and *What They Don't Want You to Know*.

The previous illustrations imply that patient reflexivity is in fact more complex than what the previously elaborated notion of "reflexive patients" would suggest. The object of reflexivity in the so-called post-truth era has been extended. In this vein, the contemporary reflexive patient is not only a proto-medical expert but also a proto-sociologist. In relation to vaccination, citizens as proto-medical experts problematise the medical knowledge. Furthermore, citizens as proto-sociologists problematise the contemporary information environment in which the debate about vaccination takes place. Through the spread of the proto-sociological perspective in society, we could observe the mechanisms already described by Giddens (1984) in his discussion of the notion of the double hermeneutic; i.e. the processes during which social scientific concepts are adopted by lay actors and contribute to the constitution of the social world that social sciences observe. The proto-sociological discussion of existing communication patterns underlying the compulsory vaccination debate are thus constitutive of the vaccination debate itself.

Reflexivity and the pharmaceutical industry
As suggested in some of the previous observations related to the media, Facebook users tended to identify the key subjects who presumably had some interest in skewing the mediated picture of vaccination. The pharmaceutical industry and the government (together with the media) were, from the perspective of political economy, perceived as mutually collaborative institutions motivated by financial profits. From this perspective, Zuckerberg's post was perceived as part of the propaganda or PR campaign of the pharmaceutical industry, wondering "how much big Pharma paid him to pose" and emphasising that "[m]illions are spent on pr campaigns and propaganda."

Proponents of vaccination were perceived as naive targets of the pharmaceutical lobby which was portrayed as a 'greedy machine [...] driven by financial interest' or an unscrupulous 'fraudulent multi-billion dollar industry,' compared to companies producing GMO plants and allegedly harmful chemicals such as Monsanto. These companies were considered to be manipulating and corrupting everyone, including governments, scientists, and the media and multiplying the numbers of vaccines recommended to people, thereby causing severe health problems endangering the population:

> ... their only studies are Pharma funded no private or third party studies, no double blind, no test for carcinogen, no test for neuro-toxins no safety studies for injecting 69 doses.

With regards to the portrayal of pharmaceutical companies, proponents of vaccination adopted a clearly defensive position – unlike in the case of the media where pro-vaccination discussants had their own specific narrative available differing completely from the narrative of vaccination opponents; in relation to 'Big Pharma', they tended to simply disprove the oppositional arguments by pointing to their illogicality, such as pointing to the incorruptibility of someone as wealthy as Mark Zuckerberg or by stressing that those blamed for poisoning other people and their children vaccinate their kids as well.

The reflexivity related to the pharmaceutical industry was sometimes encroached with the construction of broader conspiracy theories. Within this line of argumentation, links between historical events and crimes against humanity to the contemporary promotion of vaccination were developed. The pharmaceutical industry was being connected explicitly with WWII crimes through an alleged personal interconnection between the Nazi administration, research and leading pharmaceutical companies. The Facebook commentators have thereby echoed long-established conspiracy theories about powerful, often hidden elites, manipulating common people by concealing important information from them (see Oliver and Wood 2014b).

Through the lens of a conspiracist, as As Ylä-Anttila reminds, "[t]he elite holds not just secret power but secret knowledge", which the conspiracist attempts to challenge by raising him/herself "to the position of an alternative knowledge authority, a true expert instead of 'false experts leading us astray'" (Ylä-Anttila 2018: 362). While the tendencies to produce and legitimise counterknowledge or "alternative knowledge" are certainly not idiosyncratic in the so-called post-truth era, the analysed comments provide support for the claim that they are further intensified within the new communication ecosystem enabling the mass dissemination of content that provides a somewhat objectivised counter-expertise – one that is not only based on folk wisdom but also on alternative data and evidence (Ylä-Anttila 2018).

Reflexivity and politics

In line with the traditional political-economic argumentation, anti-vaccination discussants presented the role of government in the vaccination issue as one of a servant of pharmaceutical companies, rather than a desired regulator of the industry and protector of citizens:

> Unless there is enough questioning and counter-force, there is no motivation for companies to make better safer products. When government forcefully sells everyone a product (and with vaccines, unlike car seats, you don't have a range of brands to choose from), the producers are not stimulated in any way to do anything better – their product will be sold either way. Don't you see a problem with that?

The desired role of the state (government) in forcing the pharmaceutical companies to improve their products in terms of safety was ubiquitous in the argumentation of both clear opponents of vaccination and more neutral participants who stressed the importance of further research, medical and governmental independence as well as free-market competition ensuring better, safer pharmaceutical products:

> All of you ppl with negative comments, you r missing my point. I'm not against vaccines. I'm against gov't mandated vaccination unless there are massive outbreaks. There are still things to improve and more research to do to make vaccines safer. And pharm companies should not have this option of forcing their product through gov't.

On the other hand, when it came to the role of government, proponents of vaccination offered a specific narrative of governmental protection as their main argument in the discussion. Vaccination was considered important for the protection of all the people (the importance of 'herd immunity') and specifically of those who cannot be vaccinated for different reasons (intolerance/allergy to vaccines, diseases, etc.). In this logic, the government was perceived as the institution taking care of public safety and ensuring the population will not be jeopardised by irresponsible people who reject vaccination:

> They should force-inject for all the idiots who don't care enough to not infect other people and their healthy children.

Similar to the reflexivity related to pharmaceutical companies, the anti-vaccination discourse located the position of government in the context of broader conspiracies, in particular in relation to worries about personal freedom and forced governmental decisions about people's bodies. This way of thinking can be identified even in the comments of people who did not present themselves as clear opponents of vaccination:

> And WITH YOUR SUPPORT, the gov't might soon laws to FORCE MEDICAL PROCEDURES ON ALL OF YOUR WITHOUT YOUR CONSENT!!

> I think it's fine for Mark Zuckerberg to encourage ppl to vaccinate if he wants, but he adds inertia to a snowball that might soon create a situation when police will force-inject you with whatever they decide.

Furthermore, conspiratorial arguments embraced references to power interests as part of broader political objectives. In some of the comments, the 'new world order' was mentioned as a goal of these efforts and the identity of Mark Zuckerberg was compared to 'JACOB GREENBERG, GRANDSON OF DAVID ROCKEFELLER OF THE NEW WORLD ORDER.' The typical discursive strategy tended to separate 'us' (the people) from 'them' (wealthy, global elites, governments owned by wealthy people) and proposed theories in which 'they' (e.g. Mark Zuckerberg, Bill Gates, George Soros) aimed at 'de-populating', 'culling the herd', 'poisoning and sterilizing' 'us' or 'our kids':

> And of course we should just accept vaccinations, flouride and chemicals in our water, GMO food, and anything else the government (owned by people such as Zuckerberg) not his real name by the way. Because we love our government. They would never hurt us. They for sure would not hurt our children.

Again, the arguments about external political power interests are nourished by a proto-sociological hermeneutics of suspicion that aims to unmask the commercial and political interests behind vaccinations. Notwithstanding the common appearance of conspiracy plots in the Facebook discussions, the critical voice does not have to be necessarily reduced to conspiracy theories. The critical approach towards vaccinations, notably among highly educated parents, can be caused by responsibilised and reflexive citizens who react to the absence of critical debate in the context of governmental normalisation of vaccination (Hasmanová Marhánková 2014).

Discussion and conclusions

Through the analysis of the vaccination debate stimulated by Mark Zuckerberg's post on Facebook, we complement the previous scholarship on vaccination by analytically distinguishing between different layers of reflexivity, and by systematically examining those reflexive layers that focus on the context of the vaccination debate. As we suggest, the reflexivity relates to the 'post-truth' discourse in two ways. On the one hand, reflexivity can deconstruct the 'post-truth' discourse and disclose the production of counterknowledge. On the other hand, reflexivity itself can be incorporated into the post-truth discourse and reinforce the production and reproduction of misinformation and conspiracy theories, rather than deconstruct them. Therefore, contemporary reflexive agents are cognisant of medical sciences as well as of social sciences that help them understand the key mechanisms of the vaccination debate, including factors influencing the production and diffusion of biomedical knowledge.

However, the familiarity of reflexive agents with both medical and social sciences is limited, rooted in everyday life and experiences, necessarily based on selective reading and dependent on the resources of their knowledge and counter-knowledge. Thus, the epistemological capacities of reflexive agents cannot be overestimated. At the same time, regardless of the accuracy and validity of their reflexive claims, these claims continue to shape the debate. The reflexivity related to economics, politics, and the increasingly digitalised information environment can significantly influence the level of perceived certainty about vaccinations. The acknowledgement of a possible "post-truth" nature of the debate by reflexive agents, however, does not necessarily bring more certainty; although it can represent a pillar of certainty for already established opinions, it can – and often does – equally increase ambiguity and deepen the uncertainty in the debate.

The contribution of the paper is threefold. First, the paper empirically captures the debate about vaccination in the so-called post-truth era. The relatively neutral environment below Mark Zuckerberg's post, thanks to its openness to a variety of users, brought together proponents and opponents of vaccination as well as actors with a more ambiguous standpoint. The analysis suggests that participants in the global debate have increasingly taken into consideration the political and economic aspects of vaccination and the digitalised information environment.

Second, the analysis is situated within the context of previous public debates on vaccination. While we argue that the key themes and arguments mirror the previous debates (e.g. Blume 2006, Hobson-West 2003, 2007, Kata 2012), we also highlight that the vaccination debate has its own history, which has had "post-truth" attributes (e.g. conspiracy theories) since the beginning, and that this history is considered by participants in the debate. For example, the prevailing conspiracy myths about the misuse of vaccination to secure political, ideological, or religious dominance are not only reproduced thanks to social media, but are also, and once again, deciphered and problematised.

Third, this paper extends the notion of patient reflexivity, previously elaborated in a discussion of the role of the Internet and the informed patient (e.g. Adams 2011, Lupton 1997). Attempting to add to the existing scholarship while acknowledging the changes in the contemporary information environment, we have introduced the notion of multi-layered reflexivity. Through this notion we argue that the contemporary patient is still reflexive; however, this reflexivity is different compared to the previously developed sociological narratives of the "reflexive patient". More specifically, we emphasise that reflexivity is nowadays not expressed only in relation to the topic of vaccination but also in relation to the perceived 'post-truth' conditions, within which this discussion takes place and of which (at least some) of the participants are aware. In other words, mass media, the Internet and social media platforms are not viewed only as potential *vehicles* of reflexivity but potentially also as the *objects* of reflexivity, often critical ones. Furthermore, we argue that these layers of reflexivity, i.e. the layer concerning a health topic such as vaccines and the layer concerning the political, social and economic determinants surrounding vaccination, are potentially interconnected.

In this context, the dynamics between proto-medical reflexivity and proto-sociological reflexivity must be taken into consideration. Hence, the post-truth nature of contemporary debates does not only structure contemporary discussions; simultaneously, the post-truth nature of the debates increasingly represents an object of these discussions. The post-truth context has therefore further expanded the universes of social reality that represent the object of form-related reflexivity, progressively built around the content-related reflexivity. Therefore, either strategically or ingenuously used reflexivity related to the "post-truth" era re-enters the debate and influences its very nature and the position of social actors. Even if the debate about vaccination has from the beginning displayed certain features which are nowadays associated with the "post-truth" era, our findings suggest that the contemporary information environment characterised by the increasing dominance of digital communication technologies and social media platforms, the "post-truth" character of the debate is much stronger than ever.

Furthermore, while elaborating the concept of multi-layered reflexivity, rather than developing a singular notion of 'reflexive patient', the existence of a plurality of "reflexive patients" would be more appropriate. This plural notion refers to several ways in which different layers of reflexivity are potentially interconnected. In this vein, reflexive patients are potentially reflexive alongside different layers in a variety of manners. Such a variety refers to different configurations of different layers of reflexivity and to different ways in which these layers are connected, disconnected, juxtaposed, bracketed, prioritized or hierarchised. In other words, the importance attributed to different layers of reflexivity varies in a similar way to the degree of certainty or uncertainty that reflexivity, expressed in different layers and connections among them, may imply.

While this paper explored some of the most commonly appearing configurations between layers of reflexivity – e.g. the connection between anti-vaccination discourse and criticism of the pharmaceutical industry and mainstream mass media on the one hand, or the pro-vaccination stance connected with criticism of the naïve approach towards social media and counter-knowledge on the other hand – it mainly attempted to identify and describe the nature of the multi-layered reflexivity by pointing to its increasing importance in the post-truth context. The dynamics between different layers of multi-layered reflexivity could be further explored. We argue that the concept of multi-layered reflexivity has analytical utility beyond the vaccination debate and medical context and that our findings may be applied to examine contemporary controversies related to environmental issues, science more broadly or migration as well as in political debates emerging in the post-truth context. As with the topic of vaccination, debates about environmental issues, science, migration or politics have increasingly been connected with the debate about the, economic and mediated contexts in which these debates take place.

Address for correspondence: Dino Numerato, Faculty of Social Sciences, Charles University, Prague, Czech Republic. E-mail: dino.numerato@fsv.cuni.cz

Acknowledgements

This research was supported by the Czech Science Foundation (GAČR), Standard Grant Nr 17-01116S – *"Civic engagement and the politics of health care"*. We thank the editors of this Special Issue, Benjamin Marent and Flis Henwood, and the anonymous reviewers for their insightful and valuable comments on the earlier drafts of the manuscript. We thank Jakub Růžička for his assistance with data retrieval and to Tereza Sedláčková for her helpful comments on the manuscript.

Notes

1   We should add that not all of these comments concerned the vaccination debate. Many comments were regarding the appearance of Zuckerberg's daughter or simply approved the act of vaccination. Moreover, numerous actors used the visibility of the profile to address other topics (e.g. the humanitarian crisis during the war in Syria).
2   https://en.oxforddictionaries.com/definition/post-truth, accessed 6 January 2018.
3   As Ylä-Anttila reminds, counterknowledge – including conspiracy theories – should not be conflated with misinformation or "fake news"; counterknolwedge is not necessarily wrong, but it is rather difficult to falsify, which is precisely one of the reasons conspiracy theories tend to persist (Ylä-Anttila 2018).
4   As Lupton (1997) suggested, this method of individual reflexive agency is not necessarily embraced by all patients; many patients seek to eliminate any uncertainty from their treatment, and prefer to maintain a trustful and passive relationship with doctors.
5   Following Lash's (1994) distinction between "reflexivity losers" and "reflexivity winners", it should be stressed that the potential for reflexive action is not distributed equally in societies and that it is located mainly in the middle and higher social classes.
6   It was actually our analytical interest in the media representations of vaccination that brought us towards this specific post.
7   https://www.facebook.com/about/privacy/
8   For the sake of authenticity, the comments of Facebook users are reproduced in the same way they appeared in the Facebook discussion, including errors, spelling mistakes and abbreviations. Only vulgar terms were amended.
9   The recent research even suggests the involvement of Twitter bots and trolls with the aim of skewing the vaccination debate as part of wider political objectives to divide and polarise societies (Broniatowski *et al.* 2018).

References

Adams, S.A. (2011) Sourcing the crowd for health services improvement: the reflexive patient and 'share-your-experience' websites, *Social Science & Medicine*, 72, 7, 1069–76.

Beck, U., Bonss, W. and Lau, C. (2003) The theory of reflexive modernization, *Theory, Culture & Society*, 20, 2, 1–33.

Blume, S. (2006) Anti-vaccination movements and their interpretations, *Social Science and Medicine*, 62, 3, 628–42.

Boler, M. and Davis, E. (2018) The affective politics of the "post-truth" era: feeling rules and networked subjectivity, *Emotion, Space and Society*, 27, 75–85.

Broniatowski, D.A., Jamison, A.M., Qi, S., AlKulaib, L., *et al.* (2018) Weaponized health communication: Twitter bots and Russian trolls amplify the vaccine debate, *American Journal of Public Health*, 108, 10, 1378–84.

Brubaker, R. (2017) *Forget Fake News. Social Media Is Making Democracy Less Democratic*. Available at http://www.zocalopublicsquare.org/2017/11/29/forget-fake-news-social-media-making-democracy-less-democratic/ideas/essay/ (Last accessed 9 December 2018).

Corner, J. (2017) Fake news, post-truth and media–political change, *Media, Culture and Society*, 39, 7, 1100–7.

d'Ancona, M. (2017) *Post-Truth: The New War on Truth and How to Fight Back*. London: Ebury Press.

de Swaan, A. (1988) *In Care of the State*. Cambridge: Polity Press.

Dent, M. and Pahor, M. (2015) Patient involvement in Europe – a comparative framework, *Journal of Health Organization and Management*, 29, 5, 546–55.

Einstein, K.L. and Glick, D.M. (2015) Do I think BLS data are BS? The consequences of conspiracy theories, *Political Behavior*, 37, 3, 679–701.

Fuller, S. (2018) *Post-Truth: Knowledge as a Power Game*. London: Anthem Press.

Giddens, A. (1984) *The Constitution of Society*. Cambridge: Polity Press.

Giddens, A. (1991) *Modernity and Self-Identity. Self and Society in the Late Modern Age*. Cambridge: Polity Press.

Hasmanová Marhánková, J. (2014) Postoje rodičů odmítajících povinná očkování svých dětí: případová studie krize důvěry v biomedicínské vědění, *Sociologický Časopis*, 50, 2, 163–87.

Hine, C. (2011) Internet research and unobtrusive methods, *Social Research Update*, 61, 1.

Hobson-West, P. (2003) Understanding vaccination resistance: moving beyond risk, *Health, Risk & Society*, 5, 3, 273–83.

Hobson-West, P. (2007) Trusting blindly can be the biggest risk of all: Organised resistance to childhood vaccination in the UK, *Sociology of Health and Illness*, 29, 2, 198–215.

Hoffman, S.G. (2018) The responsibilities and obligations of STS in a moment of post-truth demagoguery, *Engaging Science, Technology, and Society*, 4, 444–52.

Iyengar, S. and Massey, D.S. (2018) Scientific communication in a post-truth society, *Proceedings of the National Academy of Sciences*. Published Ahead of Print. https://doi.org/10.1073/pnas.1805868115.

Kata, A. (2012) Anti-vaccine activists, Web 2.0, and the postmodern paradigm – An overview of tactics and tropes used online by the anti-vaccination movement, *Vaccine*, 30, 3778–89.

Kivits, J. (2004) Researching the 'informed patient, *Information, Communication & Society*, 7, 4, 510–530.

Kivits, J. (2009) Everyday health and the internet: a mediated health perspective on health information seeking, *Sociology of Health & Illness*, 31, 5, 673–87.

Lash, S. (1994) Reflexivity and its doubles: structure, aesthetics, community. In Beck, U., Giddens, A. and Lash, S. (eds) *Reflexive Modernization: Politics, Tradition and Aesthetics in the Modern Social Order*, pp 110–173. Cambridge: Polity Press.

Levinson, P. (2017) *Fake News in Real Context*. New York: Connected Editions.

Lewandowsky, S., Ecker, U.K. and Cook, J. (2017) Beyond misinformation: understanding and coping with the "post-truth" era, *Journal of Applied Research in Memory and Cognition*, 6, 4, 353–69.

Lupton, D. (1997) Consumerism, reflexivity and the medical encounter, *Social Science & Medicine*, 45, 3, 373–81.

Lupton, D. (2017) *Digital Health: Critical and Cross-disciplinary Perspectives*. London: Routledge.

Lynch, M. (2017) STS, symmetry and post-truth, *Social Studies of Science*, 47, 4, 593–99.

Martin, G.P. (2008) 'Ordinary people only': knowledge, representativeness, and the publics of public participation in healthcare, *Sociology of Health & Illness*, 30, 1, 35–54.

Marwick, A.E. (2014) Networked privacy: how teenagers negotiate context in social media, *New Media & Society*, 16, 7, 1051–67.

Miah, A. and Rich, E. (2008) *The Medicalization of Cyberspace*. London: Routledge.

Nettleton, S. and Burrows, R. (2002) Reflexive modernization and the emergence of wired self-help. In Renninger, K.A. and Shumar, W. (eds) *Building Virtual Communities: Learning and Change in Cyberspace*, pp 249–268. Cambridge: Cambridge University Press.

Nettleton, S. and Burrows, R. (2003) E-scaped medicine?, *Information, Reflexivity and Health, Critical Social Policy*, 23, 2, 165–85.

Newman, J. and Kuhlmann, E. (2007) Consumers enter the political stage? The modernization of health care in Britain and Germany, *Journal of European Social Policy*, 17, 2, 99–111.

Nichols, T. (2017) *The Death of Expertise: The Campaign Against Established Knowledge and Why it Matters*. Oxford: Oxford University Press.

Oliver, J.E. and Wood, T.J. (2014a) Medical conspiracy theories and health behaviors in the United States, *JAMA Internal Medicine*, 174, 5, 817–8.

Oliver, J.E. and Wood, T.J. (2014b) Conspiracy theories and the paranoid style (s) of mass opinion, *American Journal of Political Science*, 58, 4, 952–66.

Pew Research Centre (2017) *Key trends in social and digital news media*. Available at http://www.pewresearch.org/fact-tank/2017/10/04/key-trends-in-social-and-digital-news-media/ (Last accessed 9 December 2018).

Poland, G.A. and Jacobson, R.M. (2001) Understanding those who do not understand: a brief review of the anti-vaccine movement, *Vaccine*, 19, 2440–5.

Prior, L. (2003) Belief, knowledge and expertise: the emergence of the lay expert in medical sociology, *Sociology of Health & Illness*, 25, 3, 41–57.

Saurette, P. and Gunster, S. (2011) Ears wide shut: Epistemological populism, argutainment and Canadian conservative talk radio, *Canadian Journal of Political Science*, 44, 1, 195–218.

Sismondo, S. (2017) Post-truth?, *Social Studies of Science*, 47, 1, 3–6.

Skea, Z.C., Entwistle, V.A., Watt, I. and Russell, E. (2008) 'Avoiding harm to others' considerations in relation to parental measles, mumps and rubella (MMR) vaccination discussions – an analysis of an online chat forum, *Social Science & Medicine*, 67, 9, 1382–90.

Song, M. and Abelson, J. (2016) Public engagement and policy entrepreneurship on social media in the time of anti-vaccination movements. In Adria, M. and Mao, Y. (eds) *Handbook of Research on Citizen Engagement and Public Participation in the Era of New Media*, pp 38–56. IGI Global: Hershey, PA.

Strauss, A. and Corbin, J. (1998) *Basics of Qualitative Research: Techniques and Procedures for Developing Grounded Theory*. London: Sage.

Sunstein, C.R. (2017) *#Republic: Divided Democracy in the Age of Social Media*. Princeton: Princeton University Press.

Townsend, L. and Wallace, C. (2016). Social Media Research: A Guide to Ethics. Available at www.gla.ac.uk/media/media_487729_en.pdf (Last accessed 9 December 2018).

Van Aelst, P., Strömbäck, J., Aalberg, T., Esser, F., *et al.* (2017) Political communication in a high-choice media environment: a challenge for democracy?, *Annals of the International Communication Association*, 41, 1, 3–27.

Van Prooijen, J.W. and Douglas, K.M. (2017) Conspiracy theories as part of history: the role of societal crisis situations, *Memory Studies*, 10, 3, 323–33.

Williams, M.L., Burnap, P. and Sloan, L. (2017) Towards an ethical framework for publishing Twitter data in social research: taking into account users' views, online context and algorithmic estimation, *Sociology*, 51, 6, 1149–68.

Ylä-Anttila, T. (2018) Populist knowledge: 'Post-truth' repertoires of contesting epistemic authorities, *European Journal of Cultural and Political Sociology*, 5, 4, 356–88.

Ziebland, S. (2004) The importance of being expert: the quest for cancer information on the Internet, *Social Science & Medicine*, 59, 9, 1783–93.

Sociology of Health & Illness Vol. 41 No. S1 2019 ISSN 0141-9889, pp. 98–115
doi: 10.1111/1467-9566.12894

Making sense with numbers. Unravelling ethico-psychological subjects in practices of self-quantification

Jeannette Pols[1,2] ⓘ, Dick Willems[2] and Margunn Aanestad[3]

[1]*Section of Medical Ethics, Amsterdam University Medical Centre, and Department of Anthropology, University of Amsterdam, Amsterdam, The Netherlands*
[2]*Section of Medical Ethics, Amsterdam University Medical Centre, University of Amsterdam, Amsterdam, The Netherlands*
[3]*Department of Informatics, University of Oslo, Oslo, Norway*

Abstract   Prevention enthusiasts show great optimism about the potential of health apps to modify peoples' lifestyles through the tracking and quantification of behaviours and bodily signs. Critical sociologists warn for the disciplining effects of self-tracking. In this paper we use an empirical ethics approach to study the characteristics and strivings of the various types of 'ethico-psychological subjects' that emerge in practices of self-quantification by analysing how people and numbers relate in three cases of self-quantification: in prevention discourse, in testimonies from the quantified self (QS) movement and in empirical work we did with people with Diabetes type I and with 'every day self-trackers'. We show that a free subject that needs support to enact its will is crucial to understand the optimism about prevention. In the QS-movement the concern is with a lack of objective and personalised knowledge about imperceptible processes in the body. These subjects are decentered and multiplied when we trace how numbers in their turn act to make sense of people in our empirical study. We conclude that there are many different types of ethico-psychological subjects in practices of self-tracking that need to be explored in order to establish what good these practices of self-quantification might do.

Keywords: ethics/bioethics, self help/care, self-measurement, quantification, ethnography

Introduction

There is great optimism about the potential gains of improving lifestyles as a means to prevent chronic diseases, and governments and to this end health care organisations have been encouraging the use of health apps that measure behaviour or bodily signs. In June 2014 the Dutch minister of health notified Parliament about her intentions to stimulate the use of health apps amongst the Dutch population, including her aim to have 75 per cent of elderly and chronically diseased people – if they want and are able – to use health apps in 2019 (VWS 2015). The idea behind this ambitious aim is that self-tracking will lead to the prevention of disease and to better health for the trackers, and hence also to less costs for health care. These ambitions are propelled by statistical findings in population research that show that bad lifestyle habits, such as smoking, sedentariness and bad eating, cause more than half of common chronic diseases like diabetes and cardiovascular disorders (WHO 2008), and that these 'life-style diseases' are 'modifiable' (WHO 2016, 2008: 35). Lifestyles can be changed, assert prevention optimists, and this change is sought through state interventions such as agreements with the food industry and through stimulating individuals to manage their lives better. Crucial is the idea that people have a choice: it is possible for them to opt for a healthier lifestyle (Buyx and Prainsack 2012), and they may be better equipped (or 'empowered', see Constantini 2014, quoted in Owens and Cribb 2017) to do so through the use of health apps and the self-measurements they enable (WHO 2011).

Dampening this optimism is the fact that prevention programs are often ineffective. If life-styles are changeable, it is far from clear how this is best accomplished. There is a lot of quantitative research on the factors that shape the good and bad results of prevention programs. This research shows that long-term interventions work better, and that programs should involve peer-to-peer contacts, address social norms rather than focus on education alone, and suggest healthy alternatives rather than attempt to prevent 'bad behaviour' (see e.g. Dusenbury and Falco 1995, Raczynski *et al.* 2012, Tobler 1992). However, such quantitative research into 'health behaviour', we argue with Cohn (2014), often loses track of the context in which 'what people do' has meaning for them. For prevention programs, for example, it makes a difference if people understand 'eating too much' as a celebration, as self-therapy, as 'too many calories' or as a routine (de Laet 2017, Vogel 2018).[1]

In this paper we focus on the practice of using health apps in order to understand how self-quantification shapes selves, and how selves shape self-quantifications. We analyse assumptions prevalent in prevention discourse about how health apps might support individuals to change their behaviour through supporting their will. We then compare this analysis with expressions of the Quantified Self (QS) movement, and with our own research into practices of self-quantification through the use of health apps. Our question is how people relate to numbers – and numbers to people – in practices of self-quantification. What do self-trackers say they want to achieve and how does this turn out? How do numbers 'act back'? What does this imply for prevention programs that are based on the promise of health apps?

Approach

Our approach of studying the shaping of selves through quantification in prevention practices is an alternative voice alongside a rather unison chorus of certain strands in the critical sociology of technology. To a greater and lesser degree, these critical sociologists highlight how (self-tracking) devices *discipline* people into the regimes of the technologies they are using, a line of thinking that often evokes the notion of reflexive modernisation (Beck *et al.* 1994). Reflexive modernisation provides 'a context in which subjects become increasingly individualised, introspective and responsible for the project of crafting their own self-identities' (Smith and Vonhethoff 2016: 8). The freedom of this modern subject is turned on its head: power mechanisms discipline people into shaping themselves as free and modern subjects. Lupton (2013) argues that individuals are made responsible for their own health, not as a newly gained freedom but as a duty that is imposed on them, even if it is happily embraced by the individuals pursuing it. Meanwhile, the 'techno-gaze' offers 'an unprecedented opportunity to monitor and measure individuals' health-related habits in a variety of milieus' (Lupton 2012, in Smith and Vonhethoff 2016: 9, see also Rose 1999).

Although this argument is often well founded, our concern is that it imagines a too-uniform ('neoliberal') subject. A determinist understanding of technology is too limited, and reflexive modernism is too broad a concept. The ways in which subjects are positioned in different settings and engage in modes of quantification, we argue, varies in important ways. It is in this play with freedom and power, determining and being determined, acting and being acted upon, that different forms of selves emerge, as a result of the relationships they seek to engage in and are engaged by (see Moser 2005). Here we use heuristics from empirical ethics to analyse how subjects emerge in practice, through relationships amongst people, devices and numbers (Mol 2010, Pols 2015; 2017, Sharon 2015, Swierstra 2013, Willems 2010, Willems and Pols 2010). Empirical ethics combines a 'sociology of the good' (Thévenot 2001, see also Boltanski and Thévenot 2006) and a material semiotic approach that does not 'apply' theoretical concepts, but studies what these concepts come to be – or how they become enacted – in specific contexts. What is 'good', is hence an open category that needs to be substantiated through empirical study. Strictly speaking it is not a fixed methodology, but a way to study how and where particular objects – or subjects, or concepts – come into being. Our question here is about the relationships between people and their devices for self-quantification, to lean about the specific subjects that emerge.

Empirical ethics traces the intertwinement of what *is* and what is *good*. Specifically, we decipher the 'ethico-psychological selves' that are enacted through self-tracking. We unravel how such subjects are framed or enacted as having a particular (biological, sociological, psychological) way of being (a drive to chase self-interests or to reproduce, having a free will, for example), while relating to the good in particular way (say, maximising pleasure or gain, reproducing genetic material, or doing the right thing). Ethico-psychological subjects hence are described in terms of how they are made to act as well as how they make themselves act. As subjects, they are both object and agent: they are an object of study in the life – and behavioural sciences, but they are also understood as actively shaping and reflecting on themselves (as in the humanities). Psychology and ethics hence ask related questions. Why do people act as they do? The repertoires for answering them, however, differ vastly. Our empirical ethics approach brings these repertoires together by tracing particular intertwinements of facts and values in order to ask how self-tracking incorporates particular understandings of the world as well as particular 'forms of the good' (Thévenot 2001). As we will show, devices and numbers also show this intertwinement of being and valuing.

In part I and II of the analysis, we explore how people make sense of numbers in three cases. The first case is a paper that reports on prevention ideals form the health app industry. We analyse Schüll's (2016) exemplary text, in which the will of the individual is a central moral and psychological category. The second case is formed by reports from the QS movement, to show how these avant-garde number crunchers use data from self measurements to make sense of themselves as subjects. In this second part we add examples from cases from our interviews and observations with two groups of people who make sense of numbers: those we call 'everyday self-trackers', or people who do not have health problems but measure themselves for different reasons (fitness, weight-loss, out of curiosity) and people with type 1 diabetes, who measure and manage their blood glucose levels and have long experience in doing so. Within each group, 10 in-depth interviews were conducted by two master's-degree students, Liam Levy-Philipp (2017) and Floor Visser (2017). Visser and Levy-Phillip asked about the use and meaning of measuring devices and observed their use when possible. From the testimonies of the QS and the interviews, we identify two distinct styles of self-tracking. The first is the objectivist-changer style, which is oriented towards changing behaviour or outcomes based on objective measurements. The second is the semiotic-aesthetic style, which is oriented towards discovering unknown patterns in behaviour, events or bodily signs.

In part III of the analysis we use our material from the everyday self-trackers and people with diabetes to analyse *how devices and modes of quantification make sense of people.*

People may put devices and quantifications to their own use, yet numbers also 'act back', leading to effects that were out of the control of the users. This became most obvious in our interviews, as testimonies of the QS movement generally narrate individual victories and measurements that have been 'tamed' in particular ways. The activity of numbers becomes most obvious when it leads to unexpected effects or frictions in people's lives. The styles of the self-trackers are complemented by ways in which one may *become tracked* through self-quantification. In our concluding remarks, reflecting on the recommendation of the Dutch health minister, we raise some 'ethico-psychological' issues that might disturb an all too optimistic policy.

Self-tracking in a prevention logic: the importance of the will

To understand the logic of prevention – how people may change their lifestyles to prevent disease – we take up Schüll's (2016) thoughtful analysis of discussions in the app development industry. This is obviously a particular reading of prevention logic, but it is an interesting one to show how ethics and psychology may be aligned in discourses that stimulate prevention. Schüll argues that self-tracking devices are scripted by the premise that people have to constantly decide what to do. The well-being of these app users depends on the choices they make, but they are not very good at making choices. They never do the right thing, as they do not have the means to make good decisions. They tend to do what they do out of habit, lack of reflectiveness or laziness. Their intuitions, senses and automatisms are not well geared to attain what they *actually* want to achieve. They need support for this: a device that reminds them of their goals and hence 'nudges' them in better directions. Schüll (2016: 12) writes: 'The nudge is a curious mechanism, as it both presupposes and pushes against freedom; it assumes a choosing subject, but one who is constitutionally ill equipped to make rational, healthy choices'. The will of the subject here is clear and well-focused: people *want* to make healthy choices, but the *effectuation* of these choices needs improvement and outside support.

Schüll compares these ethico-psychological subjects to entrepreneurs: they need information to make better choices, and tools to provide this information. They need to see patterns over time, like correlations between the flowing inputs and outputs of stock markets that inform one's business better. And this, she argues, is what these apps provide. They support users with making better decisions by 'nudging' (rather than forcing) them in the right direction through providing them relevant information in a timely manner. Nudging, here, creates awareness, as it interrupts unreflexive, routinised or intuitive ways of acting. The app suggests the better option, what the user would prefer to do if she were not distracted by routines.

In Schüll's analysis, the goals of the users are the same as the goals of the devices, and this is crucial for their good use: they provide tools for self-induced nudging into self-prioritised activities. They help us do what we *really* want to do. Although users might have a tendency to do the wrong thing, they want and are able to follow good advice to reach long-term goals, even if these goals are in tension with immediate desires or habits.[2] The rationality of these users is that they are able to act in accordance with the goal set by the device (and hence the user).

Schüll is not explicit about the status of her analysis: is it a description, a way of theorising health apps, or a proposal for normatively understanding its actual workings? We take it to represent an understanding of the *ideal use and user* of these apps that fits with a logic of prevention and concerns of the app developers. There are no frictions or ethical concerns if people use apps to achieve goals they set themselves. Such an understanding steers clear of the 'bads' of manipulation, disciplining or coercion into goals set by governments or industry, which is the central concern in the ethical discussions around nudging (see in this context:

Owens and Cribb 2017). In Schüll's analysis of this self-tracking discourse, it is up to the individual to decide which goals to pursue.

The self of prevention logic emerges: ethico-psychological subjects are beings that may set themselves goals that are *their own,* consciously chosen goals. Once they have set their goals, they will also nudge themselves into achieving these. In this sense the individuals are *rational*; they strive for what they know or have decided they want to achieve. This implies that individuals may control the achievement of their goals – with a little help from their apps. They do this by an exertion of their will (they *want* to achieve the goals set), supported by self-set nudges built into the apps, which are tools to help enact that will. In this vision, the use of apps for self-measurement is *empowering* the individual to be enabled to better live up to self-chosen goals.

Because individuals are free to set their own goals through their rationality and will, goal-setting becomes an enactment of autonomy: it happens and has to happen outside of power relations. If force or pressure were used, the aura of will and rationality surrounding enterprise of self-tracking would disappear. Nudges would become directives to follow goals set by others, raising again the concerns of critical sociology and ethics. Where support and encouragement are possible, force will not do, nor is surveillance an acceptable means. The mechanism to change lifestyles for prevention, both because of how people are understood to act as well as from an ethical perspective, is based on individual will, however fallible.

Making sense of numbers

So now we have an understanding of the assumptions underlying an ideal 'prevention self'. Now we will turn to the question what practices of self-quantification look like and how ethico-psychological subjects position themselves in these practices by actively making sense of numbers (see also Ajana 2017). The QS movement provides a very specific avant garde practice of self-quantification. It is a popular topic amongst researchers because of this frontline position, and because self-quantifiers are very open about their practices. They post their results on the internet and organise large meetings to discuss results.

Building on the analysis of Sharon (2015) and Sharon and Zandbergen (2016), we discerned two styles of self-tracking in the texts of the QS movement, which may diverge or become linked in different ways. The first we call the 'objectivist-changer' style of self-tracking, which foregrounds an ideal of knowing the self through numbers. The aim is to produce objective knowledge about oneself, knowledge that is not disrupted by fallible perceptions or direct experience of the self (Sharon 2015, Sharon and Zandbergen 2016, Swan 2013).[3] These ethico-psychological subjects analyse their data with the aim of changing and optimising their bodies and health, by attempting to predict and control bodily processes and to act on this knowledge.[4]

The second style of self-tracking we call the 'aesthetic-semiotic' style. It betrays the roots of the QS movement in California, the breeding-ground for hippies and others averse to authority (Sharon and Zandbergen 2016). It is an anti-authoritarian orientation that experiments with different forms of self-awareness. Knowledge of the self is seen in aesthetic terms, as creating different and interesting forms of self-awareness. A different experience of the self can be a goal in itself. The artist Alberto Frigo, for example, photographs every object he takes in his right hand (ibid). This changes his understanding of himself, he writes, by providing 'some kind of DNA code of my life' (ibid: 6) through the collection of images of thousands of objects.

Aesthetic descriptions, however, may also be used to subvert dominant ways of knowing that prescribe what is 'normal' or 'common' to experience, often challenging medical or psychological modes of understanding and acting. Both tracking styles come together when these ethico-psychological subjects develop $n = 1$ experiments which are tests with one subject, here: the person conducting the experiment. They do this to gain knowledge about themselves with the aim to improve medical knowledge. They boast that, with this personalised knowledge, they will outsmart their doctors: they become the experts on their own bodies. Sharon (2015: 18) refers to Larry Smarr who diagnosed his Crohn's disease through self-measurements before his doctors were able to reach the same conclusion.

For the 'objectivist-changers', quantifications can make the body predictable, much in line with the understandings of behavioural economy. If one thinks of one's body weight as the result of the energy taken in and the energy used, for example, it becomes possible to calculate a program on how to lose weight. The body becomes calculable and predictable, or at least, that is the aim. One of our interviewees, George, a person with type 1 diabetes, exemplifies this calculability. He explained how he measures a variety of variables (blood glucose, insulin, HbAc1, calorie intake, sleep, weight, exercise, environmental temperature) with a variety of technologies (four apps that do not synchronise, an insulin pump, a sensor, his smartphone) in order to predict his blood glucose levels and influence them. George used these data as well as the continuous measurements of his blood glucose provided by a sensor. The sensor is necessary for making such measurements possible, but is too costly to be used by many.

Rather than attempting to stay within a certain range of high and low glucose levels (which would mimic 'average' glucose metabolism for non-diabetics, and is generally the aim for people with type 1 diabetes), he aimed for a *flat* line by strategically administering insulin and food at times when his blood glucose was going up or down. He explained,

> I inject insulin in the morning about 1 hour before I eat, because I have noticed that it starts to work after 1 hour. Then I see a small dent in my glucose graph, so that is when I start to eat.

By considering and calculating different variables, George could design new and clear targets. With his extensive measurements, he made the behaviour of his body predictable and controllable.

The 'semiotic aesthetes', on the other hand, are not concerned with predictability, nor with the changing of their own behaviour or bodies for the better (hence there are no type 1 diabetes subjects in this group). In our interviews, these trackers demonstrated a clear preference for recording certain variables out of interest rather than to propel change. It worked rather more like a diary than a log, and events could be traced back to what they had experienced in real life. Here is an interviewee and every-day self tracker from the semiotic-aesthetic style, Siena. She explains how she used self-tracking:

> Well, I don't look at it [the graphs from the health app] every day. But I did learn a lot from it. It gave me the amount of calories that I was using while I was biking, for instance. So it's interesting to see what's happening if the wind is blowing from the north or the south, if it takes a lot more calories. Then I have to bike against the wind. That was all new, so I think I am quite interested in the information that it gives me. It's not that I want to know how many calories I burnt during the whole day, but rather what is happening now, or see what happened then, with my heart rate ... and, oh yes, there [points at a graph] I was working in the garden. Ha ha, yes, we were cutting a tree, quite a big tree, and suddenly one of the very big branches fell down instead of going slowly down the rope.

So then in the evening I looked and saw my heart rate ... 'What happened? 180!' That was exactly at that time! [Laughs]

Siena did not use her measurements to calculate calorie intake, but to learn about the influence of the winds and falling branches on her body. The app's graphs illustrate – and interpret – her body's experience of the impact of the falling branch. Data are a way to learn how the body lives events in its own way.

The semiotic aesthetes also used results from their self-tracking to criticise existing norms. Sharon (2015: 18) describes Dana Greenfield's project about how she mourned her mother after she passed away. Greenfield did not want to mourn 'by the book', and instead registered how often she thought about her mother, what triggered that, what mood she was in at that time, and so on. In this way she developed an individual map and picture of how her mourning evolved. This was an alternative for living up to standards on how mourning should be done, when 'normal mourning' should be finished and how intense it should be. In this way she made self-measuring a constructive act to *design* mourning in a new, personalised way, providing new accents and individualised norms for how mourning is and may be done. It is a creative process rather than one aimed at controlling variables.

The mourning example shows a clear link between what is tracked, counted and archived and the ways people make sense of it. Possible modes of experience are developed through the experiment. In this style, self-tracking is not aimed at *changing* what one does, but about carving out individual pathways to *understand* what one does. This is simultaneously a critical epistemological statement on popular modes of quantification in the social and medical sciences. Calculating average probabilities across defined populations creates a norm that is not directly applicable to individuals. The mode of quantification these self-trackers put forward, however, is based on personalised calculations, and they produce a type of knowledge that is specific to the individual. It can be made relevant for others who may repeat the experiment themselves. It is a suggestion for *doing science* differently, and it shows that different modes of quantification allow for different frameworks to interpret numbers.

Another semiotic-aesthetic example can be seen in the blog by Nancy Dougherty, who registered how often she smiled in a day (Davis 2013, see also Sharon 2015: 23). Dougherty recorded a higher smile frequency when colleagues approached her, which she interpreted as her *liking* her colleagues more than she had been aware of. That her smiles represented an unacknowledged affection is a highly original interpretation, made by relating numbers to feelings. Quantifications have to be made sense of in order to be useful or mean anything at all.[5] Dougherty's conclusions are quite remote from a scientific dream of objectivity aimed at excluding the subject doing the measuring. Even when measurements exclude influences from the subject doing the measuring, interpretative frameworks are always needed to make sense of the outcomes, including when these numbers are collected without any particular hypothesis.[6]

Qualifying subjects
Even though the cases show an inseparable link between numbers and interpretations, the QS movement does not foreground an interpreting or 'qualified self' who learns about itself through direct experience. The qualified self serves as a somewhat caricaturised backdrop of imperfection, against which quantifications get their value and shine. Phenomenological tools such as sensing, feeling, memory and introspection tie the qualifying self to the here and now, in contrast to the temporalities that may be created by quantification over time. Qualified perceptions are thought of as fallible and limited, and are to be improved and complemented by quantifying the self. In contrast to the ethico-psychological subject of prevention, here it is not

the *will* that these self-trackers see as in need of support, but rather their *possibilities for knowing themselves* and what they or their bodies do. The senses are insufficient tools, too limited to adequately keep track; nor are the generalised quantifications of the sciences acceptable, as they are not specific to the individual.

If what people experience and what they are aware of is only a limited part of what informs their activities, measurements (of smiles, of glucose levels) can be a way to feed self-awareness, giving insight into what escapes everyday perceptions. There is not a 'meaningful' self, as in psychoanalysis, where turbulence is created by unconscious desires and emotions pushing and wrestling within the psyche for expression. These need extensive interpretation as a way to liberate oneself of their consequences. Self-trackers, however, battle with a more prosaic unconsciousness of bodily facts, habits, automatisms and metabolisms of which the subject is not aware. Wolf, a prominent person in the QS movement, writes:

> When we quantify ourselves, there isn't the imperative to see through our daily existence into a truth buried at a deeper level. Instead, the self of our most trivial thoughts and actions, the self that, without technical help, we might barely notice or recall, is understood as the self we ought to get to know. (Wolf 2010, quoted in Sharon 2015: 12)

Rather than representing unresolved conflicts through interpretation, these unconscious ways of acting represent physical and mental processes and events that are not under the control of the individual when they pass unnoticed. These processes simply 'happen' and do so well away from the experience of the subject, while shaping the subject through its automatic physical and physiological responses.

For self-quantifiers, measurements are ways to trap unconscious processes; objectivist-changers hope, too, to tame these automatisms. The visualisation and analysis of measurements over time makes unconscious habits and processes ready for reflection and, again for the objectivists, adaptation. Self-tracking and quantification allow one to learn about oneself by bringing to light these automatic, unnoticed processes.

Interestingly, the tracking and analysing of different ways in which they are physiologically determined as subjects, enables the ethico-psychological subject of the QS movement to insert free will in a new way. Individuals may influence their unconscious behaviours and processes, if they prudently quantify and actively manage them. By mastering different forms of being determined by one's bodily processes, space is created for agency, meaning and morality, for example to achieve a flat line on a blood-sugar graph or to observe one's own personal style of mourning. By gaining a peek into what our bodies do outside our awareness, we may find ways to control them, not by nudging ourselves towards self-chosen goals, but by getting to know the 'ways of the body', manipulating these, or understanding them better. It is not the will that needs support, but one's knowledge needs to be improved. The quantified and autonomously acting body becomes 'one's own' again.

Numbers make sense of people

In the examples above the relation between numbers, or styles of quantification, and sense-making has a clear direction: individuals, as ethico-psychological subjects, interpret numbers that represent their beings and doings. Numbers *in themselves* are not objective representatives of truth, even if they are taken to be just that. Numbers are gathered and interpreted within particular styles, sets of values and meanings (art, knowledge, activism, health, etc.). This semiotic activity, however, also works in the opposite direction: *numbers make sense of people* and act upon them.

Willems (2000) describes how, through repeated measurements, his informants with asthma came to learn to sense these quantifications, and how this changed their way of experiencing their bodies by their 'incorporating' their measurements. This also happened to some of our informants with type 1 diabetes, if their insulin metabolism was regular enough. A certain number became linked to a certain feeling that signified (too) high or low blood sugar levels. People learned to train and educate themselves and what they felt by making use of numbers.

Below, we discuss how numbers make sense of people by: (i) specifying their goals, (ii) intensifying particular concerns, (iii) suggesting coherence and predictability, and by (iv) moralising lives under the guise of 'fact collection'. We also briefly discuss a fifth way: numbers make selves transportable through their data, allowing for their re-interpretation in new contexts, but a full discussion of this remains out of the scope of this paper. Our analysis foregrounds our interviewees who enact the objectivist-changer style, as change is most visible here.

Specification: devices and quantifications translate goals
One of our informants with type 1 diabetes, Jan, told us how his experience changed when he had to quantify things he had never dreamt of quantifying before:

> I went to the dietician the first time, and she asked: 'How much do you eat?' How would I know that! I eat until I have had enough. So that was very difficult for me. [...] And what happened last time? There was a day when I had injected [insulin] and then the potatoes were burnt. And you don't realise, and you are sitting on the couch [that evening] and then, erm ... [your blood glucose level is all wrong]. And same with sports. If I plan to go out for a run in the evening, and I think later: 'Oh, I don't feel like it today', then I do not go. But I then I would have to inject more.

In this interview, Jan described how he calculated how many potatoes he had eaten, and their size, and how much insulin he would need to balance that amount out. He thus had to shift from a qualifying perception ('I have eaten enough') to making a set of quantifications. This shows how types of devices and ways of quantifying translate and hence re-interpret people's goals and self-understanding. To live healthily or to optimise one's fitness becomes a very specific target, involving, say, so many calories or exercise and so much insulin. Devices and quantifications specify general goals like fitness and health.[7]

Numbers do not come to us in an abstract form: they are produced through devices or apps that turn events into numbers. Understanding how these devices work is crucial for understanding self-quantification and concomitant different ways of living. A very clear example can be seen in the 'traditional' blood sugar measuring pen, with which measurements are taken at particular times in the day (usually 4–6 times). These discrete measurements often serve as feedback for the very short term and no particular relationship can be made between them. Our informants who wanted to minimise the impact of diabetes on their lives, including the impact from monitoring blood sugar, preferred this way of measuring (Visser 2017).

In contrast, the sensor's continuous monitoring puts measurements in relation to one another, allowing one to see trends and to relate spikes or crashes to an event or other variable that might happen to influence blood glucose levels. This was a good method of tracking for people, like George above, who wanted – and could – exert a firmer control over their diabetes. But such continuous measurements involve another set of quantifications: sensors are costly, and only paid for by Dutch health insurance for people whose blood sugar levels are hard to tame. For George, the sophisticated combination of measurements made his bloodsugar levels predictable – and their measurement prominent in his life. Even his diabetes nurse consults him as an expert when she is confronted with difficult cases.

The type of device one uses thus structures a specific form of quantification, which then opens up a specific repertoire of activities to pursue. We saw how individuals negotiated and adjusted their goals in relation to the specific affordances of the technologies they used. Melanie, for instance, wanted to stay fit and healthy:

I think that's the problem with focusing on weight loss. Because if I am exercising regularly and eating well, then I feel okay. That's why I don't like making weight loss a goal. Because if I say: 'I want to be this number by a certain time', then I feel a panic. And there shouldn't be panic. I should be enjoying things. And that's why I don't make a number goal. I have a number in my head, but I don't write it down, and I don't put all my focus on it. So, it is my goal, my motive is to lose weight, but I just think that for overall mental health, there needs to be more than that.

Melanie had to invoke the category of 'mental health' to make her general goal of 'health' feasible, which had failed when 'health' was specified as 'losing weight'. In interaction with their devices, our informants translated and kept adjusting goals in order to forge a liveable practice. Specific goals that seemed rational on the drawing board had to be fitted in with other concerns in daily life – if only to fit in the nonspecific goal of living an enjoyable life, which had not been part of Melanie's first calculations regarding weight loss. Older people with type 1 diabetes also had seen specific goals for blood sugar regulation come and go with the medical fashions of the day, moving from very strict towards to more lenient regimes.

Self-trackers reported disappointment in what goals their health apps could achieve through their specification. Gerard lamented:

There are a whole lot of things that it [the self-tracking device] is tracking but not really a whole lot of things that give proper insights. It tracks so much, but at the same time it does nothing. So, I think that is a bit of the issue that I have with it. It can do a whole lot and I don't think that the algorithms are that hard to make. Take my heart rate. It doesn't show me that I have a higher heart rate these past months or if there is a difference in months that I work out, for instance, that my resting heart rate is lower for example, or anything like that. That is data that would probably motivate people more, into actually doing [work-outs] ... But yeah, that's not available. For me it was like: well, I saw the gadget and thought: 'I want that!' Ha ha!

This aesthetic tracker's love of gadgets made him use the devices, not – or no longer – propelled by the hope that these might provide him with information to optimise his fitness, but simply because he enjoyed having them around.

Intensifying concerns
Measuring could lead to an intensification of the relevance of particular concerns in life over others. 'Becoming obsessed with numbers', as some put it, was a concern that was often articulated by our informants. Johanna described how the feeling of control the measurements provided could turn against her: 'In high school I was just doing [tracking] the steps, weight and water'. Liam, who was interviewing Johanna, prompted her to continue: 'And the reason you stopped was because ...' Johanna explained:

Well, I felt like it was fun in the beginning. I dunno, it's like: 'Oh it's new!' and then you lose concentration. And afterwards, in college I was just like: 'I don't feel like being this controlling', kind of. It felt like controlling after a while. I was like: 'I hate tracking every-thing!' It felt like I was controlling my entire life because I was tracking everything, and it's all numbers. And I was like: 'This is just too structured, and I feel like I am living day to day'. It got really like: 'I wake up, I drink this much water, I weigh this much, and I exercise …' It felt too routine, I guess.

The demands of collecting numbers could become so intense that it could seem like the only relevant thing to do. There was no pleasure, there were no surprises or unexpected events, just the routines of diligently recording and living up to one's numbers. This Johanna could not uphold. She even suggested the roles were reversed at a certain point (see also Dudhwala 2018):

Maybe I would say that it [self-tracking] gives you a little bit of control over your life. You know, life has become so complex and busy, that sometimes it gives you the feeling of sta-bility. But it can also have the other effect, like vice versa, it gives you the feeling of stress when you look into it too much. It's difficult to explain but I got it [fitbit] because I wanted to be more in control. But sometimes I feel that I am less in control because of it. That it has taken over my life.

Specification and the selectivity that comes with it worked to intensify concerns about particu-lar variables. Some things become more important than others. Piras and Miele (2017) show that pregnant women with type 1 diabetes struggled with an intensified regime to control their blood sugar levels, to protect their unborn children. Their concerns were about the 'other things in life' that mattered to them, which had to be sacrificed for intensive monitoring. They missed the freedom to improvise, for instance, to enjoy the type of meal one fancies when going out with a friend. They complained about standardised lifestyles and experienced the regime as uncaring. Tellingly, one woman said the monitoring and prescriptions made her feel sick rather than healthy. The specific aim of managing their diabetes could become so intense as to turn into an activity to live for, not a condition that allowed for doing other things in life.

Suggesting coherence and predictability in a lifeless calculable
This 'metrification' (Yates-Doerr 2015) or quantification of life comes with the suggestion that there is a calculable and controllable way of achieving a goal. Taking in X calories while expending Y calories through exercise, for example, would result in weight loss if Y is larger than X. We saw some successful and troubled examples of this above. But this predictability did not always come to be, which caused a lot of frustration. Our informants with type 1 dia-betes described their frustrations and despair when they could not link their measured blood glucose levels to their experience or to calculations of food intake and energy use (see also Hortensius *et al.* 2012). If measurements are never what they should rationally be, they pro-vide no tools to learn from and give no clues for acting. Melanie explained how this lack of reliable results from dieting spurred more binge eating:

It's kind of a weird game. Because if I cheat, or if I go out drinking all weekend, and I don't see any weight loss, I think: 'Well I expected that!' But if I am working really hard [and there's no loss], then it sucks. If I have been working out and eating well and my weight doesn't change, then that feels really bad. And that's when I start binging. I have gotten better, but I used to binge when I would behave really well all week and I didn't lose weight.

The examples show the despair that rises up when one's body does not behave in predictable ways. It challenges the very rationale for 'behaving well', however, without completely overthrowing its truth. In Melanie's case, the resulting binge was not liberating or based on an alternative hypothesis, but still felt as 'bad behaviour'.

Quantification often fails, in more or less dramatic ways. Our informants teach us that 'living' is an open-ended process in time. The potatoes may get burnt. Things may change for no understandable reason at all, as Jan described:

> For years I've injected 14 units in the morning, with a slice of bread and a glass of milk. For years. Perhaps for 10 years. And now I inject eight or nine units in the morning with the same food. Why is that! Tell me, because I don't know! And there is not much you can do about that. You can use apps and keep track of all sorts of things, but I've used 14 units for years and that used to be right. But now ...

In the end, the perfect calculation can never be carried out -the future can never be seamlessly predicted.

Moralisation through facts

As we saw in the objectivist-changer style exemplified by the QS representatives, numbers have a strong appeal of showing 'what is really there'. Measurements present people with facts about their bodies. Unless the devices are broken or imprecise, one thousand steps have indeed been taken, a blood-sugar level is 6.1, one's weight is 52 kilos and 300 g. But our informants were very clear about this: numbers are not only factual, they are also normative: they are good or bad. Numbers enforce certain ideas of the good. If the numbers are bad despair may well follow ('nothing can be done about it'), as well as feelings of being punished ('you did not behave well'). One informant told us that she set her step-counter target in such a way that she would get a daily reward rather than a punishment ('at least one thing achieved today!'). But bad numbers could also lead to unwanted moralising from others: the tracker is being tracked, just as the pregnant women felt overly controlled by their doctors. Sara recounted how she worked to avoid that critical gaze:

> You go to this doctor and he sees your readings and says: 'Well, you must be careful, this should be lower'. And then you get the entire lecture. Then I think: '*You* should try paying attention to this 24 hours a day. I am not a machine! [...] I *know* it is wrong. At a certain point I'd just time my glucose readings in such a way that it would not result in criticism anymore.

Notice the machine metaphor, pointing to the specification, intensification and rationalisation of goals, as well as to the doctor's insensitivity to the burden of moralising through numbers. In self-tracking aimed at change, the normative and the factual are intertwined.

Devices are programmed to direct how a certain good may be achieved. Schwennesen (2017) describes a case in which a woman used a device at home that gave physio-therapeutic instructions for patients recovering after a hip replacement. It was a very sophisticated device that worked with sensors, to provide feedback on motions in space ('Lift your knee higher!'). The patients could exercise at home, so they did not have to come to the clinic for rehabilitation. In this case, by sticking to the protocol of the device, the woman actually over-trained, damaged the new hip and spurred a need to replace the other hip. The clinicians had aimed to implement the good of home rehabilitation, which their patient followed. She took the instructions as the right ones to follow, but these turned out to be too unspecific, standardised and harmful. The ideal user here would have to be able to modify the device's instructions.

Making selves transportable and re-interpreting them

By generating sets of numbers, self-tracking individuals create data about themselves or what Ruckenstein (2014) calls 'data doubles'. These data doubles are the look-alikes of the selves collecting them, a snapshot presented through numbers. But, as we have seen above, these doubles are not exactly identical twins. They are selves translated into something else, selves turned into numbers that specify, intensify, moralise and attempt to make predictable. *Ceci n'est pas une pipe!* An object does not equal its representation.

One effect of translating selves, events or activities into numbers is that numbers make individuals or their data look-alikes transportable. As particular specifications and recordings of the individual, these data can travel to other places. This means that an individual's numbers may become part of different networks, where they are fit into new relationships that foreground different concerns from the ones for which the numbers were originally collected. This is what Nissenbaum (2010) points out when she shows that we experience concerns with privacy when our data travel and are used in contexts that do not seem proper. Doctors may ask us all kinds of questions, but we would feel our privacy betrayed should those answers be published on the internet. By travelling, both the factuality and normativity of numbers change (see also Mittelstadt and Floridi 2016: 321).

One reflexive user of a step-counter noted on his blog and in an interview with us that if he did not reach the set amount of steps each day, he would shake his mobile phone in order to reach and record the right amount of steps. Indeed, self-tracking here did not serve to *objectify* behaviour. The user was concerned, rather, that measurements would solidify as 'evidence' of what he had done. This evidence could travel unmediated by his explanation of it. It could be stored in databases and become unchangeable, true. Our phone shaker explained in an interview that he did not want to be recorded as a lazy person or someone with a weak mind who cannot even reach the simple goals he has set for himself.

What becomes of these data look-alikes? They change context and depart from the goals that had directed their collection and how they were made sense of. They may not even resemble the selves they are thought to represent anymore. Here's Brittany from South Africa, who got an Apple watch from her health insurance company. If she earns her points through meeting her exercise targets, the watch is free. She couldn't afford to buy it herself. And she wanted it! She explained:

> At some point I wrote an exercise schedule on my phone because I know I have to get 900 points. I have to push during the weekend, so should something happen in the week then at least I am sitting at 600 or so. It's quite important to get 900 points. So I plan. Planning is key, it's a big part of it.

Brittany gets her points, not to become healthy (is it actually wise to do all your training in the weekend?) but to obtain the watch. This has implications for how her data may or may not indicate anything about achieving health though exercise – though it does show that some people can be pushed into exercising when given a chance to own something they want, even if it is unrelated to health goals. The insurance and the user have different goals, and the insurance uses the watch to force users into the goals it finds important. The unreliability of decontextualised numbers is a concern for the validity of the knowledge created from them (Aicardi *et al.* 2016, Mittelstadt and Floridi 2016), and often very different goals need to be juggled to collect data at all (Tempini 2015).

Conclusion

What does our empirical ethics approach learn about the characteristics of psychological subjects as well as about their strivings? An obvious conclusion is that there were many different types of subjects. This nuances the extremely voluntarist ideas from prevention, as well as a technological determinist idea of the subject from critical sociology of technology. The different ways of understanding what a subject is, as well as what it wants, showed different relationships between people and numbers. We started with discussing the prevention discourse, where free will reigns, along with the discretion of self-quantifying ethico-psychological subjects to set their own, self-chosen goals. In this conception, one's will may be strong, but its execution needs support. Nudges from health apps could provide this support, as a reminder to individuals about what they really want. We found that objectivist-changers shifted the diagnosis of the problem to one in which self-quantification is an answer. The problem was not a weak will, but a lack of knowledge about processes in a body that lives according to its own rules and metabolisms, of which people are not aware. Free will remained crucial, as these unconscious processes could either be controlled or could be given pride of place to correct social or medical norms with personalised ones. Apps served as instruments to reveal hidden mechanisms that purposeful individuals could use to their benefit.

In our interviews about practices of self-tracking from people with type 1 diabetes and from everyday self-trackers, individual will was much more fragile. It was but one of the elements in the manifold, shifting relationships that influenced 'what people do' in their practices of self-quantification. A lack of knowledge that could be undone by learning about the body turned out to be complex. Modes of quantification inserted coherent, calculable and hence controllable repertoires for action into people's lives. These specified forms of the good to achieve given a specified diagnosis of the problem that intensified the search for solutions. Broad aims like health and well-being were translated into so many steps a day, or so much weight loss each week. People actively engaged with these coherences, by living up to them, by resisting them for other goals, by re-defining and adding new goals, by replacing them with new regimes, or by ambiguously accepting and rejecting them. They struggled with incalculable bodies and situations, and clashing – or failing – frameworks for interpreting these.

What people did and how was contingent on relationships amongst people, devices and contexts – of medical prescriptions, ideal body weight or aesthetic curiosity. Interpretations could be out of their influence, as when their data travelled to places unknown to their collectors. The crafting, breaking and reframing of relationships were an open-ended process. People got bored with their devices, invented new ways for how to live with them or subverted them, took time-outs or sought out fruitful combinations of health apps. There was no clear or certain line between self-quantification and health, a relationship that could also fail miserably.

Our analysis showed how numbers cannot be separated from interpretations, as interpretations are built into the technologies and regimes used, and must be translated to specific situations. Numbers are collected for specific aims. The specifications, intensifications and coherences that quantifications brought came with an aura of objectivity, because numbers seemingly erased subjective elements and interpretations. In the context of self-tracking practices, however, a strong appeal to truth in combination with clear directives on how to act made numbers double-edged interpreters of life. Numbers have a strong morality within the socio-material context in which numbers are qualified as adequate, true, boring, evidence of 'bad behaviour', or good or beautiful reporters on the wonders of the body. With our approach of empirical ethics we could show the different relations between facts and desires that are part of very different sets of self-tracking practices. Indeed, the literature about self-tracking from the social sciences that is avalanching at the moment, has important work to do to uncover many more types of ethico-psychological subjects and workings of (self) quantification (for instance the work on affective aspects of technology use and sensory aspects of digital health, Lupton and Maslen 2018, Schwennesen and Koch 2009).

Is the Dutch health minister's advice a good one for improving health? People and apps turned out to be *different beings* than speculated on in prevention discourse. Self-tracking practices were varied, and devices did not simply support an individual will to stay healthy. Apps translated goals and made people do different things than hoped for, even when striving for health or fitness. Care for health happened in relation to disease, social norms and medical regimes, which made peoples' goals less 'their own' than prevention discourse would have it. Different from QS objective changer style ideas about collecting facts about a singularly interpretable body, self-tracking practices produced multiple coherences, linking to different versions of understanding the body and what is good for it. Trackers could experience 'wrong numbers' as punishment, and this might keep the less athletic from using apps (see also Depper and Howe 2017). It is proved difficult to make apps produce *relevant* rather than merely *quantifiable* information.

Our analysis also showed that people *strived for* different things than hoped for, and that apps interpreted and translated these goals. In practice, health turned out to be an unspecific value that, when specified, emerged as just one, very specific goal between many others (enjoying life, good mental health, not being concerned by diabetes). Hence, self-tracking could lead to unintended health hazards, such as obsessive concerns (too much specification) or overtraining (too little specification).

So there is no simple (calculable!) correlation between the use of health apps and a better lifestyle. Yet one problem policy makers might be able to tackle is the risk of unwanted data travel and de-contextualisation, by supporting the production of 'standalone' apps that do not automatically send user data to companies. Rather than supporting the production of unreliable knowledge made from ill-collected data, prevention aims would be better served by investing in the development of more contextualised studies of what people are doing when they are tracking themselves or work on their health in other ways, how this interprets the aim of supporting healthy lifestyles, and how individual an population health may best be synchronised accordingly.

Address for correspondence: Jeannette Pols, Section of Medical Ethics and Department of Anthropology, Amsterdam UMC, University of Amsterdam, Meibergdreef 9, 1105 AZ Amsterdam, The Netherlands. E-mail: a.j.pols@amc.uva.nl

Acknowledgements

The research was made possible by a grant from ZONMW, The rise of consumer eHealth, grant number 70-73000-98-112. We are grateful to Else Vogel, Tamar Sharon and Marieke Bak for comments on earlier drafts. We thank Floor Visser and Liam Levy-Philip for their great interviews and the interviewees for their frankness. We thank the audiences of the preliminary talks about this work for sharing their experiences with self-tracking with us.

Notes

1   Vogel and Mol (2014: 306) ironically state that if behaviour is the target, the practical achievement would be to make people 'behave well' and 'be good' (315), rather than learn how to eat well.

2 H.G. Frankfurt (1988: 128) speaks of primary and secondary desires: 'Besides wanting and choosing and being moved to do this or that, man also may have desires to have (or not to have) certain desires and motives. They are capable of wanting to be different, in their preferences and purposes, from what they are'.

3 Daston and Galison (2007: 17) describe the historical emergence of objective knowledge in relation to a simultaneous downplaying of subjective knowledge and perceptions, holding up knowledge that does not leave traces of the knower. Rather than relying on phenomenological tools or experience, quantification through self-tracking can teach people things about the body they cannot know through subjective means. This connection of numbers to objectivity and truth to numbers is crucial.

4 This orientation towards change is also an aim for people who track themselves to make medical interventions in a third pattern that we call the 'planner' style. We discuss this elsewhere, as they are not quantifying their outcomes but planning what they need to do. This seems to be a more hopeful way to target 'good health behaviour' than health apps, as it is characterised by action rather than analysis (see Levy-Philipp 2017).

5 One could of course add that selecting the hypothesis, the instruments and the concepts is also a highly interpretive way of acting. This is however not the common understanding of quantitative research, where good methods exclude the influence of the subject.

6 This mechanism may explain how pharmaceutical industries can simultaneously use state-of-the-art methods, while still presenting results in a too-rosy fashion. Methods cannot guarantee objectivity all by themselves, and they also shape in a particular way what results will look like (see Law *et al.* 2001, Ruppert *et al.* 2013).

7 We don't use the word 'reduction', as this seems to imply that there is one 'whole' that is quantitatively lessened in one particular way. We'd rather point to the *different qualitative ways* in which specifications are made, which makes for different consistencies that do not 'add up' to a whole.

References

Aicardi, C., Del Salvio, L., Dove, D.S., Lucivero, F., *et al.* (2016) Emerging ethical issues regarding digital health data. On the World Medical Association Draft Declaration on Ethical Considerations regarding Health Data Bases and Biobanks, *Croatian Medical Journal*, 57, 207–13.

Ajana, B. (2017) *Self-Tracking: Empirical and Philosophical Investigations*. London: Palgrave MacMillan.

Beck, U., Giddens, A. and Lash, S. (1994) *Reflexive Modernization*. Cambridge: Polity Press.

Boltanski, L. and Thévenot, L. (2006) *On Justification. Economies of Worth*. Princeton: Princeton University Press.

Buyx, B. and Prainsack, B. (2012) Lifestyle related diseases and individual responsibility through the prism of solidarity, *Clinical Ethics*, 7, 2, 79–85.

Cohn, S. (2014) From health behaviours to health practices: an introduction, *Sociology of Health and Illness*, 36, 157–62.

Daston, L. and Galison, P. (2007) *Objectivity*. Brooklyn: Zone Books.

Davis, J. (2013) The qualified self. Available at: https://thesocietypages.org/cyborgology/2013/03/13/thequalified-self/ (Last accessed 31 March 2016).

Depper, A. and Howe, P.D. (2017) Are we fit yet? English adolescent girls' experiences of health and fitness apps, *Health Sociology Review*, 26, 98–112.

Dudhwala, F. (2018) Redrawing boundaries around the self: the case of self-quantifying technologies. In Lynch, R. and Farrington, C. (eds) *Quantified Lives and Vital Data*, pp 97–123. London: Palgrave Macmillan.

Dusenbury, L. and Falco, M. (1995) Eleven components of effective drug abuse prevention curricula, *Journal of School Health*, 65, 420–5.

Frankfurt, H.G. (1988) *Freedom of the Will and the Concept of a Person. What Is a Person?* New York: Springer.

Hortensius, J., Kars, M.C., Wierenga, W.S., Kleefstra, N., *et al.* (2012) Perspectives of patients with type 1 or insulin-treated type 2 diabetes on self-monitoring of blood glucose: a qualitative study, *BMC Public Health*, 12, 167.

de Laet, M. (2017) *Personal Metrics: Methodological Considerations of a Praxiographical Approach. Methodological Reflections on Practice Oriented Theories*. Cham: Springer.

Law, J., Ruppert, E. and Savage, M. (2011) The double social life of methods.

Levy-Philipp, L. (2017) The practices of every-day trackers. What does it mean to put your health in your hands, or pockets? Master's thesis, Vrije Universiteit Amsterdam.

Lupton, D. (2012) M-health and health promotion: the digital cyborg and surveillance society, *Social Theory & Health*, 10, 229–44.

Lupton, D. (2013) The digitally engaged patient: self-monitoring and self-care in the digital health era, *Social Theory & Health*, 11, 256–70.

Lupton, D. and Maslen, S. (2018) 'The more-than-human sensorium': sensory engagements with digital self-tracking technologies, *The Senses and Society*, 13, 2, 190–202.

Mittelstadt, B.D. and Floridi, L. (2016) The ethics of big data: current and foreseeable issues in biomedical contexts, *Science and Engineering Ethics*, 22, 303–41.

Mol, A. (2010) Care and its values. Good food in the nursing home. In Mol, A., Moser, I. and Pols, J. (eds) *Care in Practice. On Tinkering in Clinics, Homes and Farms*, pp 215–34. Bielefeld: Transcript Verlag.

Moser, I. (2005) On becoming disabled and articulating alternatives. The multiple modes of ordering disability and their interferences, *Cultural Studies*, 19, 6, 667–700.

Nikolas, R. (1999) *Governing the soul: The shaping of the private self*. London: Free association books.

Nissenbaum, H.F. (2010) *Privacy in Context: Technology, Policy, and the Integrity of Social Life*. Stanford: Stanford University Press.

Owens, J. and Cribb, A. (2017) 'My fitbit thinks I can do better!' Do health promoting wearable technologies support personal autonomy?, *Philosophy and Technology*. https://doi.org/10.1007/s13347-017-0266-2.

Piras, E.M. and Francesco, M. (2017) Clinical self-tracking and monitoring technologies: negotiations in the ICT-mediated patient–provider relationship, *Health Sociology Review*, 26, 1, 38–53.

Pols, J. (2015) Towards an empirical ethics in care: relations with technologies in health care, *Medicine, Health Care, and Philosophy*, 18, 81–90.

Pols, J. (2017) Good relations with technology: empirical ethics and aesthetics in care, *Nursing Philosophy*, 18, e1254.

Raczynski, K., Waldo, M., Horne, A.M. and Schwartz, J.P. (2012) *Evidence-Based Prevention*. Melbourne: Sage.

Ruckenstein, M. (2014) Visualized and interacted life: Personal analytics and engagements with data doubles, *Societies*, 4, 68–84.

Ruppert, E., Law, J. and Savage, M. (2013) Reassembling social science methods: the challenge of digital devices, *Theory, Culture & Society*, 30, 22–46.

Schüll, N.D. (2016) Data for life: wearable technology and the design of self-care, *BioSocieties*, 11, 317–33.

Schwennesen, N. (2017) When self-tracking enters physical rehabilitation: from 'pushed' self-tracking to ongoing affective encounters in arrangements of care, *Digital Health*, 3, 1–8.

Schwennesen, N. and Koch, L. (2009) Visualising and calculating life: matters of fact in the context of prenatal risk assessment. In Wahlberg, A. (ed) *Contested Categories: Life Sciences in Society*, pp 69–87. Aldershot: Ashgate.

Sharon, T. (2015) Healthy citizenship beyond autonomy and discipline: tactical engagements with genetic testing, *BioSocieties*, 10, 295–316.

Sharon, T. and Zandbergen, D. (2016) From data fetishism to quantifying selves: self-tracking practices and the other values of data, *New Media & Society*, 19, 11, 1695–709.

Smith, G.J.D. and Vonhethoff, J.D. (2016) Health by numbers? Exploring the practice and experience of datafied health, *Health Sociology Review*, 26, 1, 6–21.

Swan, M. (2013) The quantified self: fundamental disruption in big data science and biological discovery, *Big Data*, 1, 85–99.

Swierstra, T. (2013) Nanotechnology and techno-moral change, *Ethics & Politics*, 15, 1, 200–19.

Tempini, N. (2015) Governing PatientsLikeMe: information production and research through an open, distributed, and data-based social media network, *The Information Society*, 31, 193–211.

Thévenot, L. (2001) Pragmatic regimes governing the engagement with the world. In Schatzki, T.R., Knorr-Cetina, K. and von Savigny, E. (eds) *The Practice Turn in Contemporary Theory*, pp 56–73. London: Routledge.

Tobler, N.S. (1992) Drug prevention programs can work: research findings, *Journal of Addictive Diseases*, 11, 1–28.

Visser, F. (2017) Self-monitoring in insulin-dependent diabetes via health-apps; a bad influence on the perception of the self? Master's thesis, University of Amsterdam.

Vogel, E. (2018) Metabolism and movement: Calculating food and exercise or activating bodies in Dutch weight management, *BioSocieties*, 13, 2, 389–407.

Vogel, E. and Mol, A. (2014) Enjoy your food: on losing weight and taking pleasure, *Sociology of Health and Illness*, 36, 305–17.

VWS (2015) Voortgangsrapportage ehealth en zorgverbetering. Kamerbrief. Rijksoverheid Nieuws. Available at https://www.rijksoverheid.nl/onderwerpen/e-health/documenten/kamerstukken/2015/10/08/kamerbrief-voortgangsrapportage-ehealth-en-zorgverbetering (Last accessed 5 March 2019).

Willems, D. (2000) Managing one's body using self-management techniques: practicing autonomy, *Theoretical Medicine and Bioethics*, 21, 23–38.

Willems, D. (2010) Varieties of goodness in high-tech home care. In Mol, A., Moser, I. and Pols, J. (eds) *Care in Practice. On Tinkering in Clinics, Homes and Farms*. Bielefeld: Transcript verlag, pp 257–76.

Willems, D. and Pols, J. (2010) Goodness! The empirical turn in health care ethics, *Medische Antropologie*, 23, 1, 161–70.

World Health Organisation (WHO) (2016) *Global Report on Diabetes*. Geneva: WHO Library Cataloguing-in-Publication.

World Health Organisation (WHO) (2008) *World Health Report 2008. Primary Health Care (Now More Than Ever)*. Geneva: WHO.

World Health Organisation (WHO) (2011) *mHealth: New Horizons for Health through Mobile Technologies: Second Global Survey on eHealth. Global Observatory for eHealth Series*, Vol. 3. Geneva: WHO.

Yates-Doerr, E. (2015) *The Weight of Obesity: Hunger and Global Health in Postwar Guatemala*. Oakland: University of California Press.

Sociology of Health & Illness Vol. 41 No. S1 2019 ISSN 0141-9889, pp. 116–131
doi: 10.1111/1467-9566.12947

On digital intimacy: redefining provider–patient relationships in remote monitoring

Enrico Maria Piras* ⓘ and Francesco Miele ⓘ

Centre for Information and Communication Technology, Bruno Kessler Foundation, Trento, Italy

Abstract   Remote monitoring has often been thought to lead to a highly structured and standardised care process. Several studies have stressed that patient–provider communication could be hindered if mediated by technologies, leading to an impoverished relationship. We argue that while remote monitoring leads to a redefinition of the patient–provider relationship, it could also offer the opportunity to develop a more intimate acquaintance not possible via only routine visits. The study is part of a clinical trial aimed at assessing the acceptability of a remote monitoring platform for type 1 diabetes. Drawing on practice-based studies, we focused our analysis on the practice of text message exchange between patients and providers. The 396 conversations were coded with a template analysis, leading to the identification of two main categories: 'knowing the patient' and 'knowing about the patient'. The analysis reveals that the practice of messaging led to the development of a 'digital intimacy', a relationship characterised by a thorough familiarity made possible by electronic devices that extends to face-to-face encounters. Drawing on our case, we argue that remote monitoring can foster greater intimacy between patients and providers, which is made possible by the overall increase in the quantity and quality of communication between patients and providers.

Keywords: qualitative methods generally, diabetes, doctor–patient communication/interaction, E-health, emotional labour, information technology

Introduction

In recent years, the remote monitoring of chronic conditions has gained momentum due to the increasing availability of mobile technologies and self-tracking devices, leading to a debate regarding its effects on patient–provider relationships. While techno-enthusiasts consider such technologies an obligatory passage point to more efficient healthcare provision (Swan 2012) and reflective learning (Rivera-Pelayo *et al.* 2012), as well as tools to bridge healthcare

---

*The present article is the outcome of joint and indivisible work by the authors; however, if individual authorship is to be assigned, Enrico Maria Piras wrote the 'introduction', the paragraphs 'Presence at distance', 'Results' and subparagraph 'Knowing the patient' , and the discussion; Francesco Miele wrote the paragraphs 'A practice-based approach to monitoring', 'Research design and methodology', subparagraph 'Knowing about the patient', and 'Conclusions'.

Digital Health: Sociological Perspectives, First Edition.
Edited by Flis Henwood and Benjamin Marent.

providers and patients (Eysenbach 2000), others see them as embodiments of a corporate and public health agenda that will eventually lead to the medicalisation of society (Conrad 2007).

The sociology of health and illness and social studies of technology have provided more nuanced analyses, avoiding a polarisation that does not do justice to the rich phenomenology of remote monitoring. Several studies have shown how remote monitoring re-shapes health care rather than merely improving it (Pols 2012). A common trait of these studies is an emphasis on the unintended consequences of the shift from physical to digital proximity (Oudshoorn 2009), which they argue leads to more structured and impersonal patient–provider interactions, guided by protocols and constrained by the limits of the technologies, that is often perceived by patients and caregivers as an impoverished version of traditional care (Mort *et al.* 2008).

While we acknowledge the relevance of these analyses, we argue that little attention has been paid thus far to the emergence of richer forms of provider–patient relationships mediated by remote monitoring technologies. The purpose of this paper is to explore emerging forms of 'digital intimacy' between patients and healthcare providers. By digital intimacy, we mean relationships characterised by a thorough familiarity made possible, sustained or reinforced through electronic devices by means of both data sharing and personal communication. We argue that technology-mediated communication can trigger the construction and strengthening of intimacy between patients and providers that extends from online interaction to face-to-face encounters. 'Digital', in this context, refers to the locus of emerging intimacy, but this article does not intend to argue that it possesses unique features or that it is limited to computer-mediated communication.

Drawing on a practice-based approach (Gherardi 2010) we will focus on a specific practice of remote monitoring, text message exchange, to show how it can sustain the growth of digital intimacy.

The research reported here is part of a clinical trial aimed at evaluating the acceptability of a remote monitoring platform for type 1 diabetes patients. The platform enabled patients to keep track of and share information about their condition (e.g. glucose readings, insulin, diet) and communicate through an encrypted messaging system with doctors and nurses at the hospital.

The paper is structured as follows: In the next section, we briefly discuss the notion of intimacy with regard to remote monitoring. We shall then introduce the debate around practice-based studies which furnishes the theoretical foundation for the methodology adopted in this paper, the analysis of technology-mediated interactions between patients and healthcare providers. The findings are organised into two sub-sections (knowing the patient and knowing about the patients) to illustrate how intimacy develops in the intricacy of interactions and how remote monitoring practices lead to a closer relationship between patients and providers. In the discussion, we shall reflect on the idea of intimacy as knowing-in-practice and provide a tentative characterisation of intimacy.

Presence at distance: on remote monitoring and digital intimacy

Intimacy has a controversial status in the patient–provider relationship. On the one hand, emotional detachment has been regarded as critical to allowing professionals to play their role adequately (Parsons 1951). Affective neutrality is considered to shield both parties involved from an emotional involvement in the relationship. On the other hand, as the patient-centred paradigm gained momentum, a relationship based solely on clinical data interpretation became considered unsatisfactory and inadequate to unleashing the potential benefits of personalised care.

Intimacy, the feeling of deeply knowing someone and being connected to one another, is elusive in nature and defies a clear definition. In this work, we shall build on Fairhurst and May (2001) to frame it. Fairhust and May propose a distinction between 'knowing the patient' and 'knowing about the patient' (2001). 'Knowing the patient' refers to a form of deductive knowledge relying on the formulation and validation of hypotheses guided by codified knowledge (e.g. guidelines) and proceeding via the analysis of clinical data and subsequent structured patient interviewing aimed at gathering more information. 'Knowing about the patient', on the other hand, refers to the inductive process of becoming familiar with patients with a view to understanding their behaviours, habits, preferences and ways of thinking that emerge from the interactions and are elicited from the patient's own accounts. While these forms of knowledge coexist, only when providers know 'about the patient' do they develop sensitivity to the lived experience of patients and feel they have deeply understood them. Or, to use the words of Fairhust and May, only 'when doctors perceive they have discerned the authentic nature of patients as human beings they denote these patients as "known"' (2001, p. 505).

In this work, extending the notion put forth by Fairhust and May, we will also consider the 'knowing about the providers' developed by patients, considering knowing as reciprocal rather than unidirectional.

Medical technologies, including remote monitoring, are often associated with a reductionist view of medical care that favours the analysis of standardised data while disregarding context. Adopting the conceptual lenses provided by Fairhurst and May (2001), these technologies are regarded as tools privileging knowing the patient while disregarding knowledge about the patient. The debate over the introduction of remote monitoring and care is accompanied by what Jeannette Pols refers to 'inevitable nightmares', depictions of care turned into a service were the warm hands of the providers are replaced by cold technologies and alienation (Oudshoorn 2011, Pols 2012, Pols and Moser 2009). These scenarios are reinforced by somewhat simplistic representations of a health care shaped by policymakers that depict it as relying on decontextualised knowledge independent of space and time (see Mort and Smith 2009 for a critique).

These visions can partly be ascribed to the fears of professionals who are accustomed to face-to-face interactions with patients and perceive remote monitoring as a lesser service (Mort et al. 2008, Pols 2012), which may be compounded by a lack of specific training (Hart et al. 2004). However, the sociological debate around telecare has stressed other relevant dimensions. Foremost, it has been noted that, as technological devices become the cornerstone of the patient–provider relationship, they shape and limit the range of possible interactions.

Social scientists have emphasised how remote monitoring engenders a redistribution of responsibilities in the care network (Prout 1996, Willems 1995). Technologies, however, are rarely designed to support the rich set of relations among all actors involved, and they mostly focus on providing data sharing and analysis features. These limitations reflect an implicit hierarchy between hard/objective and soft data. Nonetheless, as Mark Ackersman noted, despite efforts of requirement gathering, 'there is a fundamental mismatch between what is required socially and what we can do technically' (Ackerman 2000, p. 198).

The replacement of face-to-face interaction with telecare delegates responsibilities to 'intermediary figures' like nurses (Cartwright 2000) and to technology, leading to more structured interactions (Oudshoorn 2009) and the rise of new forms of patienthood (Danholt et al. 2013). Remote monitoring technologies are designed by considering formalised representations of medical knowledge and standardised procedures, but they often fail to support the articulation work of all actors involved in their use. Such artefacts, to avoid becoming 'technological monsters', require significant articulation work which is not described nor anticipated by designers (Oudshoorn 2008).

While the programs inscribed in the technology often overlook significant portions of patient–provider communication by limiting themselves to data sharing, a shift from the artefacts *per se* to technologies in practice (Orlikowski 2000) reveals how users can adapt technologies to unanticipated needs (Joyce and Loe 2010, Pols and Willems 2011). Remote monitoring operators and patients can re-create a feeling of being together by mobilising and artfully rearranging the chronic care infrastructures, socio-material elements embedded in the everyday life of disease management (Langstrup 2013). Some studies have shown how patients and providers can manage to create an intimate and non-dehumanised or -disembodied interaction, even though this may require some emotional cost for providers (Roberts *et al.* 2012). Creating an intimate space for communication can require restricting access to parts of one's house for the duration of the consultation, as relatives might react adversely to provider suggestions (Langstrup *et al.* 2013). Other studies provide a different perspective on digital intimacy, arguing that, in some cases, the introduction of remote monitoring technologies can be perceived as too intrusive and a violation of personal space. Jeannette Pols, for instance, writes of a mutual support group of chronic obstructive pulmonary disease patients created by the clinic to sustain each other, noting that some patients refused to contact 'just anybody in the phonebook' (Pols 2013), considering the experience 'too intimate'. Similarly, Piras and Zanutto (2014) show how teenagers with type 1 diabetes can decide not to share their data with clinicians, considering it too 'personal'. In both cases, technologies are perceived by users as tools that create unwanted closeness. On the provider side, some studies have investigated the invisible work of telecare operators who attempt to create closeness at distance, showing that achieving this comes at a cost (Roberts *et al.* 2012) and that this work is often unrecognised and taken for granted (Korczynski 2009). Further, other scholars have shown how considering patients' sensations and experiences, as well as the sensibility of the practitioner, can improve the quality of clinical decisions (Barnes *et al.* 2016), but it is hard to collect this information via remote monitoring (Bjørn and Markussen 2013).

These studies provide some insight into how to frame and investigate digital intimacy. First, they suggest focusing on the socio-material practices of monitoring rather than the technical tools. Second, intimacy must be considered a negotiated and precarious accomplishment which requires experiential learning. As noted by Lopez and colleagues, 'it takes a lot of time to become acquainted with this practice of caring' (López *et al.* 2010). Third, intimacy should not be regarded as intrinsically positive or desirable for all actors involved.

Following these insights, we will discuss digital intimacy as it emerged in a remote monitoring trial concerning type 1 diabetes. We will focus on the discursive practices of patients and providers exchanged via the system. Before that, however, we shall briefly introduce the notion of practice and its relationship to knowing.

A practice-based approach to remote monitoring

Over the last 20 years, the so-called 'practice turn' (Schatzki *et al.* 2001) has involved different strands of the social sciences. It is not the purpose of this paper to provide an exhaustive account of the heterogeneous debate on practice-based studies (see e.g. Corradi *et al.* 2010, Nicolini 2012, Nicolini *et al.* 2003). We will therefore focus on the main implications of this theoretical framework for the study of the case under analysis.

The distinctive feature of a practice-based approach is that its unit of analysis is 'practice', by which is meant 'a mode, relatively stable and socially recognised, of ordering heterogeneous elements into a coherent whole' (Gherardi 2006, p. 34). Focusing on practices therefore entails considering organisational structures and roles as products of the actors' situated interactions. Every organisational process, including the use of telemonitoring technologies in health care, can be considered a practice produced, reproduced and interconnected through the everyday work of groups of actors both internal (e.g. physicians, nurses, technicians) and external (e.g. patients, familiars and other caregivers) to formal organisations. Drawing on these assumptions, several empirical studies have focused on the practices emerging around objects and technologies in health care, with special interest in the ICTs created to monitor the clinical status of chronically ill patients from a distance (Bruni *et al.* 2007, Gherardi 2010, Nicolini 2007, 2011).

From a practice-based perspective, structures are the result of 'circuits of reproduction' (Bourdieu 1972) through which practices, recursively reproduced, construct the structures and the conditions of their very existence. A practice-based perspective sheds light on the ways in which, during the reproduction of practices, social relationships and identities are enacted. Practice-based studies invite setting aside a reified view of knowledge – understood by traditional organisation studies as a cognitive activity – to embrace a view in which doing and knowing are indistinguishable (Gherardi 2010). During the reproduction of a practice, actors know about their social worlds and about other actors and, consequently, refine and redefine their ways of interacting.

The conceptual lens of practice reveals how organised activities are sustained by a shared understanding among practitioners. This shared understanding does not depend on a rigid script, but rather on a shared 'feel for the game', the logic of practice (Bourdieu 1990), which allows a 'repetition without repetition' (Clot and Béguin 2004). The recursivity of the organised activities, their regularities and the (at least partially) shared meanings attributed to them by both those who practice and those who observe from the outside, enable considering a given practice as an emic unit of analysis of a social phenomenon.

While we can define a practice (mark out its boundaries) for heuristic purposes, a practice cannot exist by itself, instead always being part of a 'texture of practices' nested one within the other (Gherardi 2006). In the case under analysis, for instance, we will focus on the practice of computer-mediated communication through a remote monitoring platform performed by patients and healthcare professionals. This practice can be singled out because it possesses some specific features (heterogeneous elements), such as the use of the technology, the constraints and affordances associated with the platform, the formal and informal rules associated with its use, the participants in the practice, the knowledge of diabetes needed to practice it and so forth. All these elements are ordered in a relatively stable way and allow practitioners to practice adequately. The practice of computer-mediated communication is connected to other organisational practices like face-to-face consultations, diabetes education in groups and ward rounds. These practices, just like computer-mediated communication, are assemblages of heterogeneous elements that practitioners and external observers can recognise as different. All these practices are interconnected and together constitute a texture of connected practices.

Practice-based approaches stress the impossibility of making a clear-cut distinction between knowing and practicing. Knowledge in not 'a set of statements about reality' (Mol 2002) but a resource for collective action. Pre-existing knowledge (e.g. protocols) is mobilised and reshaped in practicing. Knowing is practicing and participating; it is inextricably interwoven with the situated activities, or, put more elegantly, 'to know is to be able to participate with the requisite competence in the complex web of relationships among people, material artefacts, and activities' (Gherardi 2010, p. 35). From this perspective, the knowing of the patient's clinical condition occurs during the reproduction of this texture of practices, which is profoundly entangled with the communications infrastructure and leads to a definition of the clinical situation under review and the decision to be made (Mol 2002).

Research design and methodology

This work draws on a clinical trial that aimed at quantifying the effectiveness and the acceptability of TreC Diabetes, a digital platform for patients with type 1 diabetes. This larger study was conducted in the Autonomous Province of Trento, Italy (Ministero della Salute DGDFSC 0032830-P-22/04/2014, I.5.i.m 2/2014/953).

Type 1 diabetes is a metabolic disorder characterised by an instability of glycaemia (blood glucose level) caused by the destruction of pancreatic cells. The disease causes a deficit of insulin that must be corrected by injecting synthetic insulin. Type 1 diabetes cannot be cured, and patient care largely depends on self-management, holding patients or carers responsible for keeping blood glucose levels within a desired range. To this end, patients and carers operate as diagnostic agents (Oudshoorn 2008) able to 'become like a doctor' (Mol 2000). Becoming one's own doctor requires significant effort because, despite similarities across cases, diabetes is like a 'snowflake', different in every individual and also 'different every single day minute by minute' (Smaldone and Ritholz 2011). As healthcare professionals turn into educators and the empowered patients become the primary decision-makers (Funnell and Anderson 2004), the majority of care activities become intertwined with everyday activities and cannot be scrutinised by doctors. While doctors might recognise that the ability of the patient to manage the disease surpasses even their own (Piras and Zanutto 2014), telemonitoring offers healthcare professionals the possibility of re-gaining control of the condition when stricter clinical surveillance is recommended.

TreC Diabetes is a technological platform that supports both self-management and remote monitoring. The patient interface, a smartphone application, provides people with diabetes with a diary to keep track of relevant information (e.g. glucose levels, therapy, symptoms, diet) and some algorithm-based support for decision-making (i.e. a carbohydrate count, a bolus calculator, graphs, trend-tracking indexes). The providers' interface, a web-based dashboard, enables doctors and nurses to monitor at a distance patients' data through an algorithm-based alarm system triggered by specific events or recurring patterns in the patients' data.

Patient–provider communication is granted through an asynchronous messaging system (the system does not allow patient-to-patient communication). Messages are free text with no word limit and are not analysed by an automated system. The trial scheme required healthcare professionals to reply to patients within 48 h on weekdays and 72 h if messages were sent just before the weekend. In the departments under analysis, the messaging system was intended to replace emails and telephone calls for non-urgent matters.

Trials lasted 3 months and involved three hospital departments specialising in diabetes care in an Italian region. For this study, we limit our analysis to the only two departments that made use of the messaging system:

- 'DC-Adult' recruited 15 patients with poorly controlled diabetes;
- 'DC-Pregnant' recruited 10 pregnant women with previous experience of diabetes self-management (women with gestational diabetes were excluded).

These patient profiles, according to doctors, would benefit from the stricter monitoring and suggestions for disease management that the platform could provide.

As mentioned in the previous section, the unit of analysis of this study is the practice of computer-mediated communication through the remote monitoring platform. The analysis is thus focused on the messages exchanged between patients and healthcare professionals.

We analysed 396 text message conversations between patients and healthcare professionals and complemented them with semi-structured interviews conducted with all patients available (eight in DC-Adults; nine in DC-Pregnant) and with all the clinicians involved in the two settings (two doctors and one nurse in DC-Adults; one doctor and one nurse in DC-Pregnant). For the sake of this work, we have considered all the messages and interviews as a single dataset. Exploring the differences between the clinical settings is beyond the scope of the present work.

Data were coded using template analysis (King 1998, 2004), identifying categories and iteratively regrouping text segments in higher level constructs. The preliminary analysis aimed to discover the topics of the conversations (the reasons for starting the message exchange), thus uncovering the communication needs. Subsequently, drawing on Fairhurst and May (2001), we classified messages and text excerpts according to two categories, 'knowing the patient' and 'knowing about the patient', to explore the development of intimacy. The following section presents the findings structured according to these categories.

Results

Before presenting and discussing how intimacy developed through the practice of messaging, we shall briefly describe the practice of exchanging messages itself. Before the trial, the standard care consisted in programmed visits every 4 months for patients with poorly controlled diabetes and every 2 weeks for women during pregnancy. The 30-min routine visit before the trial was mostly dedicated to ascertaining an overall understanding of the trends. The retrospective analysis of data from weeks or months before the visit is a time-consuming activity and requires relying on other tools such as paper-based logbooks and memory (Piras 2018). In any case, suggestions arrive late when patients have already managed the condition. Communication in-between visits was scarce, and most patients did not recall contacting the hospital in the year before the trial. Telemonitoring makes it possible to establish a supplementary form of patient–provider communication. The trial scheme did not aim at reducing routine visits but offered a tool to increase communication.

Neither healthcare professionals nor patients had prior experience of the practice under analysis, message exchange across a technological platform. Despite some small variations between the two departments, the content of messages was similar. Besides technical issues, we identified four recurring themes: glycaemia control (through insulin therapy and diet), education (general rules for self-management), motivation (encouraging adherence) and context (information regarding patients' daily lives).

Conversations were initiated mostly by healthcare professionals (83.5% of times) alerted by reading the clinical data, and only a small fraction of interactions developed from a request made by a patient. Both patients and providers designated a time for texting. Healthcare professionals confined this practice to the late afternoon, when no visits were scheduled and they deemed it possible to dedicate their full attention to the dashboard. Likewise, patients sent messages mostly at night before bed time, when they had no family or work obligations and could dedicate their time to using the platform.

Knowing the patient

The messaging system was created to provide patients with a tool by which to receive timely suggestions for responses to specific needs and to allow healthcare professionals to be alerted in real time about blood glucose patterns requiring monitoring. Messaging is a discursive practice that emerges around the TreC Diabetes platform and through which clinicians can get a closer look at a patient's data, acquiring knowledge of her clinical conditions and gaining the ability to provide personalised prescriptions.

The platform supports healthcare providers in 'knowing the patient', drawing on clinical data entered into the diary and enabling supplemental information gathering via the messaging system. A typical exchange, presented below, is triggered by the desire of the healthcare professional to better understand some pattern.

DC-*Pregnant* [Patient name]:	We have seen your glucose pattern on Friday. They [measurements] are not within a desired range, and we'd like to understand better, but you did not specify what you had for dinner, and also there is no trace of pre-diner insulin. Post-dinner [glucose level] was low: Did you eat at all? Please, try to be more accurate in compiling the logbook.
Pregnant Woman, 32 years old:	On Friday I forgot to take my insulin, and, when I realised it, I took an extra bolus [a shot of insulin] to correct the 293 [high glucose level value], and then I checked my glycaemia at 18.30 and it was 342 [high glucose level value], so I did a 7-unit bolus. At 19.37 it was 186 [glucose level above norm], so I took the usual 8-unit dose and had some bread, fish and salad.

Glucose level measurements and therapies do not speak for themselves. Sometimes providers cannot make sense of data and require more information to fill in the gaps. The deductive reasoning of providers is guided by codified knowledge ('desired range'), hypothesis formulation ('did you eat at all?') and requests for additional information ('pre-dinner insulin'). The prescriptive attitude of the message is reinforced by the request for the patient to adhere to her role ('try to be more accurate in compiling the logbook'). While this is a good example of 'knowing the patient' by relying merely on clinical data, the response also provides an illustration of the possibility of 'knowing *about* the patient' offered by the technology. In this case, the patient does not merely offer the data requested, but she explains why she took some decisions ('I forgot to take the insulin [...] [so] I took an extra bolus'). In this circumstance, however, the provider did not enquire further, simply providing a recommendation.

Several messages show the potential of the platform to provide timely education on therapy and diet. Depending on how the conversation evolves, suggestions can be generic or tailored to the case at hand. In the excerpt below, for instance, the messaging system allows the provider to convey some basic and generic information on carbohydrate count.

DC-*Adult*:	If you eat pizza in a pizzeria, carbohydrates in a pizza vary from 140 to 180 grams … depends on the pizzeria. It is hard to tell, but 100 grams [*tracked by the patient in her logbook*] seem too few. Then, keep in mind that if you also drink a beer, you should add 7 grams. Bye.

Patient with poorly controlled diabetes, Woman, 20 years old:
Hello. The pizza was a homemade pizza. About beer, I don't drink [alcohol].

In most cases, though, the messages are more complex. A lived experience offers the opportunity to send multiple messages.

Pregnant Woman, 32 years old:	Good morning Doctor and [nurses names]. I need some information. This afternoon, 2 hours after lunch, at 5 pm, I had 188 [glucose level above norm], so I did not have

my snack, but I went for a 1 h 30 min walk (running errands). After that, I only had a [vitamin supplement brand], 1 capsule with vitamins and minerals (in the box it says 'no sugar') and 2 coffee candies (I bought them because I saw the 'no sugar' logo). Then my glycaemia was 197! How's that possible? It did not go down, not a bit, and that's strange! I measured it at 8 pm. Is it possible that after 3 hours it was still high even if I had walked a lot? Or, was there some sugar in the candies? Thanks.

Dc-*Pregnant*:   Dear [patient], taking a walk was a great idea. You need to check for carbohydrates on the candies wrapper. 'No sugar' means no sugar added, but they still have some.

In few lines, the doctor was able to do three things: provide feedback on walking to reduce glucose level ('a great idea'), offer some general education on food (meaning of 'no sugar added') and explain that what needs to be considered are not sugars but carbohydrates and where to look for information ('check [..] the candies wrapper').

The excerpts above can be considered from a different perspective. In all cases, patients provide more information than required, offering providers the opportunity to glimpse their daily life. In their responses, the providers only seem to consider the relevant clinical data: Information like the type and the quantity of insulin injected and the composition of meals are used by clinicians to explain the reasons behind out-of-range glycaemia and to rethink previous prescriptions. However, it cannot be ignored that through messaging, providers are informed of some details of the daily lives of their patients. In the next section, we shall see how sharing these data can lead to intimacy.

'Knowing the patient' through data is not a form of intimate knowledge. However, both patients and providers believe that the sharing and discussing of clinical data through messages leads to a form of 'closeness' not experienced before the use of the technology. Closeness, which is not the same as intimacy, is expressed as a feeling of 'being together' made possible by the use of the technology and leading to continuity in the relationship.

The platform is useful because you know there is someone who watches your values in real time ... above all, if there is a value that goes up or down, a message arrives to you [Interview: Adult with poorly controlled diabetes, 41 years old].

Without doubt, it is a time-consuming activity. We have had to prepare the documentation, to write the messages [. . .] ... it has been a little bit heavy. But the quality of care has changed [. . .]. If we see the patient after two weeks with the system, it is not like when we see a patient after two weeks without the system. It is like resuming something that has never stopped [Interview: Nurse, DC Pregnant].

Knowing about the patient (and patients 'knowing about the providers')

Messaging was conceived as a tool to provide timely education and feedback to patients. In this section, we shall see how the platform supported healthcare providers in 'knowing about the patient', familiarising them with the patient's way of thinking and context of life.

As described in the previous section, messages often contained more information that just strict clinical data. Sometimes clinicians investigated the reasons underpinning the 'bad' glycaemic values and the meaning attributed by the patients to their clinical condition, thereby interpreting clinical data in view of social, affective and working relations and of perceptions about the illness. Consequently, the glycaemic values are no longer just the result of therapeutic choices but are strongly interrelated with the particularities of each patient.

[Before this trial] we did not understand some things ... For example, stress increases glycaemia, and if a patient is fired, obviously this is hugely stressful. But someone could be not so stressed because, for example, he/she already hasa job offer. For another person, the same event can be much more serious, and it can be impossible to manage the blood sugar values [...]. When you go into detail, you can observe what they eat and what kind of physical activity they do. For example, [with younger patients], you can see that during the holidays they need very little insulin. Then, when school begins, it is necessary to increase the insulin dosage because with school, stress and anxiety increase. [Doctor, DC Adults]

The possibility of 'knowing about the patient' is offered by the remote monitoring scheme ('[before] we did not understand') and made possible by the practice of exchanging free text messages used by patients to provide information on their daily routines, unusual events and personal interpretations of their condition. This information allows providers to 'go into detail', understanding in depth the effects of life events on each patient.

Exchanges of messages strictly focused on self-management practices were accompanied by frequent messages aimed at understanding in depth the overall reasons for the glycaemic trends.

DC-Adult:	Yesterday was a bank holiday, and a little bit of hyperglycaemia was predictable. Everything else looks good. Bye
Patient, Man, 24 years old:	Parties and street food are not easy to manage. I do my best.
DC-Adult:	Don't worry! Take it easy!
DC-Adult:	What happened this morning? Stressful situation? :)
Patient, Man, 39 years old:	My boss was rushed to the hospital, and he had a heart surgery. Luckily, now he is ok, but in the office we've lost a valuable person. Also, consider that Christmas season is the most critical period for us. I hope that they hire someone for the next two months or it will be a living hell. I doubt, though, that someone will come to help us.
DC-Adult:	I am sorry about it; don't lose control!
DC-Adult:	Your data could be explained by some illness. I hope not ... I hope you will be ready to start the new year. [...] Happy new year!
Patient, Woman, 39 years old:	I have a 40-degree fever. Good analysis! Happy new year.
DC-Adult:	These crises are fully manageable.

In the message exchanges, various topics concerning the private lives of the patients are taken into consideration. In all the cases presented above, clinicians make hypotheses about glycaemia, asking for confirmation and/or additional information. Unlike the cases discussed in the previous section, however, the conversation leads providers to reassure patients ('these crises are fully manageable', 'Take it easy'), express their support ('I'm sorry about it') and avoid suggestions. In these and other cases, providers implicitly downgrade the relevance of diabetes management with respect to exceptional events or compelling social obligations. Also, the overall tone of the conversations is not formal, as made explicit by the use of exclamation points, emoticons and colloquial expressions.

Through the digital platform, clinicians seek explanations of anomalous values, going beyond self-management actions and examining the existence of external events. If abnormal glucose values are not ascribable to errors in self-management, the clinicians reassure patients, encouraging them not to lose motivation and to limit the damage to their health related to largely uncontrollable events. This change in the doctors' behaviours, from clinical advice to emotional support, is perceived by patients, and it paves the way to a different, intimate relationship.

DC-Adult:	'Well done! Keep going!' [analysing a perfect glycaemic trend]
Patient, Man, 33 years old:	Thanks for the technical and human support. If it [glucose level pattern] was always like this, that would be great.
DC-Adult:	It would better, but keep in mind that it is impossible also for the best diabetic patient. I do not want to demoralise you, but I want to tell you that don't have to be discouraged. Some ups and downs are normal.

When the nurse writes me 'well done!', I like it, even if I don't know who is talking with me. I don't care; I know that anyway it is someone who is knowledgeable. Therefore, she writes me 'well done', and I reply 'If it was always like this, that would be great', and she again replies 'It would not be diabetes'; she is right! They don't mislead you, they open your eyes, as it should be [interview with the patient].

Other times while messaging, clinicians come to understand emotions and perceptions that the patient has about the illness. In the dialogue above, we observe that: on the one hand, the patient is quite demoralised because he cannot reach the target glycaemic values every day; on the other hand, the ward reassures him, telling to accept even the 'bad' values since they are part of the disease. In this case, through messaging, the clinicians deeply understand the patient's relationship to the disease and, subsequently, try to change the meanings that the patient gives to their out-of-range glycaemic values. In turn, the patient expresses his gratitude for the emotional support received by 'someone that is knowledgeable' even if, in this particular case, he does not receive any specific clinical advice.

If the remote monitoring offers providers the possibility of 'knowing about the patients', this practice also allows patients to 'know about their care providers'. Patients develop a more nuanced understanding of providers in several respects. As illustrated by some excepts presented above, exchanging messages regarding unusual situations reveals the limits of codified medical knowledge and displays a provider's willingness to show empathy and support. Moreover, the situations described in this section permit the patient to gain a better understanding of the rationale behind providers' suggestions. For instance, patients experience the fact that ranges and thresholds become less compelling and can be violated with no consequences in some occasions, such as festivities or stressful situations.

In more general terms, patients reframe medical suggestions and prescriptions as not being judgemental but oriented to improving their condition and displaying the providers' willingness to go the extra mile to help—or help patients 'know that they care', in the words of a patient. This attitude is reflected in a more trusting relationship between providers and patients which imparts traits that differentiate these patients from others.

The relationships with them [patients in the trial scheme] has changed, and it is now more confidential, so to say. [. . .] Now when they come to the centre, they stop by, we talk a bit.

You don't do that with other patients. The problem we have with some patients is that they do not show up to visits. 'I can't, I do not have time right now'. Some people disappear for years. That's not what happens with them [patients in the trial scheme]. We have a bond, and we're sure they will continue ... we still have this strong relationship [doctor, DC-Adults].

Discussion: practising remote monitoring, cultivating intimacy

In the previous sections, we illustrated how intimacy between patients and providers is achieved through communication mediated by the remote monitoring platform. Intimacy is an emerging trait of the interaction made possible by the introduction of such technology into the patient–doctor relationship.

We refer to this as 'digital intimacy' to stress the primary locus of creation of such intimacy, which did not emerge in prior face-to-face interactions. Nonetheless, 'digital intimacy', despite being made possible by the use of electronic tools, is not confined to online interactions. The vocabulary of practice-based studies adopted to frame this study helps to make this point clear. The intimacy emerges in a specific practice (remote monitoring), but it trickles down into the other practices that form the texture of the patient–provider relationship (i.e. routine face-to-face clinical encounters). In the lived experience of practitioners, once an intimate knowledge of the other is achieved, there is no distinction between vis-à-vis interaction and text messaging. This is clearly expressed by the feeling of seamless connectedness that allows in-person encounters to be described as continuations of online interactions.

The lens of practice invites reflection on the continuous, multilayered and multifaceted knowing process described above. For analytical purposes, we draw on Fairhurst and May (2001) to distinguish two forms of knowing: 'knowing the patient' and 'knowing about the patient'. A third form of knowing could be introduced here: knowing to practice the practice itself. Text messaging was a new form of interaction for both patients and providers, and no strict guidelines were established beforehand. As the practice of text message exchange unfolded, practitioners recursively constructed and reconstructed the practice, negotiating a shared understanding of the rules they established as the conversation proceeded. For instance, providers learned when they had to keep asking detailed questions to gather clinical data and when it was time to show empathy and support. Each message exchange was different, but all somehow shared similarities or remained recognisable to the practitioner (Clot and Béguin 2004), and this provided an opportunity to learn about the other practitioner and about how to be a competent practitioner (Bourdieu 1990, Gherardi 2010).

To this point, we have defined intimacy as a form of knowing and an emerging trait of a recursive practice. Drawing on the data gathered, we can tentatively try to elaborate the concept of intimacy a bit more as it emerges from the interactions under analysis. While the feeling of being connected is experienced as a whole, we can single out three analytic dimensions. First, intimacy is experienced by patients as a feeling of being taken care of, as clearly expressed by the perception of continuity of care in-between visits. Telemonitoring re-creates the closeness between patients and providers usually experienced only during the first months after the onset of the disease (Piras and Zanutto 2014). Moreover, being taken care of manifests not only in the timely provision of clinical counselling but also in the form of emotional support. Second, intimacy involves feeling like more than just clinical data. The routine clinical encounter is mostly devoted to the analysis of parameters. Exchanging messages allows personal events, previously not taken into account, to be communicated and considered by providers. Salient events from the patient's perspective (e.g. troubles at work) become relevant for clinicians, contributing to the feeling of being on the same page. Third, intimacy emerges as recognising a new, more collaborative partnership. This is the cumulative effect of being taken care of and considered more than clinical data. Patients are perceived as more reliable and deserving of more trust, establishing a new alliance.

Conclusion: the making of digital intimacy

The implementation of remote monitoring schemes is often accompanied by pre-cocked and polarised expectations. Promises of efficiency and process streamlining contrast with the nightmare of a cold, impersonal care (Pols 2012). Previous research has demonstrated that remote monitoring does not inevitably lead either to a richer or to an impoverished patient–provider relationship. Rather, these relationships vary for multiple reasons, and the simplistic opposition between cold technology and warm humanity makes no sense (Pols and Moser 2009). While significant articulation work may be necessary to prevent telemonitoring devices from becoming 'technological monsters' (Oudshoorn 2008), in chronic care management with limited face-to-face clinical encounters, remote monitoring can enable moving from a logic of choice to a logic of care (Mol 2008) favouring providers' attempts to adjust knowledge to the unique and complex life of each patient.

As other authors have shown, intimacy is a practical and always-partial accomplishment (Langstrup *et al.* 2013), and it requires negotiating new thresholds in the social division of care labour between patients and providers to prevent intimacy from becoming intrusiveness (Piras and Miele 2017).

The present work contributes to this debate by investigating the redefinition of provider-patient relationships in remote monitoring, providing a processual view of how digital intimacy is created and how it permeates all interactions, both those mediated by technology and face-to-face encounters. To discuss intimacy, we have anchored this elusive and evocative construct to two distinct but complementary perspectives on knowledge. Building on the distinction proposed by Fairhurst and May (2001) between the deductive 'knowing the patient' and the inductive 'knowing about the patient', we have described intimacy as knowledge 'about each other' (knowing about the patient, knowing about the provider) developed in digital interactions. Drawing on practice-based studies (Gherardi 2010, Nicolini 2011), we have shown the impossibility of distinguishing between knowing and practicing and how, when participating in the practice of remote monitoring, the instrumental data sharing and the understanding of lived experience are inextricably intertwined.

From our perspective, thus, intimacy is to be interpreted not as an additional trait in the interaction but rather as an emerging, intimate patient–provider relationship shaped by the reproduction of textures of telemonitoring practices (e.g. sharing data, prescribing therapies, asking for advice), which are profoundly entangled with the communications infrastructure. If our study shows how intimacy develops while practicing remote monitoring, more research is needed to understand if once developed it becomes a permanent trait of the relationship or if it needs to be continuously created and re-created through interaction.

The development of intimacy is facilitated or hindered by several conditions. One of them is certainly the technology involved, as it can restrict patient–provider interaction by default to standardised and pre-structured formats. However, as we have tried to show, technologies constitute only a part of a remote monitoring practice. The outcomes of a practice can vary depending on each of the elements of the heterogeneous arrangement that constitutes that practice (e.g. time constraints, concurring task, policies of use).

The peculiarity of the trial scheme adopted in our case was that it allowed providers to decide for themselves how to fit the remote monitoring into their workflow or, to use the vocabulary adopted in this study, to reconfigure the practice of remote monitoring within the texture of other clinical practices. In the case described above, this is made possible by the overall increase in the quantity and quality of communication between patients and providers.

Address for correspondence: Enrico Maria Piras, Center for Information and Communication Technology, Fondazione Bruno Kessler, Trento, Trentino-Alto Adige, Italy. E-mail: piras@fbk.eu

Acknowledgements

This work is part of TreC (Cartella Clinica del Cittadino), a research and innovation project supported and funded by the Autonomous Province of Trento. The research presented here has been conducted as part of a clinical trial approved by the Research Ethics Committee of the Health Authority of the Autonomous Province of Trento, and written consent was obtained from the participants.

References

Ackerman, M.S. (2000) The intellectual challenge of CSCW: the gap between social requirements and technical feasibility, *Human-Computer Interaction*, 15, 2, 179–203.
Barnes, M., Henwood, F. and Smith, N. (2016) Information and care: a relational approach, *Dementia*, 15, 4, 510–25.
Bjørn, P. and Markussen, R. (2013) Cyborg heart: the affective apparatus of bodily production of ICD patients, *Science & Technology Studies*, 26, 2, 14–28.
Bourdieu, P. (1972) *Esquisse d'une théorie de la pratique*, pp 157–243. Genève: Librairie Droz.
Bourdieu, P. (1990) *The Logic of Practice*. Stanford: Stanford University Press.
Bruni, A., Gherardi, S. and Parolin, L.L. (2007) Knowing in a system of fragmented knowledge, *Mind, Culture, and Activity*, 14, 1–2, 83–102.
Cartwright, L. (2000) Reach out and heal someone: telemedicine and the globalization of health care, *Health*, 4, 3, 347–77.
Clot, Y. and Béguin, P. (2004) L'action située dans le développement de l'activité, *Activités*, 1, 1/2, 27–49.
Conrad, P. (2007) *The Medicalization of Society*. Baltimore: Johns Hopkins University Press.
Corradi, G., Gherardi, S. and Verzelloni, L. (2010) Through the practice lens: where is the bandwagon of practice-based studies heading?, *Management Learning*, 41, 3, 265–83.
Danholt, P., Piras, E.M., Storni, C. and Zanutto, A. (2013) The shaping of patient 2.0: exploring agencies, technologies and discourses in new healthcare practices, *Science & Technology Studies*, 26, 2, 3–13.
Eysenbach, G. (2000) Recent advances: consumer health informatics, *BMJ: British Medical Journal*, 320, 7251, 1713–6.
Fairhurst, K. and May, C. (2001) Knowing patients and knowledge about patients: evidence of modes of reasoning in the consultation?, *Family Practice*, 18, 5, 501–5.
Funnell, M.M. and Anderson, R.M. (2004) Empowerment and self-management of diabetes, *Clinical Diabetes*, 22, 3, 123–7.
Gherardi, S. (2006) *Organizational Knowledge: The Texture of Organizing*. London: Blackwells.

Gherardi, S. (2010) Telemedicine: a practice-based approach to technology, *Human Relations*, 63, 4, 501–24.

Hart, A., Henwood, F. and Wyatt, S. (2004) The role of the internet in patient-practitioner relationships: findings from a qualitative research study, *Journal of Medical Internet Research*, 6, 3.

Joyce, K. and Loe, M. (2010) A sociological approach to ageing, technology and health, *Sociology of Health & Illness*, 32, 2, 171–80.

King, N. (1998) Template analysis. In Symon, G. and Cassel, C. (eds) *Qualitative Methods and Analysis in Organizational Research: A Practical Guide*, pp 118–34. Thousand Oaks, CA: Sage.

King, N. (2004) Using templates in the thematic analysis of texts. In Cassell, C. and Symon, G. (eds) *Essential Guide to Qualitative Methods in Organizational Research*, pp 256–70. London: Sage.

Korczynski, M. (2009) The mystery customer: continuing absences in the sociology of service work, *Sociology*, 43, 5, 952–67.

Langstrup, H. (2013) Chronic care infrastructures and the home, *Sociology of Health & Illness*, 35, 7, 1008–22.

Langstrup, H., Iversen, L.B., Vind, S. and Erstad, T.L. (2013) Langstrup et al.: the virtual clinical encounter: emplacing patient 2.0 in emerging care infrastructures, *Science & Technology Studies*, 26, 2, 44–60.

López, D., Callén, B., Tirado, F.J. and Domènech, M. (2010) How to become a guardian angel. Providing safety in a home telecare service. In Mol, A., Moser, I. and Pols, J. (eds) *Care in Practice: On Tinkering in Clinics, Homes and Farms*, pp 71–90. Bielefeld: Transcript Verlag.

Mol, A. (2000) What diagnostic devices do: the case of blood sugar measurement, *Theoretical Medicine and Bioethics*, 21, 1, 9–22.

Mol, A. (2002) *The Body Multiple: Ontology in Medical Practice*. Duhram: Duke University Press.

Mol, A. (2008) *The Logic of Care: Health and the Problem of Patient Choice*. London: Routledge.

Mort, M. and Smith, A. (2009) Beyond information: intimate relations in sociotechnical practice, *Sociology*, 43, 2, 215–31.

Mort, M., Finch, T. and May, C. (2008) Making and unmaking telepatients: identity and governance in new health technologies, *Science, Technology & Human Values*, 34, 1, 9–33.

Nicolini, D. (2007) Stretching out and expanding work practices in time and space: the case of telemedicine, *Human Relations*, 60, 6, 889–920.

Nicolini, D. (2011) Practice as the site of knowing: insights from the field of telemedicine, *Organization Science*, 22, 3, 602–20.

Nicolini, D. (2012) *Practice Theory, Work, and Organization: An Introduction*. Oxford: Oxford University Press.

Nicolini, D., Gherardi, S. and Yanow, D. (eds) (2003) *Knowing in Organizations: A Practice-Based Approach*. New York: ME Sharpe.

Orlikowski, W.J. (2000) Using technology and constituting structures: a practice lens for studying technology in organizations, *Organization Science*, 11, 4, 404–28.

Oudshoorn, N. (2008) Diagnosis at a distance: the invisible work of patients and healthcare professionals in cardiac telemonitoring technology, *Sociology of Health & Illness*, 30, 2, 272–88.

Oudshoorn, N. (2009) Physical and digital proximity: emerging ways of health care in face-to-face and telemonitoring of heart-failure patients, *Sociology of Health & Illness*, 31, 3, 390–405.

Oudshoorn, N. (2011) *Telecare Technologies and the Transformation of Healthcare*. Basingstoke: Palgrave Macmillan.

Parsons, T. (1951) *The Social System*. London: Routledge.

Piras, E.M. (2018) Kairotic and chronological knowing: diabetes logbooks in-and-out of the hospital, *Data Technologies and Applications*, 52, 1, 148–62.

Piras, E.M. and Miele, F. (2017) Clinical self-tracking and monitoring technologies: negotiations in the ICT-mediated patient–provider relationship, *Health Sociology Review*, 26, 1, 38–53.

Piras, E.M. and Zanutto, A. (2014) "One day it will be you who tells us doctors what to do!". Exploring the "Personal" of PHR in paediatric diabetes management, *IT & People*, 27, 4, 421–39.

Pols, J. (2012) *Care at a Distance: On the Closeness of Technology*. Amsterdam: Amsterdam University Press.

Pols, J. (2013) The patient 2. Many: about diseases that remain and the different forms of knowledge to live with them, *Science & Technology Studies*, 26, 2, 80–97.

Pols, J. and Moser, I. (2009) Cold technologies versus warm care? On affective and social relations with and through care technologies, *ALTER-European Journal of Disability Research/Revue Européenne de Recherche sur le Handicap*, 3, 2, 159–78.

Pols, J. and Willems, D. (2011) Innovation and evaluation: taming and unleashing telecare technology, *Sociology of Health & Illness*, 33, 3, 484–98.

Prout, A. (1996) Actor network theory, technology and medical sociology: an illustrative analysis of the metered dose inhaler, *Sociology of Health & Illness*, 18, 2, 198–219.

Rivera-Pelayo, V., Zacharias, V., Müller, L. and Braun, S. (2012) Applying quantified self approaches to support reflective learning. In *Proceedings of the 2nd international conference on learning analytics and knowledge*, 111–4.

Roberts, C., Mort, M. and Milligan, C. (2012) Calling for care:'disembodied'work, teleoperators and older people living at home, *Sociology*, 46, 3, 490–506.

Schatzki, T.R., Knorr-Cetina, K. and Von Savigny, E. (2001) *The Practice Turn in Contemporary Theory*. London and New York: Routledge.

Smaldone, A. and Ritholz, M.D. (2011) Perceptions of parenting children with type 1 diabetes diagnosed in early childhood, *Journal of Pediatric Health Care*, 25, 2, 87–95.

Swan, M. (2012) Health 2050: the realization of personalized medicine through crowdsourcing, the quantified self, and the participatory biocitizen, *Journal of Personalized Medicine*, 2, 3, 93–118.

Willems, D.L. (1995) Tools of care: Explorations into the semiotics of medical technology (Doctoral Dissertation, Maastricht University).

Sociology of Health & Illness Vol. 41 No. S1 2019 ISSN 0141-9889, pp. 132–146
doi: 10.1111/1467-9566.12943

Temporalities of mental distress: digital immediacy and the meaning of 'crisis' in online support

Ian M. Tucker[1] and Anna Lavis[2]

[1]School of Psychology, University of East London, London, UK
[2]Institute of Applied Health Research, Birmingham University, Birmingham, UK

Abstract   The Internet is increasingly used to seek support by those suffering with mental distress (Bauman, S. and Rivers, I. *Mental Health and the Digital Age.* Basingstoke: Palgrave Macmillan; 2015). Drawing on research on a major online peer support forum, we analyse discussions around acute distress, self-harm and suicide. The paper argues that new temporalities of mental health 'crisis' are emerging through the intersection of the immediacy of online support, the chronicity of underlying distress and the punctuated nature of professional support. Online support adds a layer of temporal immediacy that does not traditionally feature in other forms of support (e.g. professional in-person services). This shifts the meaning of a mental health 'crisis' from acute to processual, and can lead to definitions of 'crisis' being used when not desired nor necessarily accurate. By attending to the layering of temporalities at the intersections of professional in-person, and online support, we demonstrate how parameters of crisis support are set – by whom, for whom and in relation to whose bodies. This has implications for professional clinical practice internationally in relation to the increased digitisation of support and the meanings of 'crisis' that emerge.

Keywords: Mental Health Crisis, Digital Immediacy, Online Forums, Temporality

Introduction

Since its advent, the Internet has become increasingly medicalised (Ferguson 1996, Miah and Rich 2008), and it now offers many opportunities to seek information, care and support for mental ill health (e.g. specialist online forums, conversational chat bots, health information, access to clinical services, 'therapeutic' mobile apps) (Bauman and Rivers 2015, Lupton 2018). The unpredictable nature of living with mental health problems means that support is often required outside of the availability of professional services (Tucker and Smith 2014), which can make the availability of digital support appealing (Trnka 2016). Coupled with funding pressures causing reduced provision of mental health services, people may find themselves seeking help online (Naslund *et al.* 2016, Tucker and Goodings 2017). Using digital forms of support can involve moving across boundaries between professional and more 'informal' support, e.g. from in-person contact with mental health services to accessing online forums that operate outside of mainstream services. This is not to suggest a simplistic distinction between formal–informal, and online–offline. There are multiple ways in which these overlap and intersect in healthcare practices and help seeking (Lupton 2018).

Digital Health: Sociological Perspectives, First Edition.
Edited by Flis Henwood and Benjamin Marent.

In the current paper, the analysis focuses on support sought online and the temporalities and meanings of 'crisis' that such online support creates and questions. The specific online forum under focus operates outside of mental health services and does not link, nor provide access to, in-person services. It is an online forum designed to facilitate peer support. As we will show, people's use of online forums often operates outside of professional services and usually against a backdrop of engagement with professional in-person services. For instance, support may be sought through an online forum at a time when in-person support is not available (e.g. overnight) or to discuss or query something that has happened during a contact with professional services. Indeed, it is often reported that online support is being increasingly relied upon because of the limited availability of professional in-person services (Tucker & Goodings, 2018). The content of online support does not necessarily follow clinical parameters and can run counter to clinical advice or even illness categories, while also being valued and becoming embedded in everyday life (Lavis 2016).

Attempts are being made to provide digital support within professional services, with the National Health Service (NHS) in the UK increasingly looking to develop digital services (its Beta NHS Health Apps site currently has eighteen apps, although none has yet been fully endorsed with the 'NHS Approved' badge). Regulatory requirements can lead to commissioning being a slow process, particularly given the perceived need for randomised controlled trials as the gold standard of evidence-based interventions (Slade and Priebe 2012). Consequently, digital health technologies often operate outside of professional services (Lupton 2018). One key area to do so is online forums, with their 24/7 availability making them important sites for support when professional in-person services are unavailable.

Online peer support can involve any aspect of life, from managing day to day tasks, discussing formal support, through to sharing experiences of various treatments (Repper and Carter 2011). Existing research has identified the ways that online forums have been used by people with long-term health conditions (e.g. Diabetes, Chronic Fatigue Syndrome), in terms of the benefits of connecting with others who have similar experiences (Allen et al. 2016). In an analysis of young people's use of online forums, Prescott et al. (2017) pointed to the power of sharing similar experiences (what they refer to as 'non-directional' support), which Internet forums make possible in ways in-person settings do not. Online forums have also been reported to facilitate empathic support through the creation of online communities of people with similar experiences who are prepared to share their stories. The anonymity of forums is seen as creating disinhibition effects, which help users to open up and share their experiences, in what they perceive to be a safe space. Trust develops through engaging with others with similar experiences and perspectives as yourself (Wang et al. 2008). Existing literature has identified some of the complexities of online and offline communication and support. To date though, there has not been a specific focus on how 'crisis' features in communication in online forums, and therefore how online spaces may be shifting accepted meanings.

Online forums are not designed to be part of crisis intervention (beyond suggesting users contact their mental health teams if feeling acutely distressed), and yet their availability means that people can use them at times of acute distress, or perceived crisis (Tucker and Goodings 2017). While clinical definitions of crisis exist, in online forums operating outside of formal services, there is not a unified sense of what a mental health crisis is, how it should be identified and what forms of support can help (Winness et al. 2010). Against this background, in this paper we explore the mechanisms through which 'crises' come to be labelled as such, and how this may impact on the community and user. Online forums lack the clinical oversight through which crises are commonly defined, and as such can define these in forum-specific ways that are reflective of users' lives. As the current paper will argue, this can lead to uncertainty as to what constitutes a 'crisis' and who gets to define this: Is it the person them self, the wider community, forum moderator or new, perhaps transient, meanings that emerge through interactions among these actors? Distress takes many different forms and intensities; what one person experiences as a crisis another may not. Specific behaviour can be perceived as a sign of crisis (e.g. self-harm, suicide), and/or it may be one element of a more long-term mode of being or (lack of) coping. Its embeddedness in the everyday points to the need to reflect on whether crisis is a 'one moment event' or something more processual that ebbs and flows across online/offline boundaries.

Digital immediacy

This paper's focus is the temporality of both crisis and support, as these emerge online. Digital technologies are claimed to have the potential to transform temporal and spatial practices of health care (Trnka 2016), particularly in relation to their 'always-on' and 'always-there' operation. This makes them an immediate source of potential support at times of need, particularly when in-person services are unavailable. Immediacy though is only one temporality of the experience of using online forums. We explore how crisis and support operate simultaneously in relation to lived corporeality as well as the online interactions of individuals and the community. This analysis thereby also poses a challenge to prevalent assumptions regarding digital immediacy as a one-directional speeding up of life through increasingly networked worlds, with information, connections and media always available through the tap of a keyboard or the swipe of a screen (Sprenger 2014). More nuanced accounts have emerged that provide scope to consider ways in which the digital may slow life down, to stabilise and calm (Wajcman 2015, Duclos *et al.* 2017, Reading, 2012). These are important points in relation to analysing the meanings of 'crisis' that emerge through the immediacy of online support. They help to elucidate complexities around role expectations and responsibilities, such as the closeness of seeking and/or providing support in a digital context in which others can feel quite distant, or vice versa. By exploring crises as both ephemeral snapshots of distress felt and embodied 'elsewhere' and yet also tangibly experienced (and/or re-experienced) within the 'real time' of digital interaction, we demonstrate how participants experience and define responsibilities of support online. Paying attention to temporality thereby offers a way to critically scope the boundaries of crisis moments, as these are shaped by the specific operation of digital platforms, individuals' experiences of distress, and the wider online community.

This analysis intends to draw forth the potential clinical implications of the impact of online forums in relation to seeking and providing 'crisis support'. Addressing the temporal multiplicities of experiences of distress and online forums highlights how the 'present' intersects with dimensions of past and future, both in terms of the interactional operation of the platform, and the fluctuating reality of users' underlying distress. Experiences of distress can have particular relationships to the past through a rootedness in traumatic life events, the effects of which may ebb and flow in the present and also impact on decisions made about the future (Brown and Reavey 2015). Considerable literature supports the idea that past and future life experience can bear heavily on present levels of distress, and that living with ongoing mental health problems can often involve remaining connected to past life events, and concerns and anxieties about what the future may hold (McWade 2015, Read *et al.* 2018, Van der Kolk 1987). Analytically connecting the already-overlapping temporalities of distress with immediacy of online forums is key to revealing how crisis moments come to be labelled, supported and experienced online.

Digital immediacy can operate in multiple ways and intersect with the temporal practices that constitute other parts of life (e.g. engagement with professional in-person services). As such, in this paper, we are focused on analysing digital immediacy in relation to support for ongoing mental ill health, and the challenges that arise in relation to meanings of crisis. For instance, seeking support at a time outside of the availability of professional services may gain responses that categorise an individual's distress as 'inherently' a form of crisis, even if the person does not consider it to be. To unravel these challenges, an approach is required that highlights the impact of the intersections of the multiple temporalities of chronic distress, professional in-person support, past trauma and the immediacy of digital communication. Tracking these resonances and their impact provides important insight regarding how we should support people at times of significant need both within and beyond the clinic.

Elefriends

The forum under focus in this paper is Elefriends (www.elefriends.org.uk), a specialist online community designed and run by the UK mental health charity Mind to facilitate peer support for people experiencing ongoing mental distress. It is not designed to provide clinical guidance or information, but to utilise the power of social media to connect people to other 'experts by experience' (McLaughlin 2009), thereby facilitating peer support. Elefriends is similar to other social media platforms, e.g. Facebook, as people create a profile, can post comments, upload visual images and videos, private messages as well as press 'thinking of you', 'I like this' and 'I hear you' buttons (similar to the 'like' button in Facebook). Elefriends is a major online community in the UK, with registered users numbering in the tens of thousands at the time of writing.

The data drawn upon in this paper come from a broader project analysing the impact of online forums on peer support practices (Tucker and Goodings 2017, 2018). Ethics approval was gained from the University of East London's Research Ethics Committee, after which an online post was placed on www.elefriends.org.uk inviting participants to take part in the study. An online recruitment process was used, in which interested users could 'click through' a series of screens with all the participant information and consent information. Online posts and comments of participants were collected over a 3-month period (March–May 2014), with all participant information subsequently anonymised. As a specialist mental health forum, support on Elefriends typically involves discussions about interventions, formal care, periods of acute distress and more general discussion of a range of issues in relation to living with ongoing mental health problems. No visual data were collected, and neither were private messages.

Analytic approach

The digital research approach developed in this paper involves analysing how experiences of crisis are shaped by the specifics of the online platform. We are wary of avoiding the ambiguity that can arise with digital platform-based research, namely whether it is a social phenomenon, or the platform itself, which is being researched (Marres 2017). Attention will therefore be paid to the temporal shaping enacted by the forum as a digital technology, namely by recognising that digital temporalities are not homogenous, nor necessarily linear, but can fluctuate through different rhythms and speeds (Reading, 2012). In terms of 'crisis support', we are focusing on how online forums like Elefriends, as digital technologies, have "occasioned potentially complex changes in its associated practices and forms" (Marres 2017: 25). This analysis will consequently focus on how crises are constituted or disrupted in and through the complexities of fluctuating digital temporalities and the layered multiplicities of the *lived presents* of times when crisis is labelled, reacted to, supported and experienced in and through an online forum.

This was not an online ethnography in 'real time', as data were only accessible once collected. The online posts and comments were originally subject to a systematic familiarisation and coding stage, which followed the principles of thematic analysis (Braun and Clarke 2006). A theme development stage followed, which included several stages of checking emergent themes, in advance of a final set of themes being confirmed. This process identified 'crisis support' as an important part of peer support in Elefriends. However, the theme of 'crisis' was not fully analysed in previous publications that focused on other themes (Tucker and Goodings 2017; 2018; Tucker in press). Given the importance of 'crisis', and the meanings associated with it, a dedicated analysis was identified as needed. The analysis in this paper signifies a secondary thematic analysis of the data, undertaken by the two authors, which focused specifically on the meaning of 'crisis'. This analytic process demonstrated the need to attend to temporality in order to understand how crisis moments emerged online, as well as their individual and collective impact. Online forums do not operate through a universal temporality, and therefore our analysis tracks and traces multiple temporalities in relation to online communication. This is grounded in a concomitant recognition of the reality of living with ongoing mental distress as involving fluctuations in terms of acuteness and chronicity.

Online temporalities of 'crisis'

This section focuses on the ways that crises come to be defined and responded to by forum users and the wider Elefriends community. This begins to illustrate the paper's central argument that paying attention to temporality reveals how crisis, support and participants' ongoing experiences of distress overlap, drawing the past into the present and shaping future interactions and experiences. Temporality, therefore, emerges not as a singularity, but rather as multiple, with crises unfolding across these multiple temporalities. Crucially, temporalities are not viewed as separate to support and distress, but rather are argued to be the forms they take, i.e. time is not an external shaping force; support, crisis and distress *are* temporal. We begin this discussion by exploring how the temporalities of professional in-person support intersect with online support in relation to episodes of acute distress.

Waiting online: filling temporal gaps in formal care
The immediacy of online support means people can seek support in relation to concerns they have about the support they receive through professional in-person services. Elefriends is present at times when this in-person support is not, and as such interaction online operates in relation to the different temporal configurations of in-person and online support:

Extract 1
  Bridget (POST) Went to see my doctor. Seen a new one, and he seemed really good, im not normally good with male doctors but he seemed ok. And I told him about what happened on Sunday where I self harmed. And I asked for a crisis team number, so he rang up my CPN. And turns out she's nothing to do with me anymore! So the doctor said ill speak to her and see what to do, and he's made me a app to see him tomorrow. Feeling very lost and stressed now. Don't know what's happening. Feeling suicidal and lost and alone do you know what i can do?

  Sue (COMMENT) Big hugs to you Bridget. Please try and keep safe in the meantime. It looks live you've got a good GP there and pleased that he made an appointment for you to see him again tomorrow.

(COMMENT) The Elephant is sorry to hear you feel like that Bridget - is there an appointment today then? If so can you talk to your GP about how this is making you feel? Hugs x

For Bridget, online support provides a momentary stop gap between access to the in-person support provided by her mental health team. Bridget is in need of support in the present moment, she is feeling "very lost and stressed now", and without Elefriends she faces waiting until the following day's appointment with her doctor. The immediacy offered by Elefriends can respond to this need, in terms of facilitating support when it is needed, providing Bridget with a temporal closeness to support, rather than the feeling of distance caused by waiting between doctor appointments. Moving between the contrasting temporalities of in-person and online support can impact on individuals' experience of distress. The professional support provided by her doctor (General Practitioner (GP) in the UK) is marked out as the main source of support, but unavailable at this time. The online support through Elefriends is more empathically focused because it is immediate, and as such responds to Sue's distress in the present, as it is experienced. A challenge can arise through this interconnection, when the forms of support shift between online and in-person domains.

Bridget's expression of suicidal feelings is not something the immediacy of Elefriends offers support for in a clinical sense. Both Sue and the 'Ele' (the collective name used by moderators) offer words of reassurance that the GP appointment will provide support, rather than engaging in more detailed support, e.g. in terms of exploring possible ways of helping Bridget deal with her suicidal feelings. This is despite Bridget's cry for help of asking whether anyone in the Elefriends community can offer specific guidance as to what she can do to overcome the perceived failings of the support through her mental health team. Bridget's GP is presented as proactively trying to organise support from the community mental health team. As such, Sue and the Ele encourage Bridget to hold tight and await the following day's appointment. At this time, Elefriends does not substitute for professional in-person support but can help participants to endure the gaps between mainstream provision. This is important as such gaps can become filled with ongoing distress; a heightening of which can lead to crisis that can be attributed to the wait itself. The immediacy of Elefriends can help here. However, during periods of acute distress users can feel they are not providing sufficient support to others (a central tenet of peer support), which itself adds to the overall experience of distress.

Extract 2

Kirstie (POST) Haven't been on here in a while; had a really bad week and to be honest have been considering S. Haven't felt that bad in a long time, but I think I'm slowly coming out of it now. Though, I'm still feeling depressed and anxious, I don't want to end up being sectioned again. Trying to resist curling up forever in this black hole I seem to be in is really hard. I've cried so much this week. Waiting on another letter with an appointment with my psychologist sometime soon, I really hope I can get one. I can't carry on with this burden on my own any more. I feel bad for being such a bad elefriend (If I can even call myself one anymore) I haven't provided anyone any support recently, but I've felt I was simply unable to, because of how bad I was feeling myself. I'm sorry.

Temporality is central to Kirstie's post, in which she describes not having used Elefriends in a 'while' due to having experienced a period of increased distress that involved suicidal thoughts. Kirstie's return to Elefriends is described temporally in terms of 'slowly' coming out of the period of crisis. She is faced with gaps between appointments with her psychologist, which are 'filled' by seeking support through Elefriends. In a sense Elefriends acts like a 'digital waiting room', in which peer support can be sought and provided for people during the periods between access to professional services.

Kirstie's post refers to the responsibility to provide as well as seek support. This give and take aspect of peer support will shift according to levels of distress but can lead to users feeling as if they are not fulfilling their responsibility, primarily in terms of taking and not giving enough support to others. In the above extract Kirstie presents an identity of a "bad elefriend" through claiming that she has not been providing enough peer support to others recently. This is an additional layer to online support. Its immediacy can fill the gaps between in-person care, but it comes with felt responsibilities to reciprocate, to engage with the peer support made possible by Elefriends. This requirement to support others is not usually part of the support provided by professional services (unless they include a peer support element). The felt need to reciprocate in the potentially 'acute' present moment, however, contrasts to the issue that what may look like a moment of crisis requiring immediate response can in fact be a space away from one's distress, to reflect on it, as Kirstie's return to Elefriends *after* a crisis suggest. Elefriends can thereby provide the opportunity for supporting oneself by gaining a moment of stillness, or temporal halting through the narrating of experience. Although this is not about supporting others, but rather about a space that is immediately at hand that allows for a 'positioning' of experience, it can leave others not knowing how to respond as multiple temporalities and diverging interpretations of crisis come together:

Extract 3

Anth (post) I don't really need a reply to this. I just need to write it and somewhere to post it. It's just a therapy thing, self soothing, writing it out to help me process my emotions.

Anth's words suggest that not only is the temporality of the digital slow rather than fast here but also that this halting slowness has a particular relationship with other parts of Anth's life away from Elefriends. Narrating experience allows Anth to strategically 'post' it somewhere else, which positions online as distant, and thereby separate from, 'crisis' moments. This would seem to set up a binary between offline and online, in which crisis moments take place 'elsewhere'. Turning to explore self-harm support on Elefriends demonstrates this sense of a crisis as processual and lived rather than an event, and yet it also cautions against binary interpretations, by elucidating how crises may be experienced online and offline, in the virtual and corporeal, simultaneously as two elements of experience rather than fundamentally distinct realities.

"The rush stops but the thoughts don't" – temporalities of self harm
With Elefriends, online support is not infrequently sought in relation to moments of self-harm, which are often discussed though the abbreviation s/h or SH. Content around self-harm can involve descriptions of specific acts just completed, in process or planned, as well as of the ongoing distress of which self-harm may be a part. Often such posts are signposted with 'trigger warnings', to identify them as potentially anxiety provoking for others with experiences (past or present) of self-harm. Here an additional temporal layer to crisis emerges, in terms of the injured body, and how this is discussed and negotiated online:

Extract 4

Olivia (POST) Feeling weak right now - I just can't stop it - why can't I just live without SH - why do I have to go so deep - why can't my mind just stop the thoughts - I so hate me

.....

Olivia (COMMENT) I wish they would pass but they never seem to .... I still need to do more but I know I already need stitches ..... My head is so screwed up

.....

Olivia (COMMENT) Still so there - i need stitches but it will wait - i can't go and leave my son - i dont have anybody - can't risk him being put in care xx

Julia (COMMENT) Do you need medical attention friend. The rush stops after while but the thoughts don't. so sorry my friend. If you are bleeding profusely, hold a piece of clean material like a tea towel or shirt over the wound and hold firmly, and call for help. Keep in touch yeah. xxxx

Self-harm can be presented as a compulsion, in terms of being the focus of an enduring pressure to engage. It can operate as the physical manifestation of underlying distress, something users wish would end. It can also be framed as a temporal relief, in terms of offering a moment of intensity that halts, albeit briefly, underlying distress. In the above extract Julia states "the rush stops after a while but the thoughts don't". Multiple temporalities work here to denote the boundaries between crisis and support; firstly, the enduring underlying distress (the non-stop thoughts). Secondly, the short intensive rush of physical pain. And thirdly, the potential permanency of the scars left behind. These temporalities of self-harm itself, moreover, are overlaid by the temporalities of narrating the short-term and long-term pain online as well as the future act of reading this post on the part of others. While it may be tempting to assume that the act of self-cutting that Julia describes is *the* crisis, the coming together of these many temporalities questions that.

Furthermore, the support of other forum users is fragmented across this temporal multiplicity. Priority is often given to the physical impact of harm, with support focusing on seeking medical assistance or tending to the wound in the present moment. The immediacy of this particular form of online support therefore focuses on the 'here and now' concerns at play, in this case Olivia's physical injuries. The underlying distress is not discussed. At this moment, it is the wounds that need to be attended to, which is what Julia's support focuses on. Yet, across Elefriends, it can be seen that once wounds are dealt with, support is refocused elsewhere, as crisis moments emerge within the ebb and flow of ongoing distress.

Temporalities of self-harm also relate to periods during which service users manage to avoid self-harm. These can take a temporal significance, even if they concern seemingly small periods of time in relation to the durations of underlying distress (e.g. which can span weeks, months and years); as such they deconstruct crisis, positioning this as 'elsewhere', absented by an, albeit perhaps transient, lack of self-harm.

Extract 5
Emily (COMMENT) The ridiculous thing is that I've not hurt myself in almost 3 weeks which is a MASSIVE achievement for me with how things have been ....

Extract 6
Sophie (POST) I resisted for two whole weeks but old friend sh has visited. I guess I can be glad I made it so far and can do again. Truth is I wish I could do a lot more but my compromise is to do a little. To stay safe. Night night eles. I am tucking myself up now. xxx

. . ...

. . ..

Chloe (COMMENT) Awwww hunni . . .. i know how difficult it is to stop s/h . . . i often beat myself up over it . . .. but it's our way of coping my darling when things feel so impossibly difficult . . . u will stop, when u are ready and when you aren't hurting so much inside . . . don't be too hard on yourself . . .. you don't deserve it. We don't judge u my lovely, we just take u as the lovely person you are . . . Stay safe . . .. Night xxxx

The above extracts feature descriptions of time without self-harm (3 and 2 weeks respectively). These periods are presented as significant. Achieving such periods can be positive, providing confidence and a potential sense of control over injurious behaviour. In doing so, they construct crisis through its opposition to self-harm. Extract 6 draws this polarity out in terms of presenting a necessity to self-harm; after 2 weeks "the old friend is back". Yet, Sophie also shows an ambiguity of crisis as we cannot assume a crisis moment to simply be one in which self-harm occurs. Rather, Sophie expresses a minor episode as a positive compromise, something to help her "stay safe", and thereby avoid crisis. This formulation is maintained by a response from Chloe, whose support works to present self-harm as a coping strategy set *against* crisis, something that echoes existing accounts of self-harm (Favazza and Favazza 1987). In professional services, on the other hand, such an episode may well be defined as a crisis, and elicit certain responses (e.g. engagement with crisis team, admission for in-patient care). Online support does not necessarily define self-harm as a crisis and can instead seek to reassure that such activity is part of coping with underlying distress and the haunting of the present by difficult pasts, and as such should not be viewed as a sign of not coping by those who self-harm.

Re-living difficult pasts in the present: across times and spaces
The need to address the impact of difficult pasts on current distress has become increasingly recognised (see Brown and Reavey 2015). Doing so in an online forum presents new challenges. On the one hand, utilising the power of social media technology in the form of an online community provides participants with multiple opportunities to connect with others to seek and provide peer support. On the other hand, becoming part of an online community can be constraining in terms of managing one's difficult past, e.g. the awareness that one's online activity is visible to the whole community shapes the expression of life and distress in the present:

Extract 7
   Hannah (COMMENT) I wish things were better for you as well Chloe, are there things you could makes steps towards changing when your feeling a bit stronger? Xxx

   Chloe (COMMENT) i can't say on here...too triggering...but i want so much for things to change...but i've been hurt so badly, i'm struggling to get passed it all...i tried to move forward...i try ....in my head i think i'm ready .. in my heart, i'm not, i can't. too painful. too scared. xx

   Hannah (COMMENT) Sorry Chloe, didn't mean to delve, it sounds as if you have been through a lot, I really hope that given time you will heal and find a way to move forward, keep taking baby steps Chloe, you will come out the other side of this stronger than you are now xxx

   Chloe (COMMENT) you don't need to apologise ... it's ok hun .... i really need to talk ... but instead i s/h. i'm just hurting so much xxx

   Hannah (COMMENT) we all find our own way of dealing with stuff Chloe, be it s/h alcohol or otherwise, they are all coping mechanisms, maybe at this time your not ready to talk about things, you'll get there xxx

Extract 8
>   Chloe (POST) A few tears escaping. . .i have all this emotion tangled up inside, i'm trying desperately to unravel it, everyday i'm fighting to keep it at bay and it always wins one way or another. . .the pain and anxiety inside, feels like a heavy weight on my chest and i try and choke back the tears. . .swallow them back. All i'm doing is pushing the pain deeper inside, so no one can touch it, feel it or see it . . . . cos if they do, then i need to face it and i can't.

The online community of Elefriends provides multiple opportunities to connect with the similar experiences of other users, which can lead to discussions of one's own needs in relation to managing distress. Underlying distress can be referred to as being "deep inside", and something very difficult to open up about. This relates to the sheer difficulty of expressing underlying trauma. But it also points to the fact that online forums may not only facilitate a narrating of trauma but also a re-experiencing of it through that narration. Crisis moments coincide and become enfolded as they are re-lived across multiple temporalities.

This crisis-as-multiplicity may also be disseminated across spaces, as well as times. In extract 8 Chloe articulates this: A few tears are a visual embodied articulation of the pain 'inside', which takes a material form in terms of feeling like 'a heavy weight on my chest', as well as through the words on the screen. Expressions of the underlying distress emerge, but it is difficult to move beyond these in terms of trying to address the deep-seated issues. The statement of "pushing the pain deeper inside" sounds spatial, the idea that distress can be buried or submerged deep within. This suggests the underlying distress can be hidden from view, but is ever present. We can think of this as the pressing of the past on Chloe's life. Bergson framed this overlapping as the past constantly 'gnawing' into the present (he uses his famous cone diagram to illustrate this) (1988). The idea being that as life persists the present is a plane at the tip of an ever-increasing past, any of which is available to the present. This renders short- and long-term equal. An event from many years ago is no 'further' away from the present than an event that occurred last week. For Chloe, it is the incessant pressure of her 'traumatic past' that she is trying to suppress and keep control of. The challenges of trying not to express the presence of the past can lead to a temporal stickiness. Chloe talks about wanting to move forward/passed her present difficulties but struggles to do so.

The 'living present' is consequently shorn of its past and future elements. And yet, it is the past and future elements of the living present that can feature in the emergence of crisis. The feeling that one cannot cope anymore with chronic underlying distress. Crisis tends to manifest in relation to present concerns, which is not, in itself, surprising. It cannot manifest in any other temporal form. However, without expression of past and future elements, the present online can become a 'narrow' temporality, a bounded present cut away from the past and present. This goes against the common views that being online, by definition, expands connections. Chloe's struggles are presented as the slowing down of time, creating a fixed present full of distress without a sense of time passing, and with it a reduction in distress. Support is focused on restoring a sense of time for Chloe, that her current acute distress is temporally specific, it will pass. Its severity though makes it difficult for Chloe to feel it as temporary. In Extract 7 Hannah responds to an earlier post of Chloe's, and does not encourage Chloe to avoid self-harming, which is not a direction typically taken by formal mental health services. The self-harm is not deemed to be the problem. It is a symptom of temporal stickiness; if support can be provided to help Chloe regain a sense than things can (and will) improve, then the desire to self-harm may diminish. Other members of the community can see (and potentially feel) the signs of underlying distress, which shape their responses.

Living through such crisis moments online poses a further difficulty to participants as they widely recognise the possibility that their own discussion of traumatic histories can trigger distress in others. Chloe's comments in Extract 7 express a need to release the pain inside, but that she "can't face it", and that it would be "too triggering". The reality of the potential to trigger distress in other members of the community shapes the support in the above extracts. Periods of acute distress can provoke an immediacy to support in others that renders the present as potentially manageable, and a sense that care and support is 'on tap'. However, this instantaneity also means that crises can potentially spread through online communities.

Contagious crisis and temporal overlaps: fear of triggering others
The challenge of seeking support for underlying distress relating to traumatic past can operate across individual and collective temporalities. Chloe's extracts above demonstrate a challenge at an individual level to express the underlying distress in its entirety. To do so would be to attempt to flood the present with the past, which feels too overwhelming; it has too much *potential* for crisis. Even if Chloe were able to discuss her underlying distress in terms of its traumatic history, she fears spreading distress through the community, and thereby triggering 'crises' elsewhere.

Extract 9
> Chloe (POST) i feel like no one believes me …. no one believes this pain inside and how it can last so long, these feelings of worthlessness. If i could share what i'd been through they'd understand … but i can't …. the silence is killing me.

Extract 10
> Vicky (POST) Apology time, I'm really sorry if I triggered or upset anyone earlier by what I posted (ele has taken it off). I guess I was in such a bad place I didn't think, and that was wrong. I'll try and be more careful in future.
> Natalie (COMMENT) I don't know what it was Vicky, but *hugs* xxx

Extract 11
> Ellie (POST) "Avoiding this site for a bit. Whilst I appreciate that there are times when people may feel the need to want to end their lives at the moment, it is too much for me. This Sunday marks the 14th mothers day where I haven't been able to give my mother a mother's day card, and also I am planning a wedding, again without my mum who should be here as my best friend and my mum. She committed suicide 14 years ago and it breaks my heart to hear other people say that's how they feel. I don't know whether it's sheer luck or the fact I have lost my mum to suicide but I have never felt like that, probably because I know first hand the pain it causes, it still hurts/angers/scares me/sickens me even after all these years, and that's before you even account for the grief. So I'm sorry guys, but I'm just going to give this site a wide berth for now because it's a little bit too much"

Support provided through online forums relies on connecting with the body of collective lived experience, rather than expert knowledge through mental health services. These extracts illustrate a widely held fear among users of Elefriends of the potential of individual distress to be transmitted to others; through its narration it becomes concrete and therefore uncontained – or uncontainable. As such, we see how a crisis – in oneself or others – may be produced through the narrating of another, or an other's, crisis. The concern not to trigger contagion through the community can also emerge following an intervention by a moderator, which can act as an external signifier of crisis possibility. For instance, Vicky's post is an apology for posting something a moderator deemed potentially triggering, which had subsequently been removed. This is a formal marker of acceptability of post content, something that Vicky has now learned, and states she will try to avoid falling foul of in the future.

Ellie's post highlights the issue of contagion from the side of a receiver. She posted at a time when lots of other community members were discussing upcoming Mother's Day. Online discussion can exacerbate the distress of other members, particularly if it relates to a significant issue in relation to their own distress (e.g. the fact Ellie's mother took her own life). Elefriends facilitates this emotional contagion, which can involve the spread of positive support, e.g. coalescing around a specific topic (e.g. medication), but can also lead to raising levels of distress in others, as we see for Ellie.

It is this entangling of emotion, as participants are drawn close to others' crises, that poses a challenge to prevalent understandings of the digital as facilitating connection. Here the instantaneity of re-living a crisis can give rise to disconnections as well as connections; people can leave forums when others' distress becomes "too much" as Ellie puts it. This sense of contagion can therefore lead to members of the group taking time away from the site. This can be seen as a form of resilience, of being self-aware enough to recognise when to move away from online support if it starts to negatively impact one's own distress. This does not need to be permanent, just until such time a member feels able to re-engage. However, users' lives online are indelibly integrated, and as such when a user departs Elefriends, it can create anxiety among those left behind. The memory of crisis remains online, and a new collective crisis focused on the absent participant can emerge. If a person in crisis leaves, the community can be left not knowing what has happened, with the 'crisis' both enduring in the community and potentially in the individual user's body elsewhere.

Thus, the temporality of online life with Elefriends can lead to users reaching a point of feeling they need to move away from the site, which suggests that life with Elefriends, while providing multiple benefits, can come to feel too restricted. The idea that being online is not a 'full life' is not new, and yet with Elefriends this is not a spatial concern. The narrowing is temporal, through the pressure to render past and future absent on the site, despite their clear influence in the living present of distress. Chloe and Vicky's extracts present two instances of this at work. For Chloe, it is a difficulty of expressing her past. A potential solution is offered ("if I could share what I've been through they'd understand"), but the online support is not seen as a way to facilitate the solution ("the silence is killing me"). This introduces an additional temporal layer, or seeking support in the present for not being able to express the force of the traumatic past.

On Elefriends, thus, past and future do not feature as distinct temporal categories, but as dimensions of what constitutes present experience. A non-chronological sensing of time emerges, in which time is not experienced in a linear way, as the one-way movement from past, through present, to future, but as a temporal experience of varying configurations of past–present–future, in singular form. The past and future are never disconnected from the present. Rather, they are thought of as dimensions of the present. They are not successive instants that can be divided according to the quantitative logic of chronological 'clock time'; the passing of temporally consistent units of time (e.g. seconds, hours, days). Instead, time is thought of as a *qualitative multiplicity* (Bergson 1988) made up of elements of past, present and future. The specific configuration of their dimensionality depends on the material structure at the time under focus. This breaks the chronological idea of succession, and in doing so, recruits past and future as constant features of what Deleuze (2004) calls the 'living present'. As such, crisis moments do not take place in a singular slice of chronological time, but across an enfolded mixture of what may be traditionally thought of as different temporal elements. This sense of temporal co-existence, rather than successive chronology, elucidates that participants are never disconnected from previous life events, which do not gain quantifiable distance with the passing of time. Indeed, present distress involves living in direct connection with past and future, they are dimensions of the present. In relation to mental distress, what this approach does is to recognise that past experiences are always-already 'carried' with the present. Levels of distress can then be thought to relate to *duration,* the ways that present experience involves memories of the past and anticipations of the future. At times, these may be relatively passive, and distress deemed manageable, at other times, distress may increase due to the active nature of the past and/or the future in the 'living present'.

Concluding remarks

The temporal approach taken by this paper has highlighted how issues of crisis, support and distress unfold online at the intersection of multiple temporalities, including the immediacy of the forum as a digital platform, the chronicity of participants' underlying distress, the interaction with the community, as well as the past and future as agents in the present. This is not to suggest these are all distinct temporal entities, but rather dimensions of the temporal operation of the platform, and users' interactions with it. The reality of increases in distress often arising during periods when people feel overwhelmed by past experiences and/or anticipations as to what the future may hold means that traumatic past experiences can weigh heavily on the present (Read *et al.* 2005). Indeed, it can be at these moments that support is sought. These periods are not necessarily predictable, and as such the immediacy of digital forums can be welcome, particularly if distress rises at times when contact with professional services is not possible (e.g. overnight). The immediacy of online support is a new part of the experience of living with ongoing mental ill health and provides additional temporalities of support.

What comes to be felt or interpreted as a 'crisis' is not fixed; instead, experiences of distress, including periods of acute ill health, arise through the intersections of the different temporalities of in-person professional, and online support that operates outside of mainstream services. While this does illustrate the need to reflect on mental health crises as processual rather than, necessarily, acute events, it is not to suggest a clear distinction between online and offline support. Rather, the temporal layers that emerge through intersections with new forms of online support and the immediacy it facilitates suggest the need to reflect on the meaning of crisis more widely, offline as well as online. Elefriends operates outside of formal (NHS) services, and without clinical oversight, so the support on the platform does not fit the parameters of professional health care (e.g. clear programmes of treatment, specific appointment times). The punctuated temporality of professional support can leave service users seeking additional support through the immediacy of online forums such as Elefriends. While we have argued that these support gaps, such as overnight, might be crisis triggers, the support given on Elefriends has highlighted how such moments may be a worsening of an ongoing existing crisis. It is important, thus, to consider how crises may be processual as experiences of distress, and associated difficulties, may unfold through multiple temporalities, which are not always predictable or stable. Additional temporal layers can emerge in relation to behaviours that are often used as signs of crisis, e.g. self-harm. Here, the harmed body introduces immediate concerns in terms of attending to wounds, which then feature as a more long-term presence in the form of scars.

The power of online support to connect people is significant, and brings many benefits. One important consideration though is what constitutes a 'trigger' online. While posts disclosing self-harm behaviour and suicidal thoughts often feature trigger warnings, the definition of them as provoking 'crises' does not always come from the individual them self, but from the community and/or moderator. However, the tendency for online support to focus on the present means that underlying issues that can contribute to the development of instances of acute distress, or crisis, e.g. living with traumatic pasts, are rarely supported in the forum, as to do so would be a risk to the wider community. People are fearful of expressing underlying distress for fear of triggering others. Our contention is that a temporality that facilitates such expression, perhaps in a less 'immediate' forum, would be beneficial. This could result in fewer 'times of crisis' being labelled, as others would come to see spikes in distress as part of the fluctuating expression of living with ongoing mental health problems. The past needs to feature in a meaningful way in the present. Without this, the problem is not just a temporal one, it is an experienced one in which the living present feels too narrow, too focused on the manifestation of underlying distress in the present.

The use of digital technologies for support is likely to increase, and with it, new forms of support will emerge. Such technologies are not just tools for providing support but come to shape the experience of distress of those who engage with, and connect through, them. Digital technologies offer significant power to seek a range of support, largely due to the immediacies they offer. There are clear benefits to accessible support, and digital options such as online forums can provide an immediacy often not found in formal in-person services, particularly given the increased rates of access to digital devices. Understanding what is at stake temporally is valuable in terms of highlighting what support may be needed, and how best to provide it. For instance, identifying that self-harm is not necessarily a crisis in the present, but as a complex phenomenon linked to traumatic past experience. Online support can be useful for recognising this but can be limited in terms of helping people to discuss and try to unravel what can be very entangled and traumatic pasts, of which self-harm is a manifestation in the present. The idea that past, present and future are not linear chronological forms, but are actually dimensions of present experience helps to shed light on what is needed from support. It can also potentially help to identify periods of acute distress (crisis), and the temporal issues at play. Online support can help here, and will no doubt become more developed. Understanding how online forums operate in terms of support and associated meanings of crisis is important for mental health service providers and stakeholders such as those who provide access to online support outside of professional services (e.g. charities such as Mind). The immediacy provided has defined benefits but can also limit support to practical issues in the present rather than enduring issues relating to the development and maintenance of distress. The digitisation of mental health support is a global phenomenon, and as such the findings here have potential to inform policy and practice internationally, particularly as the digitisation of mental health support continues apace.

Address for correspondence: Ian Tucker, University of East London, School of Psychology, Water Lane, London E15 4LZ, UK. E-mail: i.tucker@uel.ac.uk

References

Allen, C., Vassilev, I., Kennedy, A. and Rogers, A. (2016) Long-term condition self-management support in online communities: a meta-synthesis of qualitative papers, *Journal of Medical Internet Research*, 18, 3, e61.

Bauman, S. and Rivers, I. (2015) *Mental Health and the Digital Age*. Basingstoke: Palgrave Macmillan.

Bergson, H. (1988) *Matter and Memory*. New York: Zone Books.

Braun, V. and Clarke, V. (2006) Using thematic analysis in psychology, *Qualitative Research in Psychology*, 3, 2, 77–101.

Brown, S.D. and Reavey, P. (2015) *Vital Memory and Affect: Living with a Difficult Past*. London: Routledge.

Deleuze, G. (2004) *Difference and Repetition*. London: Continuum.

Duclos, V., Sanchez Criado, T. and Nguyen, V.-K. (2017) Speed: an introduction, *Cultural Anthropology*, 32, 1, 1–11.

Favazza, A.R. and Favazza, B. (1987) *Bodies Under Siege: Self-mutilation and Body Modification in Culture and Psychiatry*. Baltimore: Johns Hopkins University Press.

Ferguson, T. (1996) *Health Online: How to Find Health Information, Support Groups, and Self Help Communities in Cyberspace*. Reading, MA: Addison-Wesley.

Lavis, A. (2016) Social media and anorexia: a qualitative analysis of 'pro-anorexia', *Education and Health*, 34, 2, 57–62.

Lupton, D. (2018) *Digital Health: Critical and Cross-Disciplinary Perspectives*. London: Routledge.

Marres, N. (2017) *Digital Sociology*. Cambridge: Polity Press.

McLaughlin, H. (2009) What's in a name: 'client', 'patient', 'customer', 'consumer', 'expert by experience', 'service user' – what's next?, *The British Journal of Social Work*, 39, 6, 1101–17.

McWade, B. (2015) Temporalities of mental health recovery, *Subjectivity*, 8, 3, 243–60.

Miah, A. and Rich, E. (2008) *The Medicalization of Cyberspace*. London: Routledge.

Naslund, J.A., Aschbrenner, K.A., Marsch, L.A. and Bartels, S.J. (2016) The future of mental health care: peer-to-peer support and social media, *Epidemiology and Psychiatric Sciences*, 25, 2, 113–22.

Prescott, J., Hanley, T. and Ujhelyi, K. (2017) Peer communication in online mental health forums for young people: directional and nondirectional support, *JMIR Mental Health*, 4, 3, e29.

Read, J., Harper, D., Tucker, I.M. and Kennedy, A. (2018) Do mental health service find out about child abuse and neglect? A systematic review, *International Journal of Mental Health Nursing*, 27, 7–19.

Read, J., van Os, J., Morrison, A.P. and Ross, C.A. (2005) Childhood trauma, psychosis and schizophrenia: a literature review with theoretical and clinical implications, *Acta Psychiatrica Scandinavica*, 112, 5, 330–50.

Reading, A. (2012) Globital Time: Time in the Digital Globalised Age. In Keightley, E. (ed) *Time, Media and Modernity*, pp 143–64. Palgrave: Basingstoke.

Repper, J. and Carter, T. (2011) A review of the literature on peer support in mental health services, *Journal of Mental Health*, 20, 4, 392–411.

Slade, M. and Priebe, S. (2012) Conceptual limitations of randomised controlled trials. In Priebe, S. and Slade, M. (eds) *Evidence in Mental Health Care*. London: Routledge.

Sprenger, F. (2014) Global immediacy. In Birkle, C., Krewani, A. and Kuster, M. (eds) *McLuhan's Global Village Today: Transatlantic Perspectives*, pp 31–46. London: Pickering & Chatto.

Trnka, S. (2016) Digital care: agency and temporality in young people's use of health apps, *Engaging Science, Technology, and Society*, 2, 248–65.

Tucker, I.M. and Goodings, L. (2018) Medicated bodies: Affection, distress and social media, *New Media & Society*, 20, 2, 549–63.

Tucker, I.M. and Goodings, L. (2017) Digital atmospheres: affective practices of care in elefriends, *Sociology of Health and Illness*, 39, 4, 629–42.

Tucker, I.M. and Smith, L.-A. (2014) Topology and mental distress: self-care in the life spaces of home, *Journal of Health Psychology*, 19, 1, 176–83.

Van der Kolk, B.A. (ed.) (1987) *Psychological Trauma*. Washington, DC: American Psychiatric Publishing.

Wajcman, J. (2015) *Pressed for Time: The Acceleration of Life in Digital Capitalism*. Chicago: University of Chicago Press.

Wang, Z., Walther, J.B., Pingree, S. and Hawkins, R.P. (2008) Health information, credibility, homophily, and influence via the Internet: web sites versus discussion groups, *Health Communication*, 23, 4, 358–68.

Winness, M.G., Borg, M. and Hesook, S.K. (2010) 'Service users' experiences with help and support from crisis resolution teams. A literature review, *Journal of Mental Health*, 19, 1, 75–87.

Sociology of Health & Illness Vol. 41 No. S1 2019 ISSN 0141-9889, pp. 147–161
doi: 10.1111/1467-9566.12871

Smart textiles: transforming the practice of medicalisation and health care

Kelly Joyce

Sociology Department, Center for Science, Technology and Society, Drexel University, Philadelphia, PA, USA

Abstract   Smart textile medical devices are forms of clothing that use sensors and fabrics to monitor bodily processes and communicate with data systems through wireless transmission. To investigate the co-evolution of digital technologies and health care practices, this study draws on focus group and fieldwork data to analyse the sociological implications of the creation of two smart textile devices: one – the bellyband – will replace the tocodynamometer and foetal heart rate monitor during labour and birth in hospitals and the other – the babyband – will replace the cardiopulmonary monitor in neonatal intensive care units. Analysis of potential users' views of smart textiles demonstrates the contemporary contours of medicalisation and surveillance medicine. Smart textiles blur the boundary between hospital/medicine and home/daily life. In this blurring, medicalisation becomes "cozy" or "comfortable" and surveillance takes on a friendly form. Smart textile medical devices thus fit into broader trends in health care in which hospitals are designed to be homelike and intimate even as patients and devices become fully integrated into data systems.

Keywords: medical technology, medicalisation, pregnancy

The creation of smart textile medical devices that aim to replace plugged-in, hospital machines is part of the digital health revolution. Although this effort has received less public attention than digital health applications or consumer tracking devices, both the private and public sectors are investing in research that aims to create smart textiles that monitor one's heart rate, oedema, respiration rate and other physical processes and send the data to the patient and/or clinicians' digital knowledge systems.

Smart textiles are fabrics that draw on innovations in electrical engineering, computer science and fashion design to create fabrics that can sense, communicate and change. Such fabrics incorporate properties into the material itself so that particular threads may act as antennae or create coolness or heat (Gaddis 2014, Syduzzaman *et al.* 2015). Sensors and radio-frequency identification (RFID) chips may also be embedded in the fabric to both sense and transmit data. Smart textiles are thus part of the internet of things, connecting individual users to larger digital knowledge networks.

In this study, I investigate potential users' understanding of two smart textiles in the making – the bellyband and the babyband, which are devices that could be used in hospitals, clinics and homes. Users is a term used in science and technology studies (STS) to describe people who interact with or use a technology. Imagined as knowledgeable, creative actors, users are considered to be a critical part of the innovation process (Kline and Pinch 1996, Oudshoorn and Pinch 2003). In this study, intended bellyband and babyband users include physicians, nurses, midwives, doulas, women who gave birth in the last 5 years and birth partners who had supported a woman during birth in the last 5 years. Analysis of potential users' expertise demonstrates how smart textiles encourage the continued acceptance of medical monitoring of pregnant women and infants. Potential users resist, though, the extension of monitoring across time (during pregnancy and children's first year of life) and space (in the home). Attention to the expertise of potential users draws on STS insights into the importance of attending to and including users' views early in design processes (see, e.g. Epstein 1996, Joyce 2006).

Combining STS with research in the sociology of health and illness, this article provides insight into the co-evolution of digital health and medical practice. In particular, I pose the following research questions: How can analysis of potential users' expertise and views provide insight into the contemporary contours of medicalisation and surveillance medicine? How does the rise of smart textiles as medical devices relate to broader shifts in hospital design? And, finally, how does the study of smart textiles provide insight into the social factors that might promote or hinder the blurring of medical and consumer markets for monitoring devices? In answering these questions, the article demonstrates how smart textiles represent a new way of practicing medicalisation and surveillance medicine – one that holds the potential to further blur boundaries between the medical and consumer markets as well as reconfigure the distribution of data and workload during pregnancy and early childhood.

Making monitoring fashionable

Research and development laboratories, primarily in Europe and North America, are investing in the development of smart textile devices that incorporate innovations in electrical engineering, computer science and fashion design. The European Union Horizon 2020 research initiative, for example, funded laboratories in Italy, France and Portugal with the aim of developing smart textiles. The United Kingdom, Canada, the Netherlands, the United States and Singapore also house laboratories dedicated to this endeavour.

The roots of this effort are in fashion, computer science and engineering. The public became aware of smart textiles when fashion designers began to integrate electronics such as lights and sensors into clothing. In the early 2000s fashion designers created an emergent, hybrid technology by designing dresses that lit up and clothes that communicated to other clothes (see, e.g. CuteCircuit's Hug Shirt that uses sensors to allow wearers to send electronic hugs to other wearers) (Ryan 2014). The desire to integrate these diverse domains of knowledge has further expanded into a range of arenas including the military, medicine, consumer goods and protective gear for emergency responders. All of these devices are part of the internet of things, creating connections among smart textiles, mobile devices, and institutional digital knowledge systems (Want *et al.* 2015).

Smart textiles differ from wearable technologies, such as Fitbit or the Apple watch, in that the goal is to fully integrate electronic elements like sensors and RFID chips into textiles, making them part of the clothing, not something worn in addition to clothing. Such a move transforms a tracking device from being a visible accessory to one that is integrated into fabric. In this move, the device has the potential to disappear by being woven into clothing.

There are two main categories of smart textiles related to health and illness, both of which are available for purchase and use in select markets. First, there are smart textiles to be used in medical practice. In this category of smart textiles, the aim is to replaced plugged-in medical devices with wireless smart textiles that can be integrated into broader digital knowledge networks. These are prescribed by clinicians to be used in clinics, hospitals or patients' homes. Although slower to enter the market because of the need to undergo national regulatory review processes, research and development efforts are underway to bring such products to medical practice. Edema ApS, a company in Denmark, for example, is developing what they call the Edema Stocking. The Edema Stocking monitors swelling in a person's leg and then sends this information to a user's mobile phone and the user's hospital's computer system. Clinicians can advise medical treatment or adjustments while users can make personal adjustments via exercise or leg elevation.

Second, within the broader health domain of fitness tracking, there has been an explosion of smart textiles marketed directly to consumers, with the promised goal of tracking one's heart rate and other bodily processes. These smart textiles, which include washable socks, sneakers, underwear, shirts and yoga pants, send information from the smart textile to other devices such as phones, computers, smart thermostats and lighting. The companies that produce these devices are also able to store and analyse these data. Because these smart textiles are marketed directly to consumers (bypassing the hospital, clinicians and insurance companies), they do not have to undergo review by the US Food and Drug Administration or other national medical device review processes. It is projected that this market size will grow to USD 4–5 billion worldwide by the early 2020s with compound annual growth rates of 35–50% (Dishman 2015, Global Market Insights, Inc. 2017; Research Nester 2017).

In this study, I focus on two smart textiles – the bellyband and the babyband – that aim to replace medical devices in the hospital, clinic *and* home. The bellyband, as the name suggests, is a band of cloth that covers a pregnant woman's lower abdomen and is worn like a "tube top". The threads in the bellyband act as antennas, sending information about uterine contractions and foetal heart rate to other computer knowledge systems (e.g. the nurses' station in hospitals or a smart phone) via a tiny RFID chip that is sewn into the device.

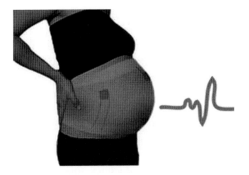

The Bellyband. [Colour figure can be viewed at wileyonlinelibrary.com]
Source: Drexel Center for Functional Fabrics and Drexel Wireless Systems Lab

The research team is exploring two possible uses for the bellyband. First, the primary goal for the bellyband is to replace two devices currently used in hospital births – a foetal heart rate monitor, a device that tracks the foetus's heart rate during labour and delivery, and a tocodynamometer, a device that monitors and records uterine contractions before and during labour. Both devices connect birthing women to the machines and the birthing room via wires, plugs and outlets. Second, the research team aims to explore the use of the bellyband in the home, which would increase monitoring to include the months prior to labour and delivery. In this

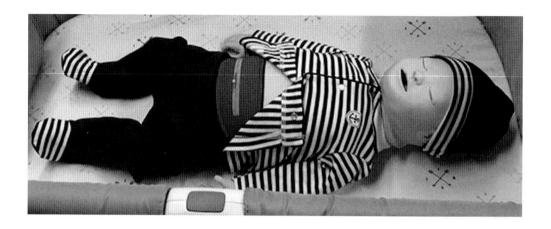

scenario, the data could be sent wirelessly to the pregnant woman's smart phone or to a clinician's data systems.

The babyband, which is the red fabric around the mannequin's stomach in the picture below, is another smart textile in the making. As with the bellyband, the babyband incorporates threads that act as antennas in combination with RFID chips to send information wirelessly to other computer systems. The babyband's design is still in progress. The designers are exploring different garments such as a band (as shown below), vest or onesie.

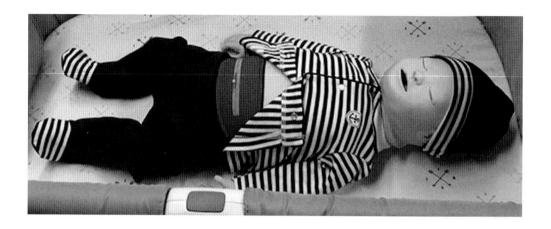

The Babyband. [Colour figure can be viewed at wileyonlinelibrary.com]
Source: Drexel Center for Functional Fabrics and Drexel Wireless Systems Lab

As with the bellyband, the research team imagines two potential markets for the babyband. First, the team's primary goal is to replace the cardiopulmonary monitor, a device that monitors infant respiration and heart rate in neonatal intensive care units (NICUs). The cardiopulmonary monitor requires electrodes or leads to be placed on a baby's chest, which are connected to wires that send heart rate and respiration data to a monitor's screen. The cardiopulmonary monitor is in turn plugged into walls or floors, creating a system of cords and outlets that connect patients to machines in the NICU. Second, the research team is considering a secondary market in which the babyband would be used in the home to monitor newborns. In this scenario, the data from the babyband could be sent to parents' smart phones, to a baby monitor or to hospital data systems and staff. In all, the bellyband and the babyband offer the potential to integrate two realms – medical monitoring in hospitals and clinics with the tracking of a woman's or baby's body in the home and in everyday life. Investigating how potential users make sense of smart textiles provides insight into the contemporary contours of medicalisation and the co-evolution of digital health and medical practice.

Research methods

This research project primarily draws on focus group data with 10 groups of differently positioned intended users. Focus groups were selected as an innovative way to bring future users' expertise into the design process and allow each participants' ideas to build together in dialogue. The author and two graduate research assistants conducted 10 focus groups with 97 participants during an early stage of design. Focus groups were conducted with doctors, nurses, midwives, doulas, women who had given birth in the last 5 years and birth partners who had supported a woman during birth in the last 5 years. The team expanded traditional understandings of stakeholders (which typically emphasise doctors, nurses and birthing women) to include the perspectives of certified nurse midwives, lay midwives, doulas and birth partners in data collection. Doulas are trained professionals who support women and their families during and after birth. They are in the hospital during delivery and advocate for pregnant women's emotional and physical wellbeing (Morton and Clift 2014). Birth partners were defined as a friend or family member who assisted a woman during birth (e.g. a spouse, a sister, a mother and a friend). The breakdown of participants is included in Table 1.

Participants were recruited from the eastern Pennsylvania and southern New Jersey region in the US. Due to the hectic schedules of doctors, midwives and nurses, focus groups were scheduled at locations and times that were convenient for each professional group (e.g. a conference room in a hospital or birthing centre). In many cases, we identified an interested participant (e.g. a nurse or a physician) who then recruited others from their field to a focus group. The focus groups with birth mothers, birth partners and doulas were held at Drexel University where there was ample parking and accessible public transportation. Recruitment for the birth mothers, birth partners and doula focus groups was done through parenting and doula listservs, flyers and snowball sampling.

Each focus group lasted 45–60 min. The same open-ended questions about the smart textiles' design and use were used in each focus group with small variations to account for participants' profession or role in birth and infant care. All focus groups were recorded, transcribed and analysed. Analysis focused on identification of areas of agreement across groups and moments where users' expertise and input could impact device design or use. Separate focus groups were held for each stakeholder group so that participants would be encouraged to speak openly and freely as well to build upon one another's thoughts and ideas given their shared position. The one exception to this occurred with nurses and midwives. Due to the fact that both professions work together in clinics and hospitals and shared weekly meeting times, two focus groups included both nurses and midwifes.

Focus group size ranged from 3 to 24 people. Recruiting doctors, midwives and nurses required flexibility. These professionals work long shifts that have little (if any) built-in free time. Without an invested participant from their professional world, they were reluctant to make time to participate in focus groups. For example, when an invested participant shared information about the focus group, 24 doctors showed up for the physicians' focus group. Although this was more than for a typical focus group, the larger number of participants

Table 1 *Focus group participants*

Number of participants	Potential users	Number of focus groups
6	Birth partners of women who gave birth in last 5 years	2
15	Doulas	2
32	Midwives & Nurses	2
4	Nurses	1
24	OB/GYN Doctors	1
16	Women who gave birth in last 5 years	2
97		10

allowed for a lively, engaged discussion in which areas of agreement and disagreement became visible. On the lower end, one focus group comprised solely of nurses had four participants. Although it was smaller than a typical focus group, we conducted the session in order to be able to include nurses' perspectives and accommodate their work schedules. Of the three groups – birth mothers, doulas and birth partners, recruiting birth partners was the most challenging. Even though we tried to schedule focus groups at times and dates convenient for each group, we found that birth partners were the most difficult to recruit. Due to this, we ran two focus groups, each with three birth partners.

The focus group data are supplemented with participant observation of weekly research team meetings, meetings of subsets of the team and practice research presentations given by team members, which was conducted for the 16-month duration of the project. I was invited to be on the research team because the team valued the perspective a social scientist could bring to the study, that is, the systematic investigation and integration of potential users' expertise and knowledge into the design process. The research team was university based and was comprised of faculty and students; it included three electrical engineers, three engineering PhD students, a design scientist, an obstetrics and gynaecology physician, a sociologist, two science, technology and society graduate students and an engineering undergraduate research design team. I took notes at each team meeting, practice presentations and meetings of smaller subsets of the team.

This project was approved by the university's Institutional Review Board (IRB) and names and other potentially identifying information have been altered to protect the identities of participants.

Creating mobile patients

Across all user groups, participants fully supported the use of bellyband and babyband in hospitals and clinics. They overwhelmingly liked the wireless dimension of the smart textiles, noting that this feature would better support patients and their caregivers by eliminating the cords required by current devices. The use of fabric was also important in the social shaping of the device; fabric was perceived as more comfortable and homey than the metal, plastic and wires that comprise current machines.

Focusing first on the bellyband, participants from all groups highlighted how the device supported birth processes by allowing the woman in labour to move around. A birth partner exemplified this view when he said, "If you're going to give birth, it's so much easier and nicer if you can move. There's exercises you can do to ease our pain, to help the baby move down. There's all kinds of things you can do and if you're attached to a bed, you can't. So, it's a huge deal." Or as a doula noted, "I like the fact that one is wire-free, and it allows the mother mobility. So, that would be the plus for me. That she can finally walk around." For users, the wireless feature of the bellyband created a patient who could move, which in turn supported women as they laboured to give birth. This emphasis on movement is part of a larger cultural fascination with and positive valuation of mobility (Salazar and Smart 2011). In the 21st century, mobility has become an organising metaphor for contemporary life (Cresswell 2006, Urry 2007).

The use of soft fabrics was important in imagining the mobile woman. Fabric samples were distributed in focus groups to get user feedback on the types of qualities needed in the fabric (e.g. breathable, soft). As participants looked at prototypes of the bellyband and touched fabric samples, they repeatedly used the words "comfortable" to describe the combination of wireless and soft fabrics. Across participants, a soft fabric that allowed people to move evoked ease and comfort.

A majority of participants in all stakeholder groups agreed that the more functions that could be included in the bellyband, the better. Although recognising the scientific and design challenges, such an aim may represent, most participants spoke of the need to include maternal heart rate, foetal heart rate, foetal contractions and baby movement in the bellyband. The key reason for this was to decrease the number of machines attached to women in labour. As one doula noted, "Get rid of the finger monitor. Get rid of all that. As many wires as you can remove is great and that one is a biggie." Or as a doctor said, "If the smart people who were working on this, engineers and everybody, if they could just figure out a way to have maternal pulse that transmits to the same external hub, that would kind of solve that whole problem of letting mom move and also knowing what the maternal heart rate is. I don't know how that plays into what we're monitoring on the band but that would be a good solution." In the aim of eliminating machines and cords, the integration of more surveillance and monitoring was encouraged to increase a woman's ability to move.

Participants' enthusiasm for the bellyband was generated in part by comparing it to their experiences with existing machines. In the US, routine pregnancies, not just births perceived as risky, are monitored with foetal heart rate monitors and uterine contraction monitors during labour and birth in hospital settings (Davis-Floyd 2004, Lothian 2014). Participants were well aware of this, expressing frustration about how the devices "tether" labouring women. Exemplifying this point, a doctor described the potential of the bellyband, noting that, "It's great that the patients are not tethered to the unit anymore because a lot of patients feel like they're stuck in the bed and can't move around, can't use the bathroom. They constantly need a nurse to get unplugged and get re-plugged in to have the monitors refocus on the baby again. It's just a big headache so it would be great to kind of get to end all that." Further exemplifying this emphasis on tethering, a nurse explained how women in labour are "strapped to the monitor. I think this technology would be more comfortable because they wouldn't have two huge bulky ultrasound pieces on them. They wouldn't be tethered with wires to a box." Comfortable and uncomfortable were two metaphors of contrast. Across all focus groups, participants described the smart textiles as "comfortable" and contrasted these devices with the current machines, which are "uncomfortable."

In addition to the language of tethering, participants used language like "tied down" or "restrictive" to describe current systems of monitoring. A midwife stated, for example, "If the mom is stuck in a bed, stuck to a machine, you feel like you're tied down." Further illustrating this view, a doula explained that current technologies have a "restrictive nature. Like they hold the mom – it, it makes her feel very restricted, in movement. it just creates a little distress for mom." For participants, being "tethered" to machines and cords confined or bound women in labour and, as some described it, turned them into what looked like a "science experiment."

Dispensing with the cords and using clothing as the technology form were equally important in imagining the babyband's use. The babyband consistently evoked a positive, visceral reaction as participants imagined a baby in cloth instead of hooked up to wires and machines in the NICU. The picture of the baby in the babyband pajamas (see above) elicited a strong positive emotional response, in the form of many non-lexical "oohs" and "aahs". Participants imagined the baby being able to move freely and to be touched more easily without the encumbrance of cords. A quote by a doula illustrates the enthusiastic response from participants. She exclaimed, "It allows mobility for the baby. It's just wonderful. Great idea." As with the bellyband, the babyband offered the possibility of a hospital experience that emphasised movement.

Resisting the expansion of monitoring into the home

Although participants were enthusiastic about the devices' use in hospitals, they overwhelmingly rejected the proposed expansion of monitoring into the home during routine pregnancies or a baby's first year or two of life. As noted earlier, the research team was interested in exploring potential users' perspectives on the bands' use at home. The portability of smart textile medical devices extends the possible reach of monitoring into pregnancy (not just the birth experience) by imagining 24 h use throughout pregnancy, not just at wellness or prenatal care visits or during the birth experience at hospitals. Similarly, the imagined use of the babyband extends the reach of infant monitoring into the first year or two of a child's life at home.

Participants' reaction to over-the-counter (OTC) products was loud and clear – many participants groaned or sighed. The following quotes demonstrate the general reaction to OTC, extended use of bellybands and babybands. "Sounds horrible," said one midwife. "Big thumbs down," another stated. "Disaster," a doula noted.

Participants highlighted three main reasons for this position. First, across all groups, participants thought using the device at home without clinician oversight would increase prospective and current parents' anxiety. Drawing on her experience during pregnancy when she learned that it is normal for a foetus's heart rate to fluctuate, one recent mother noted, "If this is something that people are wearing all the time, is there going to be this increased panic that they're constantly seeing their baby's heart rates fluctuate, which is a normal thing, but we didn't know that because nobody was paying attention … if it is for a commercial market, if that is something – it's almost like those things that monitor the babies' breathing in their sleep. Like it's almost too much information."

Another mother highlighted how the OTC babyband would increase the anxiety or what she called "the crazy." She noted, "It's only because it would make me crazy. And you're already sleep deprived. Information overload on top of that, and then you, I don't know that it would make me feel any better. I think that I would still check to see the technology was working, which is crazy too. Like, you're a little crazy when you're a new mom." Routine use of a babyband at home would intensify the already anxious experience of new parents.

Second, participants who worked in the health sector were concerned that OTC sales would create more work for clinicians who would get called when people thought there was an unusual reading. A doctor, for example, stated, "I don't really want to get calls from patients like, 'I'm on the monitor now and my baby's … ' It'll be just a lot of time." Further illustrating this point of view, another doctor said, "It opens up this Pandora's box. What are we going to do with all these patients that are calling in that they've done home monitoring and they're finding these findings?" Or as a doula explained, "People would buy this and go home. Using it improperly, they'd be running to emergency room or any of their doctors and calling us up. There are certain medical technologies that are meant to be operated by only medical people." Doctors, doulas, nurses and midwives were concerned that at home use would expand clinicians' workload to include responding to parents' responses to device output.

Finally, doctors, doulas, midwives and nurses emphasised that there is no medical evidence that monitoring would have any impact on pregnancy or infant outcomes. In their view, there is no medical reason for constant surveillance of routine pregnancies or healthy newborns. Illustrating this point of view, a doctor explained, "As an outpatient product, this would be terrible. Honestly that would be my opinion because patients always knowing more, especially when it's half knowledge, is never a good idea. It just leads to a lot more panic and a lot more monitoring for 9 months which helps nobody because more monitoring is not showing an improved outcome. It just increases intervention."

Although participants wholeheartedly rejected at home, OTC use, participants across all user groups were interested in bellybands and babybands that could be prescribed by a clinician and then taken home for use when warranted. Exemplifying the support for the use of the babyband at home *with a clinician's prescription*, one birth partner explained that he preferred, "a prescribed take-home situation, where you know, you went home after the hospital and you needed to have more-more anything, more monitoring. Then that would be nice to take home with you rather than having to go back, or worse, leave the baby there for monitoring." In all, participants accepted home use when there was the provision of medical oversight and evidence of impact.

The contemporary contours of medicalisation

The smart textile design of both the bellyband and babyband offers an opportunity to think about contemporary configurations of medicalisation, the increasing tendency to define mental, physical and emotional processes as diseases (Bell and Figert 2012, Busfield 2017, Clarke *et al.* 2003, Conrad 2007). Medicalisation pathologises processes previously considered normal, and thereby increases the scope for medical knowledge and practice to intervene in everyday life (Zola 1972). This trend has positive aspects, such as potentially destigmatising behaviours previously thought to be under one's personal control and choices (e.g. addiction) (Lupton 1997). Yet, this move has also been criticised because it transforms life processes previously considered normal, such as shyness or ageing, into medical diseases in need of treatment and management.

Birth has been highly medicalised in contemporary medicine (Barker 1998, Oakley 1984, Riessman 1983). As an example of medicalisation, routine births that could potentially take place in homes at low cost are transformed into expensive, risky practices that are managed by medical professionals in hospitals (Davis-Floyd 2004, Martin 1987, Morris 2013, Rosenthal 2013). Surveillance, via monitoring, is an important way that medical management is enacted (Armstrong 1995). The development of smart textiles fit into an already established practice of monitoring labour, birth and infants (Burton-Jeangros 2011). Defining most births as at-risk and most pregnant women as at-risk bodies co-produces technologies, such as smart textiles, as the best approach to manage this risk. Analysis of participants' responses to smart textiles brings six insights about the contemporary practice of medicalisation forward.

First, smart textiles change the delivery and experience of medicalisation by transforming the monitoring devices from machines recognised as clinical or medical into devices that participants repeatedly described as comfortable or cozy. The following quotes illustrate this way of understanding the design and use of the bellyband and babyband. A woman who recently gave birth, for example, noted, "It's more comfortable if you can move. I mean, that's the big thing." A birth partner explained that the bellyband is "more comfy for the baby." Or, as a doula noted, "It's cozy."

Participants repeatedly discussed how the wireless clothing design of the bellyband and the babyband made monitoring seem less medical. Exemplifying this point, a birth partner noted, "You still feel like you have something on that is, you know you have something on, but it doesn't feel like medical, like old school medical equipment. Like this feels like light and new and, you know, not invasive." Or, as a woman who recently gave birth noted, "This feels much less clinical than having things stuck to you." The social shaping of the technology, and by extension monitoring, as comfortable and cozy reconfigures the experience of medicalisation in medical practice.

With the arrival of smart textiles, surveillance, which is an important element of medicalisation, takes on a friendly, even intimate form. Cozy medicalisation, or monitoring via fabrics, facilitates the possibility of touch, skin to skin contact and activities like bathing. Illustrating the emphasis on intimacy, when shown the bellyband, a doula stated, "My initial, like visceral, reaction was like, aw that's so much nicer. Like, it feels like a hug." Another doula explained, "It [the bellyband] looks reassuring, nurturing." Transforming monitoring from an activity perceived as medical to one that "feels like a hug" or is perceived as "nurturing" recasts surveillance medicine into a friendly, familiar practice – the line between medical and non-medical is blurred.

Second, participants highlighted how smart textiles had the potential to transform hospital experiences into ones that they described as more "natural," "normal" and "human." Throughout the study, participants articulated what may initially seem like a contradictory claim – that use of smart textiles might allow for a natural birth. A birth partner, for example, explained, "That's really nice … if there's a way to not be attached to cords, you know, because my wife was pretty much attached to the bed for 36 h through cords. It sucked super bad. If you're having a natural birth you're not going to be attached to anything, which was our goal, you know, to not be hooked up to a bunch of monitors and tubes and whatever. So this would be a really nice solution for people to not have, you know, if it's like a normal birth. One less wire." In this example, the appearance of a "natural" birth is achieved through the lack of visible cords and machines. The invisibility and intimacy of smart textiles is crucial to this achievement.

Participants also emphasised how the babyband's design made the device and the experiences of seeing a baby in the NICU seem more human and normal. Exemplifying this point of view, a doula noted, "Having a onesie on a baby who is in the hospital being monitored for whatever reason just feels so much more dignified to me, keeping them warm, making them feel more like a baby." A woman who recently gave birth explained, "It [the babyband] normalises it. It brings less stress. It looks homey." As with the bellyband, the babyband's design transformed the practice of monitoring from a medical one to one that, according to participants, allowed the infant to look more like a baby. Technological mediation, in other words, when enacted as wireless clothing, reconfigured the image of babies in the NICU as human instead of, as one participant described it, as "a test."

Third, user input pushed the technology away from the medical/clinical into a device that evokes the everyday and mundane. Across all groups, participants insisted that the designers stay away from white, pink or blue. Instead, they suggested providing a variety of colours such as purple, sage green, and turquoise. Clarke *et al.* (2003) show how multiple actors and factors participate in medicalisation processes. In this study, patients and medical professionals encouraged the use of colourful fabrics instead of colours that recreate the appearance of a medical device or stereotypical colours associated with gender. In their discussion of fabric choices, participants thus reinforce the blurring of what is perceived as medical/clinical and as everyday/mundane. Fashion designers are key actors in this process. Their involvement in research and development initiated the discussion of colours and fabrics as part of the devices' design. As new actors in processes of medicalisation, they are shaping its contemporary contours.

Fourth, in the US, where this study took place, the turn to what I call cozy or comfortable medicalisation is consistent with broader trends in hospital care in which hospitals are designed to be more homelike. In the US, design practices highlight how what is perceived as medical or signals illness should be kept hidden (Less 2004). Natural lighting and other features of homes are integrated and encouraged in hospital clinics (Moon *et al.* 2017, Siddiqui *et al.* 2015). This is part of a broader move to conceptualise patients as consumers, and it is often done under the banner of patient-centred care (Bromley 2012). The belly and baby bands fit into the hospital as homelike paradigm by being comfortable, intimate and small even as they gather and transmit an array of information that links patients to hospital data systems. Although part of the "datafication of health," the design, size and appearance of smart textiles transforms the experience of being monitored and surveilled into one that is perceived as creating a more "normal" and "natural" experience of birth (Ruckenstein and Schull 2017). The development of smart textile medical devices mirrors the shift from the hospital as clinical, beige/neutral colours, and a temple of science to one that is intimate, colourful and homelike – in this setting, technologies become invisible and integrated at the same time.

Fifth, the transformation of monitoring medical devices into cozy or comfortable ones meant that very few participants challenged the medicalisation of pregnancy and birth. Doulas, the professionals one might think as most likely to challenge these trends given their role as advocates for pregnant women, were the most concerned that monitoring is overused in the US. As one doula explained, "They're very overused. That's one of my only issues with potentially endorsing a new technology is that they are so overused. But, there will always be the women who do need them, so there is going to have to be some kind of technology. My only concern about this being easier and more convenient, is it will continue to be overused ... I think that the research is pointing towards higher C sections, because of the overuse of the monitor, more so than inductions and all the other things that woman have been concerned about." This viewpoint was a minority one in this study.

Finally, although most participants embraced the new delivery forms of medicalisation that smart textiles offered in the hospital, these same participants resisted the potential expansion of medicalisation and surveillance into new domains. The encroachment of monitoring during routine pregnancies and early childhood is not new (Barker 1998, Martin 1987). In the US and UK, for example, health care professionals have tried to expand the time period of a healthy pregnancy from 9 months of medical surveillance to include what is called preconception care, that is, the cultivation of conditions and behaviours related to having a healthy baby throughout a woman's reproductive years (CDC 2006). In the US, some health care professionals have tried to expand the time period women are under maternity care from 9 to 12 months by creating the category of "zero trimester" to describe the 3 months prior to becoming pregnant (Waggoner 2017).

Devices that monitor newborns are also available in the OTC consumer marketplace. In addition to OTC foetal heart monitors, two US companies offered textile baby monitors – the Owlet and Mimo – in 2015 (McRobbie 2014). The Owlet's smart sock aims to monitor a baby's heart rate and oxygen levels. Mimo is a bodysuit that aims to track infants' respiration, heart rate, skin temperature, sleep quality and position. Both devices (initially sold for approximately USD $200 and $300, respectively) send information to parents' smart phones so that parents can track an infant from a distance. These OTC devices take advantage of the belief that constant monitoring will lead to changes in health outcomes, even though there is little evidence to suggest this. Although marketing materials make it clear that the devices will not prevent sudden infant death syndrome, the manufacturers of baby monitors take advantage of first time parents' anxiety about parenting in general and baby's breathing patterns, offering the belief that they are doing something to take care of their child. The devices are sold over the counter and therefore do not need the US Food and Drug Administration (USFDA) approval, making it easier for manufacturers to bring such products to market.

Although the bellyband and babyband hold the possibility of joining the two smart textile markets (OTC and Rx), participants resisted this move. Drawing on personal experiences with birth and infants as well as use of OTC monitoring devices, participants pushed back on what

Natasha Schull (2016) calls "data for life." For Schull (2016, p.319), data for life are "a related, complimentary response to the notion that we are all potentially sick in which wellness depends on the continuous collection, analysis and management of personal data through digital sensor technologies." Health, no longer simply the state of being free of disease, has become something that must be monitored and cultivated (Dumit 2012). The availability and use of health tracking digital devices is increasing as more people monitor their mental, emotional and bodily processes (Lupton 2013a,b, Neff and Nafus 2016). Although the portability and design of smart textiles offer the potential of joining these two markets, participants greatly resisted this move, challenging the wisdom of the further production of anxious parents, an increased workload for clinicians and interventions that had no evidence of positive impact on outcomes.

Conclusion

Analysis of potential users' views of two technologies in the making contributes to the sociological literature on digital health. Smart textiles change the delivery and experience of medicalisation because, when the medical device is woven into clothes, the technology becomes perceived as invisible, mundane and familiar. This change, from clinical, plugged-in machine to familiar/clothing, blurs the line between hospital/medicine and home/daily life. In this blurring, smart textiles become a "cozy" or "comfortable" form of medicalisation. In this study, users overwhelmingly liked the way smart textiles removed cords, promoted women and infants' ability to move and enabled the ability to make skin-to-skin contact with babies in the NICU. The product design transforms the act of surveillance into a friendly form of surveillance that recasts medical monitoring as a familiar, more natural process.

The smart textile medical devices discussed in this study illuminate a broader turn to the homelike hospital in which technologies perceived as medical are pushed into the back stage and are "hidden from view" (Bromley 2012, p.1060; see also Less 2004, Sloan 1994, Suess and Mody 2017). Smart textile medical devices are the technology exemplar that illustrates the transformation of hospitals into homelike, and at times even hotel like, spaces (Moon *et al.* 2017, Siddiqui *et al.* 2015). Smart textile medical devices are perceived as comfortable, intimate and cozy, which in turn fit in with the broader project of homelike hospitals. Cozy medicalisation and friendly surveillance mark new configurations of these processes that sociologists must attend to in order to better understand the politics of medical practice in a digital era.

The imagined use of smart textiles throughout pregnancy and during the first year or two of a child's life holds the potential to extend medicalisation to new processes of life (the duration of pregnancy and early childhood) and new sites (the home). Although there have already been moves in this direction (e.g. OTC foetal monitors, the zero trimester), smart textiles would add to the monitoring of daily life. Smart textiles hold the potential to become another lifestyle technology used in the optimisation of life or the practices of the worried well (Dumit 2012, Schull 2016). In this study, participants overwhelmingly rejected the extension of monitoring into OTC devices for use at home, noting that it would add to the production of anxious parents and that it would create more work for medical professionals. Given the profitability of OTC markets, it is not clear that participants' concerns about home use will drive innovation and use.

The smart textile field is in formation, sitting at the crossroads of fields such as engineering, computer science and fashion. It is a hybrid technology that through its design and use blurs boundaries between the medical and the non-medical, potentially extending the reach of medicalisation into more contours of daily life. The move to smart textile medical devices also opens up the possibility of the creation of big data about patients' bodies and lives. Although companies with OTC devices are aware of the big data potential in terms of sales and revenues, academic research teams focus primarily on identifying the fabric, engineering and computer science innovations needed to measure what they hope to measure. Future research should follow smart textiles in the digital health arena to investigate how and when they become part of data analytics. Future research should also take up smart textiles' use in locations outside the US that have different birthing traditions, systems of device regulation and health care financing to better understand how digital health and medical practice are co-produced in particular and varied contexts.

Address for correspondence: Kelly Joyce, Sociology Department, Center for Science, Technology & Society, Drexel University, Philadelphia, PA 19106, USA.
E-mail: kaj68@drexel.edu

Acknowledgements

This material is based upon work supported by the United States National Science Foundation under grant no. 1430212. I would like to thank the anonymous referees, Susan Bell, Ann Jurecic, Laura Mamo, Susan Sidlauskas and participants in Rutgers University-New Brunswick's Medical Humanities Seminar for their thoughtful comments on earlier versions of this study.

References

Armstrong, D. (1995) The rise of surveillance medicine, *Sociology of Health & Illness*, 17, 3, 393–404.
Barker, K. (1998) A ship upon a stormy sea: the medicalization of pregnancy, *Social Science & Medicine*, 47, 8, 1067–76.
Bell, S. and Figert, A. (2012) Medicalisation and pharmaceuticalization at the intersections: looking backward, sideways and forward, *Social Science & Medicine*, 75, 5, 775–83.
Bromley, E. (2012) Building patient-centeredness: hospital design as an interpretative act, *Social Science & Medicine*, 75, 6, 1057–66.
Burton-Jeangros, C. (2011) Surveillance of risks in everyday life: the agency of pregnant women and its limitations, *Social Theory & Health*, 9, 4, 419–36.
Busfield, J. (2017) The concept of medicalisation reassessed, *Sociology of Health & Illness*, 39, 5, 759–74.
Centers for Disease Control and Prevention (CDC) (2006) Recommendations to improve preconception health and health care—United States. *MMWR Recommendations and Reports*, 55, RR-06, 1–23.
Clarke, A.E., Fosket, J.R., Mamo, L., Shim, J., *et al.* (2003) Biomedicalisation: theorizing technoscientific transformations of health, illness, and U.S. biomedicine, *American Sociological Review*, 68, 161–94.
Conrad, P. (2007) *The Medicalisation of Society*. Baltimore: John Hopkins University Press.
Cresswell, T. (2006) *On the Move: Mobility in the Modern Western World*. New York, NY: Routledge.
Davis-Floyd, R. (2004) *Birth as as American Rite of Passage*. Berkeley: University of California Press.
Dishman, L. (2015) Here's why you will be wearing 'smart' workout clothes soon, Forbes, September 11
Dumit, J. (2012) *Drugs for Life: How Pharmaceutical Companies Define our Health*. Durham, NC: Duke University Press.
Epstein, S. (1996) *Impure Science: AIDS, Activism, and the Politics of Knowledge*. Berkeley, CA: University of California Press.
Gaddis, R. (2014) What is the future of fabric? These smart textiles will blow your mind, Forbes, May 7
Global Market Insights, Inc. (2017) *Smart Clothing Market Size By Product (T-shirts, Pants, Shoes, Undergarments, Jackets, Socks), By Application (Sports & Fitness, Healthcare, Military & Defense,*

Industrial, Entertainment), Industry Analysis Report, Regional Outlook (U.S., Canada, UK, Germany, France, Italy, France, China, Japan, South Korea, Australia, Brazil, Mexico), Growth Potential, Price Trends, Competitive Market Share & Forecast, 2017 – 2024. Selby, DE: Global Market Insights, Inc.

Joyce, K. (2006) From numbers to pictures: the development of magnetic resonance imaging and the visual turn in medicine, *Science as Culture*, 15, 1, 1–22.

Kline, R. and Pinch, R. (1996) Users as agents of technological change: the social construction of the automobile in the rural United States, *Technology and Culture*, 37, 4, 763–95.

Less, F. (2004) *If Disney Ran Your Hospital: 91/2 Things You Would Do Differently*. Bozeman, MT: Second River Health care Press.

Lothian, J. (2014) Healthy birth practice #4: avoid interventions unless they are medically necessary, *Journal of Perinatal Education*, 23, 4, 198–206.

Lupton, D. (1997) Foucault and the medicalisation critique. In Petersen, A. and Bunton, R. (eds) *Foucault, health and medicine*. New York: Routledge.

Lupton, D. (2013a) The digitally engaged patient: self-monitoring and self-care in the digital health era, *Social Theory and Health*, 11, 3, 256–70.

Lupton, D. (2013b) Quantifying the body: monitoring and measuring health in the age of mHealth technologies, *Critical Public Health*, 23, 4, 393–403.

Martin, E. (1987) *The Woman in the Body: A Cultural Analysis of Reproduction*. Boston, MA: Beacon Press.

McRobbie, L. (2014) Selling fear: smart monitors cannot protect babies from SIDS, so what are they tor?, Slate, February 18.

Moon, L., Nebby, C. and Stanton, B. (2017) Making hospitals feel more like home, Iowa Public Radio, July 12

Morris, T. (2013) *Cut it Out: The C-Section Epidemic in America*. New York: New York University Press.

Morton, C. and Clift, E. (2014) *Birth Ambassadors: Doulas and the Re-Emergence of Woman-Supported Birth in America*. Amarillo: Praeclarus Press.

Neff, G. and Nafus, D. (2016) *Self-Tracking*. Cambridge, MA: MIT Press.

Oakley, A. (1984) *The Captured Womb*. Oxford: Blackwell.

Oudshoorn, N. and Pinch, T. (eds) (2003) *How Users Matter: The Co-Construction of Users and Technology*. Cambridge, MA: MIT Press.

Research Nester. (2017) Smart Clothing Market: Global Demand Analysis & Opportunity Outlook 2024. https://www.researchnester.com/reports/smart-clothing-market-global-demand-analysis-opportunity-outlook-2024/444

Riessman, C.K. (1983) Women and medicalization: a new perspective, *Social Policy*, 14, 1, 3–18.

Rosenthal, E. (2013) Paying until it hurts: cash on delivery, New York Times, June 30

Ruckenstein, M. and Schull, N. (2017) The datafication of health, *Annual Review of Anthropology*, 46, 261–78.

Ryan, S. (2014) *Garments of Paradise: Wearable Discourse in the Digital Age*. Cambridge, MA: MIT Press.

Salazar, N. and Smart, A. (2011) Anthropological takes on (im)mobility: an introduction. *Identities: Global Studies in Culture and Power*, 18, 6, https://doi.org/10.1080/1070289X.2012.683674.

Schull, N. (2016) Data for life: wearable technology and the design of self-care, *BioSocieties*, 11, 3, 317–33.

Siddiqui, Z.K., Zuccarelli, R., Durkin, N., Wu, A.W., *et al.* (2015) Changes in patient satisfaction related to hospital innovation: experience with a new clinical building, *Journal of Hospital Medicine*, 10, 3, 165–71.

Sloan, D. (1994) Scientific paragon to hospital mall: the evolving design of the hospital, 1885-1994, *Journal of Architectural Education*, 48, 2, 82–98.

Suess, C. and Mody, M. (2017) Hospitality healthscapes: a conjoint choice modeling approach to understanding patient responses to hotel-like hospital rooms, *International Journal of Hospitality Management*, 61, 59–72.

Syduzzaman, P., Farhanaz, K. and Ahmed, S. (2015) Smart textiles and nano-technology: a general overview, *Journal of Textile Science and Engineering*, 5, 181.

Urry, J. (2007) *Mobilities*. Malden, MA: Polity Press.

Waggoner, M. (2017) *The Zero Trimester: Pre-Pregnancy Care and the Politics of Reproductive Risk*. Berkeley, CA: University of California Press.

Want, R., Schilit, B. and Jenson, S. (2015) Enabling the internet of things, *Computer*, 48, 1, 28–35.

Zola, I. (1972) Medicine as an institution of social control, *American Sociological Review*, 20, 487–504.

Sociology of Health & Illness Vol. 41 No. S1 2019 ISSN 0141-9889, pp. 162–175
doi: 10.1111/1467-9566.12870

'Built for expansion': the 'social life' of the WHO's mental health GAP Intervention Guide

China Mills[1] and Eva Hilberg[2]

[1]*School of Health Sciences, City, University of London, London, UK*
[2]*Sheffield Institute for International Development, University of Sheffield, Sheffield, UK*

Abstract   The focus of this study is the WHO's mhGAP-Intervention Guide (mhGAP-IG) 2.0 (2016), an evidence-based tool and guideline to help detect, diagnose and manage the most common mental disorders, designed for use by non-specialists globally but particularly in low- and middle-income countries. This research is a starting point in tracing the multiple 'doings' of mhGAP-IG – connecting questions of how it is 'done' and what does it 'do' – to the living histories and wider global mental health assemblages that make the tool possible and shape its global circulation. We examine the conditions of possibility that produce and legitimate mhGAP-IG, and the ways these are 'black boxed' through casting mhGAP-IG in technical rather than epistemological terms. The study illuminates how its explicit design for global expansion positions mhGAP-IG as open to questioning from those who are technical 'insiders' and setting the epistemological parameters of its own critique. It analyses mhGAP-IG as an 'inscription device' that inscribes and materialises algorithmic imaginaries of mental health that impact on design and local implementation. This study is one attempt at initiating dialogue with the WHO from perspectives and methodological approaches not usually included in the conversation.

Keywords: mental health and illness, public health, sociology of scientific knowledge, ethnography

Introduction

The World Health Organization's (WHO) (2008) Mental Health Gap Action Programme (mhGAP) aims to mitigate the 'treatment gap' between need for mental health interventions and availability of specialist care especially in low- and middle-income countries (LMICs). A key component in closing this gap is the WHO's mhGAP-Intervention Guide (mhGAP-IG), developed in 2010 as 'a simple tool to help detect, diagnose and manage the most common mental, neurological, and substance (MNS) use disorders' (Department of Mental Health and Substance Abuse, WHO 2011: 2), specifically addressing non-specialist audiences (i.e. doctors, nurses, other health workers, without mental health specialism, as well as health planners and managers, WHO 2016). The Guide is now in version 2.0 (2016) and is also available as a smartphone application (app) (e-mhGAP).

Digital Health: Sociological Perspectives, First Edition.
Edited by Flis Henwood and Benjamin Marent.

The WHO describes the mhGAP-IG as 'an evidence-based technical tool aimed at supporting non-specialised healthcare providers to redistribute clinical tasks previously reserved for mental health specialists' (WHO 2017a: 75). mhGAP-IG is an evidence-based guideline using an algorithmic protocol designed for 'streamlined and simplified clinical assessment', where one moves through a flowchart of questions, eliciting yes or no answers from the person interviewed, with the input of answer they give determining the next questions asked (from a predetermined list) (WHO 2016). The IG is part of a larger portfolio of products including training materials and implementation and operations manuals (WHO 2015: 13).

The choice to focus on mhGAP-IG in this study lies in its global significance, evident in the fact that the 'first mhGAP-IG was used in over 80 countries and translated into more than 20 languages' (Keynejad *et al.* 2017: 1). mhGAP-IG is the 'principal clinical tool being used as part of the scaling up strategy of the mhGAP programme in countries', and provides 'a definitive platform to define "what" should be scaled up' (Dua *et al.* 2011: 9). The IG is framed as providing 'the ingredients for scaling up mental health services in LMICs' (Petersen *et al.* 2011: 319) – a 'robust foundation for scaling up by answering the key question of what should be scaled up' (Patel 2012: 8). Some argue that the mhGAP-IG 'should become the standard approach for all countries and health sectors' (Patel *et al.* 2011: 1442).

As algorithmic tools become an increasingly common state of the art (see Jasovic-Gasic *et al.* 2013), and given the global significance of the mhGAP-IG, it is important to question the conditions of production of these tools and guidelines, their underlying theories and assumptions about mental health, and how the kinds of knowledge that they create have implications for the governance and experience of mental health globally. According to the WHO the development of mhGAP is seen as an iterative process and feedback is encouraged. This study is then one attempt at initiating dialogue with the WHO from perspectives and methodological approaches not usually included in the conversation. This study aims to extend and somewhat disrupt the 'official' story that is told by the WHO about mhGAP-IG by making a first step in tracing its 'social life'.

Methodology: the 'social life' of mhGAP-IG

This study is an early stage in a larger research project documenting how the mhGAP-IG is 'done' in multiple sites by different actors who coalesce around the guidelines, from crafting its design to implementing in the field. Our methodological approach traces the social life of the mhGAP-IG, building upon ethnographic work into quantification (Merry 2016), medical technologies (Hardon and Moyer 2014) and pharmaceuticals (Ecks and Basu 2009). We understand the mhGAP-IG as a culturally constituted object, aiming to highlight it's conditions of its production as well as its 'social uses and consequences' (Whyte *et al.* 2003: 13 & 3).

The focus our research is the 'doing': (Mol, 2002) of mhGAP-IG – how is it 'done' and what does it 'do', particularly with regard to its design for global expansion. In this study, the 'doing' of mhGAP-IG is organised around an analysis of its contemporary and historical conditions of possibility; how it is made and how it is performed across different sites. Our analysis begins by focusing on the 'conditions of possibility' (a Foucauldian approach widely used in Critical Global Health, for example, by Bell (2017) to trace the history of evidence-based medicine [EBM]) of mhGAP. We explore the context in which mhGAP-IG developed and was made to make sense (i.e. conceptions of mental 'illness' as universal, commensurable and measurable; metrics that construct mental illness as chronic, disabling and burdensome but also as treatable; and technical conceptions of care).

We then give a detailed account of the methodological approach to the production of mhGAP-IG and the (partial) story behind its construction. We are interested in how the mhGAP-IG and e-mhGAP act as 'inscription devices' (Latour and Woolgar 1979), in the wider quantification of mental health, diverting attention from their material processes of production, and constituting 'the domains they appear to represent' (Rose 1999: 198). We aim to explore how mhGAP operates as part of 'the knowledge-power processes that inscribe and materialise the world in some forms rather than others' (Haraway 1997: 7), and makes possible certain understandings of mental health over others. The significance of this approach lies in making visible the 'black box' (Porter 1995) of the mhGAP-IG and its associated products, i.e. the social, cultural and political processes, that produce systems of classification but are often obscured in technical language (Mills and Hilberg 2018).

In talking about performance, our focus is on the 'doing' (Mol 2002) of the mhGAP-IG, and the ways the mhGAP-IG 'does' mental health (e.g. as 'illness'). This approach understands the mhGAP-IG as multiple, meaning that despite its algorithmic approach to decision-making, we are interested in how the guidelines are done differently in different contexts, and the alignments and contrasts between these different ways of doing. For example, how mhGAP-IG is done at the annual WHO Forums is different from how mhGAP-IG is done during implementation in one country to another, which is different again to how a government Ministry does mhGAP-IG. Our methodological approach in this study includes participant observation into the performative aspect of mhGAP, and specifically here, one of the author's attendance at the 2017 mhGAP Forum; ongoing discussion with some of the main architects of mhGAP-IG; and engagement with the extensive reports produced by international organisations.

Our focus on 'social life' extends to explore the historical and political forces that produce and legitimate mhGAP-IG. In this analysis we are interested in how the history of classification and quantification of mental health for international comparison 'lives' on (Stoler 2002) – shaping present algorithmic conceptualisations of mental health. In doing this, the study draws upon postcolonial analysis of quantification and technology (Appadurai 1993) and Haraway's (1997) feminist technoscience, aiming to situate the knowledge that has made mhGAP-IG possible and to show how this knowledge risks displacing other situated knowledges about mental distress. Situating the mhGAP-IG in this way contrasts with WHO framings of it as universal, where design is explicitly for global expansion.

The mhGAP-IG does not operate in a vacuum and its historical conditions of possibility are 'alive' in the present (Stoler 2002). Therefore, these histories and the wider global assemblage of mental health in which mhGAP is embedded are woven throughout the analysis, which focuses on how mhGAP-IG is made and how it is performed across different sites. Our analysis and findings are organised as follows: first, we set the scene with a foundational condition of possibility for mhGAP-IG – the construction of a 'treatment gap'; next, we detail the making of mhGAP-IG; we then explore the expansionary logic built into the tool; followed by tracing its living history; and analysing it as an 'inscription device', before we conclude.

Analysis and findings

The 'gap' in mhGAP

A key condition of possibility and a central narrative trope for the development of mhGAP and its products is the construction of a 'treatment gap'. A statistic illustrating this gap was oft repeated at the mhGAP Forum: That 45 per cent of the world's population lives in a country where there is less than 1 psychiatrist per 100,000 people (WHO Global Health Observatory Data 2014). The mhGAP programme's conception of the treatment gap relies on burden of disease metrics, and very frequently references them (see WHO 2015: 13, WHO 2018, 2008) as does glo-bal mental health literature (Lund *et al.* 2012: 1). This reifies Global Burden of Disease calcula-tions as an important 'rhetorical resource' within global (mental) health (Weisz *et al.* 2017: 520).

The statistical construction of a treatment gap enacts a performative function in spurring action (Applbaum 2015) and constructing a sense of urgency to close the 'gap'. For example, Dua *et al.* (2011) claimed that guidelines were 'urgently needed' to tackle the 'large treatment gap' (of around 75%) in LMICs. Metrics have been central in making visible and constructing the lack of availability of mental health care as a 'hidden emergency' (WHO 2009), where failure to act is framed as a 'failure of humanity' (Kleinman 2009). Thus, mhGAP mobilises a moral call for action made on the basis of a quantified notion of the scale of the 'problem', which has been hugely successful in increasing global visibility of mental health. The mhGAP-IG emerged as a solution to this 'emergency', a way for Governments, clinicians and others to 'act' on mental health to reduce the quantified burden. Partly made possible through metrics, the mhGAP-IG has since come to be used in the production of metrics, such as for economic modelling to highlight the economic burden of mental disorders and to make a case for 'return in investment' of interventions (Chisholm *et al.* 2016: 415, Summergrad 2016).

The underlying assumptions of mhGAP's 'treatment gap' have not gone without critique. Some critique the WHO's 'use of alarming statistics' as being too heavily biomedical and overly focused on 'treating individual conditions', paving 'the way for further medicalisation of global mental health' (UN Human Rights Council 2017: 5). Similarly, concerns have been raised that the mhGAP-IG disregards 'ongoing debate about the cross-cultural validity of psy-chiatric diagnoses' and suggests 'an overreliance on psychotropic medication' (White and Sashidharan 2014: 415); that it overlooks grass-roots approaches (Kirmayer and Pedersen 2014); and that it constructs mental health as being largely a technical problem of delivery of services (Applbaum 2015) – a 'problem' amenable to treatment using packages of care.

How mhGAP-IG was made

For many in our ongoing expert interviews and personal communication with some of the actors who crafted mhGAP-IG, the above arguments around cross-cultural validity of diagnosis had created stagnation within mental health governance. The idea of mhGAP-IG grew in oppo-sition to this nihilism – a practical response to show something could be done. The original Guideline Development Group for mhGAP-IG was formed in 2007, led by Shekhar Saxena (then Director of the Department of Mental Health and Substance Abuse, at the WHO). A grant was applied for to enable the Group to hold a workshop at the Rockefeller Foundation's Bellagio Center in Italy, and it was here, next to Lake Como, that ideas were 'hashed out' for the first IG (what would need to be done?; what format would it take?; who would be the audience?). The concept of task sharing (Hanlon *et al.*, 2016) was central throughout. The Group consisted of professionals who work in the field (including psychiatrists, psychologists and NGO representatives), but did not include services users. According to one of our expert interviews, the 'process was very congenial and collegial,' with a 'clear sense of cause, per-sonal relationships and friendship'. This workshop was then followed by larger workshops at the WHO, with Graham Thornicroft taking on leadership of the Guideline development, while Corrado Barbui led the systematic review process.

The methodological process of developing the original mhGAP guidelines is outlined in a number of places: an article by Dua *et al.* (2011) published in PLoS Medicine and widely cited; and in WHO documents (all available online through the WHO mhGAP Evidence Resource Cen-tre http://www.who.int/mental_health/mhgap/evidence/en/) (WHO 2009). The development of the mhGAP-IG firstly began with the identification of its 'priority conditions' – 'depression, schizophrenia and other psychotic disorders (including bipolar disorder), suicide prevention, epilepsy, dementia, disorders due to use of alcohol and illicit drugs, and mental disorders in children' (WHO 2009: 2). These were 'identified on the basis of high mortality and morbidity, high economic costs or association with violation of human rights within the area of MNS disorders' (WHO 2009: 2), showing the centrality of metrics to the development of mhGAP (Mills 2018).

The guidelines were 'based on systematic reviews of the best available evidence and consideration of values, preferences, and feasibility issues from an international perspective' (Dua *et al.* 2011: 2). This process exposed the fact that little evidence on mental health interventions was available from LMICs, in which cases 'new systematic reviews were commissioned' (WHO 2009: 5). Once the priority conditions were identified, the formulation of scoping questions began, in consultation with an international expert panel using the PICO framework (Population, Intervention, Comparator, Outcome, Time) (WHO 2009: 4). The evidence was then graded using the Grading of Recommendations Assessment, Development and Evaluation (GRADE) approach, which synthesises the scientific evidence on the effectiveness of clinical interventions (Dua *et al.* 2011, WHO 2009, 2015). GRADE methodology includes only data that meet specific predetermined scientific criteria (from systematic reviews and Randomised Control Trials [RCTs]). This means that smaller-scale qualitative data were excluded from the development of mhGAP-IG from the start (Cooper 2015). According to Cooper, who details the methodological development of the mhGAP-IG and explores its significance for African countries, the

> elision of more qualitative data has time and time again been shown to lead to misleading accounts that overlook certain crucial dimensions … [because] there may be potentially important aspects of the social world that cannot so easily be captured by the scientific processes of abstraction, reduction and standardisation and prediction. And yet these more qualitative 'things' end up being excluded or silenced within the current evidence-based edifice (Cooper 2015: 532–3).

Evidence-based medicine is a key condition of possibility for mhGAP-IG, meaning that debates about EBM are also applicable to the mhGAP-IG. Central to EBM and mhGAP-IG is the standardisation of decision-making processes (Timmermans and Berg 2003). This is linked to wider 'audit cultures' (Strathern 1992), where medical expertise is configured in statistical and epidemiological terms seen by some as a democratising force that remedies a growing distrust in professional opinion and autonomy (Bell 2017). Others point out that hierarchies of evidence established within EBM (and in the making of mhGAP-IG), with systematic reviews and RCTs seen as the gold standard and an emphasis on rationality, frame ways of conceiving of and doing health and care that are not amenable to being measured as 'irrational', thus discrediting and delegitimising them within global health (Bell 2017: 75). This is evident for the mhGAP guidelines, which Vikram Patel (a key figure in the Movement for Global Mental Health) says 'should become the standard approach for all countries and health sectors', meaning that 'irrational and inappropriate interventions should be discouraged and weeded out' (Patel *et al.* 2011: 1442). 'Irrational and inappropriate' here seems to mean those interventions lacking an evidence base as defined by the parameters of EBM, which conceptualises other frameworks as being 'non-scientific' in a hierarchy where biomedical and psychiatric knowledge is privileged (Mills 2014). The displacement of indigenous forms of healing as being 'irrational' was also a colonial strategy, for example in British colonised India, that occurred simultaneously alongside the recruitment, and co-option, of indigenous healers to extend public health strategies into rural areas (Khalid 2009). Thus, the logic of 'task-sharing' alongside conceptualisation of 'rationality' has a colonial history.

By setting the parameters of what counts as evidence, and not including users and survivors in the early formulation of mhGAP, the makers of mhGAP-IG craft the epistemological parameters of critique for the guidelines, excluding alternative conceptualisations from different worldviews of distress (such as different cultural understandings and/or user/survivor/Mad epistemologies) (LeBlanc and Kinsella 2016, Rose 2017, Russo and Sweeney 2016). Sociological research into the production of guidelines show that it is common for them to create their own parameters for debate, which often allow technical debate but no political debate (Timmermans and Berg 2003). This, alongside the technical accounts of how mhGAP-IG was made, risks positioning the mhGAP-IG as only open to questioning from those who are technical 'insiders'. This practice stands in contrast to the stated intentions of the WHO, where development of mhGAP is seen as an iterative process and where feedback is encouraged.

There are also critiques from within the methodological paradigm. Dua *et al.* identify a number of challenges in creating the guidelines, including no or very poor-quality evidence 'insufficient to make any recommendation', for example, this was the case for some psychosocial interventions (p. 2); and a majority of evidence from high-income countries, raising issues of applicability because of feasibility issues and lack of infrastructure. Dua *et al.* give the example that 'full cognitive behavioural therapy may be hardly feasible in many low- and middle-income settings considering the training, supervision and time needed for this intervention, and taking into consideration the need for local adaptations' (pp. 2–3).

The WHO's strong emphasis on evidence-based guidelines (Dua *et al.* 2011) means that the mhGAP-IG will undergo revisions every 5 years, hence the launch of version two of the guidelines in 2016 (WHO 2015). In 2015, a 'WHO mhGAP Guideline Update' was published and used to inform development of the mhGAP-IG version 2 (2016). The review of version 1.0 focused on evaluating the efficacy of different interventions, balancing evidence, for example, between drug-based treatments and psychosocial interventions. A number of changes were made: from more strongly emphasising the 'General principles of care', to the inclusion of more low-intensity psychological interventions (thanks to availability of more evidence). This links to a simultaneous increase in the evidence base around the implementation of mhGAP, especially through the PRIME (Programme for Improving Mental health carE) project (Lund *et al.* 2012).

Furthermore, the development of e-mhGAP (the app and increased online availability) impacted the structure of the second IG, leading to a change from a horizontal flowchart into a vertical decision-making model, which is more compatible with the format of smartphone apps. While this has the advantage of reducing printing costs and being easier to update, a vertical format impacts use through requiring the user to navigate the flowchart in a predetermined order, and thus is more prescriptive as to how it is administered.

Building mhGAP-IG for expansion

In October 2017, the ninth meeting of the mhGAP Forum took place at the WHO in Geneva, and was attended by China Mills. The Forums, and other such events, operate as a performative space where mhGAP is 'done', including providing an opportunity for those who use mhGAP products, including Member States and ambassadors, to network and to feedback to the WHO.

Multiple issues were discussed at the 2017 Forum, but for the purposes of this study, we will focus on two topics: the explicit rationality of expansion underlying the development of mhGAP and its link to digitisation, and the tension between the local and global enacted at the Forum. The 2017 Forum saw the launch of the mhGAP-IG 2.0 app (e-mhGAP, WHO 2017c), alongside launching mhGAP Training Packages and an Operations Manual (WHO 2017a; see also Forum Report WHO 2017b). The app, like the mhGAP-IG, uses an assessment algorithm of yes/no answers to produce suggested treatment outcomes which vary from psychoeducation to psychopharmaceuticals. However, the app is not simply a digitised version of the IG, it also 'adds value' through a note taking and feedback function, which tracks previous answers, meaning it can be used as a learning tool and has the potential to link to electronic health records.

Digitisation was framed as a central issue at the Forum. Tarun Dua (a key figure in the design of the app at the WHO) emphasised the importance of digitisation of mhGAP products to reach more people. Similarly, Shekhar Saxena, in talking about 'the road ahead', emphasised the need for digitisation in 'every part of the world' so that e-mhGAP gives 'you the material you need to scale up mental health'. Dua explained that a complex design lies underneath the app's easy use, with a similar layout to the IG. She explained that the app is 'built for expansion'.

'Expansion' and 'scale' invoke a spatial orientation of mental health, where knowledge and practices are seen as extendable though a geographic plane. This expansionary logic has epistemological effects, shaping the idea of local context, the interaction between the global and the local, and impacts design. Designing mhGAP-IG for expansion necessarily requires the decontextualisation and simplification (Lingard 2011, Merry 2016) of mental health, framed as largely universal and commensurable, in order for the guidelines to travel. Building for expansion also means that more contextualised 'local' interventions that are not as amenable to being 'scaled up' are somehow made not to count (even though they may be more effective) (Bell 2017).

At the Forum, implementation and training were conceived as key to expansion, with pre-publication Operations Manuals given out to attendees, showing step-by-step implementation of mhGAP-IG. The guidelines cover the assembly of mhGAP, including forming an operations team, carrying out situational analysis, planning and budgeting, and templates for plans are included. There is an expectation in the Manual that components will need 'adapting' to local contexts, including translation, and many of the tools are described as being 'adaptable'. Tarun Dua explained that a key feature of this process is that trainers can choose modules depending on local relevance and context. The Forum was also the stage for the launch of new Training Manuals – Training of Trainers and Supervisors (ToTS) and Training of Health-Care Providers (WHO 2017a). The WHO provides extensive and comprehensive training materials for the mhGAP-IG, all available online for free. These materials include: session-by-session outlines for a full week's training, each including learning outcomes, activities and evaluation exercises; powerpoints and videos; and pre- and post-training multiple choice questions for assessment.

The ToTS manual states: 'When adapting the ToTS training to local context, care should be taken to avoid adding or removing slides, eliminating activities or interactive components, or removing the opportunities for participants to practise these skills' (WHO 2017a: 6). Although we cannot know from the manuals how training takes place in practice (and indeed this would make for fascinating ethnographic research into another component of mhGAP-IG's social life), local context is acknowledged as a matter of translation and having a choice between predetermined training components (although not adding and removing slides in training activities). There is, however, a growing literature documenting the development of country-specific versions of mhGAP-IG, where the guidelines are seen as a 'generic template that requires adaptation and contextualisation to suit the particular needs of the health system in a given country' (Abdulmalik et al. 2013 on implementation in Nigeria). Much of this conceives of local context through differing organisation of health systems, availability of resources and different models of training. However, this literature and WHO training manuals do not tend to conceive of how localised understandings and practice might disrupt or question the underlying logic and epistemology of universal tools such as the mhGAP products. Kenneth Maes (2017) documents similar cultural models of training practices within Africa's AIDS industry, where well-intentioned programmes provide narrow training (often through manuals providing detailed 'scripted minutiae') in 'technical forms of care' and interpersonal skills that risk reorienting localised forms of care to more clinical conceptions (76–7) and that overlook 'the political economies that shape the global health industry' (72).

Expansion was mentioned throughout the Forum, showing the WHO's long-term ambition in terms of the globalisation of mental health services. Devora Kestel (Unit Chief for Mental Health and Substance Use, at the Pan American Health Organisation and the WHO) talked about mhGAP training in the Americas, and the 'gradual expansion' in Central America as the region adopts mhGAP as a key strategy. E-learning has been helpful to reach islands with limited resources, and a mental health 'virtual clinic' is under development. A key objective of this work is to 'identify, diagnose and treat' MNS because 'mhGAP trainees need to develop diagnostic skills based on ICD 10' (Kestel, WHO mhGAP Forum 2017; see also Forum Report WHO 2017b).

The living history of mhGAP-IG
mhGAP-IG is based on the WHO's International Classification of Diseases (ICD-10), now in its 11th version. Discussion of the social life of psychiatric classificatory systems (how they are made and how they circulate) is important because these criteria are programmed into and performed globally through diagnostic algorithms, such as mhGAP-IG, and are thus key conditions of possibility. While diagnosis through mhGAP-IG is predetermined by an algorithm, it is also likely a fluid social process (Nissen and Risør 2018) that is 'done' differently in different contexts. However fluid, diagnostic texts have global significance in setting the terms for debate and their creation has long created controversy over what gets included in the criteria and who gets to decide. This reflects both the social life of diagnostic texts and the 'importance of diagnosis to the governance of social and clinical life' (Pickersgill 2013: 521).

Up to its fifth version, the ICD was produced by the French Government, coming in its sixth revision to be published in 1948 by the newly formed WHO. Due to low rates of adoption outside of France, the WHO established a commission to put together ICD-8 – said to be the first symptom-based model of classification, and conceptualised as a public classification useful for epidemiological work to compare findings across countries through promoting uniformity in usage (Fulford and Sartorius 2009). The nomenclature from ICD-8 was adopted by the American Psychiatric Association (APA) in the Diagnostic and Statistical Manual of Mental Disorders (DSM) II, replacing earlier psychodynamic and theoretical frameworks.

The aim to 'improve the comparability of statistical information about rates of mental disorder between different parts of the world' (Fulford and Sartorius 2009: 39) was written into the ICD from an early stage. But further homogenisation of reporting systems and evaluation was seen as necessary. The APA, after much publicised critique of DSM I and II, set up a taskforce – headed by Robert Spitzer – to create a radically different classification system – DSM III using rating scales and structured diagnostic interviews, specifically designed to systematise how people report 'symptoms', to enable commensurability between diagnosis in different contexts, and ultimately to make psychiatric decisions more data driven (Orr 2006: 226, Whooley 2017). Before his work on the DSM III, Robert Spitzer experimented with the computer simulation of psychiatric diagnosis, aiming to 'replicate in the realm of code' what clinicians practice daily, 'transforming mental disorders into patterns of information that can be manipulated by computer algorithms' and leading to the development of computerised diagnostic programmes: DIAGNO I, II and III (Orr 2006: 243–4).

DIAGNO was based not on a statistical model but on a logical decision-tree model, consisting of a series of true or false questions on a standardised interview scale (based on the Psychiatric Status Schedule), where the output is '1 of 25 standard APA diagnoses' (Spitzer and Endicott 1968: 747). Thus, from the 1970s onwards, the pressure to find ways for non-specialists to produce statistics for international comparison about mental disorder shaped the design of psychiatric nosology and classification systems (Orr 2006) and drove their increasing digitisation. Here, in DIAGNO, we can see an early predecessor of the WHO's mhGAP-IG, with its algorithmic decision-making models and management tools designed for use by trained non-specialists.

This shows that expansionary logic (including the conceptualisation of mental disorders as universal and the desirability of uniformity in usage globally) was built into diagnostic criteria from its early formulations, thus making mhGAP-IG thinkable and do-able. In fact, psychiatric classificatory systems, and the imaginary of what is now known as 'mental disorder' as being universal, date back further than the beginnings of the DSM, ICD and cybernetics. 'Colonial political arithmetic' (Appadurai 1993: 133) was a critical component of colonial biopolitics, where invasive investigations of poor people, 'lunatics' and criminals carried out domestically were transposed to whole populations of the colonies. More specifically, from censuses carried out in the USA in 1840 and in India in 1871, a colonial concern with calculating prevalence rates of insanity started to emerge. This provided in the US early claims of the statistical link between blackness and madness (Gilman 2004: 11), while in British-colonised India insanity was framed as an illness of civilisation, meaning India (whose population was understood by the colonisers to be uncivilised) had one-eighth the level of insanity of England and Wales (Sarin and Jain 2012). The measurement of mental health for purposes of international comparison, then, has a long and complex genealogy that links calculation and enumeration to domestic and colonial forms of governance. Here, it becomes apparent that not only do techniques quantifying mental health constitute that which they measure (Hacking 1982, 2006), enumerative logic also serves a justificatory role – justifying the colonial biopolitical logics and moral economies of the times in which the calculations occur.

This 'living' history of the conditions that make mhGAP-IG possible is significant to its social life, as it situates the guidelines within a long-articulated impetus to create data on mental health for international comparison that is written into contemporary global north understandings of what constitutes mental distress. This frames mhGAP-IG as only one of the most recent manifestations of a long-standing project aiming to develop a universalised understanding of mental health, to some extent questioning ways of talking about the globalisation of psychiatry, and algorithmic health interventions, as 'new' phenomena.

mhGAP-IG as an 'inscription device'

The above discussion of the historical and contemporary production of mhGAP-IG is significant to the ways mhGAP-IG operates as an 'inscription device'. For Latour and Woolgar (1979: 63) a feature of 'inscription devices' (in the laboratory) is that once the inscription has been produced (the end product) 'the intermediary steps which made its production possible are forgotten ... and the material processes which gave rise to it are either forgotten or taken for granted as being merely technical matters'. While mhGAP-IG is designed explicitly for use in non-laboratory contexts, we can see how once the 'inscription' (the diagnosis and resultant interventions) has been produced, the material processes of production that made the device possible (the controversial history of diagnostic criteria, the development of guidelines and the other factors documented above) are forgotten or seen only as technical matters. This contributes to the 'black boxing' – the rendering invisible and hence incontestable – of the complex array of judgments and decisions that go into the creation of classificatory systems and the data they produce (Porter 1995: 42). This makes the inscriptions of mhGAP-IG (its diagnoses and interventions) appear as facts that seem only open to challenge from technological insiders and inscribes subjective decisions and culturally specific rationalities of diagnostic criteria deeply into the project of global mental health. Also inscribed but rendered invisible are the discriminatory prejudices (ableism, classism, heterosexism, racism, sanism and sexism) themselves threaded deeply within the classificatory politics of diagnostic criteria (Fernando 2010, Metzl 2009, Ussher 2017). This process of black boxing should be of importance to the WHO as it goes against its stated aim of eliciting feedback for its mental health products.

The reconfiguring of epistemological issues as technical issues and related black boxing of mhGAP-IG is evident in Patel's identification of future 'roadblocks' for the guidelines, seen to 'lie on the path between knowing what works (as synthesised in the mhGAP-IG) and how it will be delivered 'to scale' – that is, to entire populations' (Patel 2012: 8). Here, it is taken for granted that mhGAP-IG provides the recipe for what works, shifting the debate to focus only on more seemingly technical questions of how to optimise the scale of implementation.

Black boxing also enables another key element in the production of mhGAP-IG to be side-lined – its funding architecture. The WHO acknowledges financial contributions in the development and production of the mhGAP-IG (2016) from a number of Governments, charitable organisations (such as Autism Speaks) and the corporation Syngenta (WHO 2016: vi). The intermingling of corporate interests and public health agenda setting is a marker of a number of global health programmes, as Sunder Rajan shows for example in the co-production of corporate value and public health knowledge through international clinical trials (Sunder Rajan 2017). Yet this merging of health, business and philanthropy, its impact on the development and use of technology in global mental health, and its multiple (and sometimes uneasy) effects has so far attracted minimal scholarly attention. A closer look at Syngenta's financial contribution to the mhGAP-IG reveals a complex relationship to the global mental health agenda. Syngenta is a Swiss biotechnology and agribusiness company owned by ChemChina. Syngenta has been widely critiqued for contributing to India's agrarian crisis through restrictive seed patenting practices, and to high rates of farmer suicides linked to debt (Münster 2015, Perspectives 2009). The corporate practices of Syngenta sit somewhat uneasily alongside their sponsorship of the WHO's World Suicide Prevention policies (WHO 2014) and of the mhGAP-IG – which includes suicide as one of its priority conditions and has management and prevention strategies written into its algorithm.

At the e-mhGAP app's launch at the Forum, the National Institute of Mental Health was acknowledged for providing technical and financial support, and Universal Doctor (a private health technology company based in Spain)[1] as the app developer. Here then not only does the app use global north diagnostic classifications but it is also developed using global north expertise in technological production. This is not an isolated case in the field of digital health, as most market leaders are based in the UK or US, and work in LMICs is often based on innovation in the global north.[2]

Conclusion: algorithmic inscriptions of global mental health

This short and partial journey through some aspects of the social life of the mhGAP-IG focused on how the tool was made, its sites of performance, its conditions of possibility and its living history. In tracing the living colonial history of mhGAP-IG, the study argued that the measurement of mental health for international comparison (and expansion) is already written into contemporary understandings of what constitutes mental distress, for example, in the historical development of universal psychiatric nosology. These deep historical roots spanning colonial biometrics and censuses of insanity underlie the conditions of possibility for the expansionary logic of mhGAP and the wider Movement for Global Mental Health. mhGAP could be seen to operate, like EBM more generally, as a 'technology of capture, synthesis and dissemination' (Broom and Adams 2012: 2).

Part of the social life of mhGAP-IG is the wider global mental health assemblage (crafted through metrics, funding, EBM, etc.) in which the tool is embedded and circulates. The study showed how quantification (including systematisation and commensuration), decontextualisation, epistemological exclusivity and digitisation converge to construct a globalised notion of mental health, out of which a particular algorithmic imaginary of mental disorder emerges. We saw how the relationship between the mhGAP-IG as a global tool and local context is mediated through a choice of predetermined modules and training packages (that also always entail some fluidity in practice). Importantly, this preselection of possible inputs is part of an algorithm's influence on the data it creates. Critical studies have focused increasingly on epistemological effects of algorithms (see collection in Amoore and Piotukh 2015), and how digital technology and data have a fundamental influence on 'ways of seeing the world' (Beer 2017: 8).

The analysis throughout this study was written in the spirit of engaging in dialogue with the WHO. We argue the importance of paying closer attention to the epistemological underpinnings of mhGAP-IG's algorithmic imaginary, in order to open the 'black box' of its production. An important element in this process is to take seriously critique of mhGAP-IG both from within its own paradigm and from other epistemological standpoints, particularly the multiple perspectives of and critiques from what might broadly be termed user/survivor/ Mad, as well as situated, localised and indigenous, epistemologies (LeBlanc and Kinsella 2016, Rose 2017). This would also need to take seriously what algorithmic approaches miss, i.e. those understandings and practices 'not easily rendered in the language of standardisation and [that] may lie outside of scientific metaphysical realities' (Cooper 2015: 532).

The study has highlighted how mhGAP and its products operate as part of 'the knowledge-power processes that inscribe and materialise' (Haraway 1997: 7), i.e. 'do', mental health in particular ways (as an illness, as universal and as measurable) rather than others. In this way, the mhGAP-IG acts as a global 'inscription device' that reifies specific theories and practices (Latour and Woolgar 1979) of mental health, and constitutes 'the domains [it] appear[s] to represent' (Rose 1999: 198). This means that the 'ethnospecific narrative field' (Haraway 1997: 4) of mhGAP-IG is made to seem universal, while the guidelines function as a device that enables different manifestations of distress to be connected up and conceived of in ways already determined by Euro-American specifications (Strathern 1992: 17).

The mhGAP-IG is only one of an increasing number of diagnostic algorithms used for mental health, and the social lives discussed in this study are far from the only sites that exert an influence on the formulation of its content. The examples here are only a beginning of a necessarily and always partial account of the social life of mhGAP-IG, given that it is done differently in different contexts. Therefore, much was missing here, including the relationalities that make possible mhGAP and that mhGAP make possible – the relationships and power dynamics between 'non-specialists' administering the tool and those whose answers are inputted; within the WHO; and between the WHO and those who use mhGAP but have no say in its design. Also missing here, but part of our ongoing larger research, are accounts of how mhGAP-IG is done in different contexts, i.e. how people actually use it in the field, and the ways different actors understand, implement, appropriate and/or resist these guidelines. This study has marked a starting point in tracing the multiple 'doings' of mhGAP-IG – connecting questions of how it is 'done' and what does it 'do' – to the living histories and wider global mental health assemblages that make the tool possible and shape its global circulation.

Address for correspondence: China Mills, The University of Sheffield, 241 Glossop Road, Sheffield, S10 2GW, UK. E-mail: china.mills@sheffield.ac.uk

Notes

1 http://www.universaldoctor.com/sect/en_GB/9004/Our+team.html.
2 Much of the work around mental health innovation is brought together by the Mental Health Innovation network, based at the London School of Hygiene and Tropical Medicine (www.mhinnovation.net).

References

Abdulmalik, J., Kola, L., Fadahunsi, W., Adebayo, K., *et al.* (2013) Country contextualization of the Mental Health Gap Action Programme intervention guide: a case study from Nigeria, *PLoS Medicine*, 10, 8, e1001501.

Amoore, L. and Piotukh, V. (eds) (2015) *Algorithmic Life: Calculative Devices in the Age of Big Data*. Abingdon; New York: Routledge.

Appadurai, A. (1993) Number in the colonial imagination. In Breckenridge, C.A. and van der Veer, P. (eds) *Orientalism and the Postcolonial Predicament*. Philadelphia: University of Pennsylvania Press.

Applbaum, K. (2015) Solving global mental health as a delivery problem. In Kirmayer, L.J., Lemelson, R. and Cummings, C. (eds) *Re-Visioning Psychiatry: Cultural Phenomenology, Critical Neuroscience, and Global Mental Health*, pp 544–74. Cambridge: Cambridge University Press.

Beer, D. (2017) The social power of algorithms, *Information, Communication & Society*, 20, 1, 1–13.

Bell, K. (2017) *Health and Other Unassailable Values: Reconfigurations of Health, Evidence and Ethics*. London and New York: Routledge.

Broom, A. and Adams, J. (2012) A critical social science of evidence-based healthcare. In Broom, A. and Adams, J. (eds) *Evidence-Based Healthcare in Context: Critical Social Science Perspectives*, pp 1–22. Surrey: Ashgate.

Chisholm, D., Sweeny, K., Sheehan, P., Rasmussen, B., *et al.* (2016) Scaling-up treatment of depression and anxiety: a global return on investment analysis, *The Lancet Psychiatry*, 3, 5, 415–24.

Cooper, S. (2015) Prising open the 'black box': an epistemological critique of discursive constructions of scaling up the provision of mental health care in Africa, *Health*, 19, 5, 523–41.

Department of Mental Health and Substance Abuse, WHO (2011) mhGAP Newsletter. WHO. Available at: http://www.who.int/mental_health/mhGAP_newsletter_jan2011.pdf (Last accessed 6 January 2018).

Dua, T., Barbui, C., Clark, N., Fleischmann, A., *et al.* (2011) Evidence-based guidelines for mental, neurological, and substance use disorders in low- and middle-income countries: summary of WHO recommendations, *PLOS Medicine*, 8, 11, e1001122.

Ecks, S. and Basu, S. (2009) How wide is the 'treatment gap' for antidepressants in India?, *Journal of Health Studies*, 2, 68–80.

Fernando, S. (2010) *Mental Health, Race and Culture*. London: Palgrave Macmillan.

Fulford, K.W.M. and Sartorius, N. (2009) The secret history of ICD and the hidden future of DSM. In Broome, M. and Bortolotti, L. (eds) *Psychiatry as Cognitive Neuroscience: Philosophical Perspectives*, pp 32–47. Oxford: Oxford University Press.

Gilman, S.L. (2004) *Seeing the Insane: A Visual and Cultural History of Our Attitudes toward the Mentally Ill*. Re-issue 1982. Battleboro: Echo Point Books & Media.

Hacking, I. (1982) Biopower and the avalanche of printed numbers, *Humanities in Society*, 5, 3/4, 279–95.

Hacking, I. (2006) Making up people, *London Review of Books*, 28, 16, 23–6.

Hanlon, C., Alem, A., Medhin, G., Shibre, T., *et al.* (2016) Task sharing for the care of severe mental disorders in a low-income country (TaSCS): study protocol for a randomised, controlled, non-inferiority trial, *Trials*, 17, 76.

Haraway, D.J. (1997) *Modest_Witness@Second_Millennium.FemaleMan©_Meets_OncoMouse™*. New York & London: Routledge.

Hardon, A. and Moyer, E. (2014) Medical technologies: flows, frictions and new socialities, *Anthropology & Medicine*, 21, 2, 107–12.

Jasovic-Gasic, M., Dunjic-Kostic, B., Pantovic, M., Cvetic, T., et al. (2013) Algorithms in psychiatry: state of the art, *Psychiatria Danubina*, 25, 3, 280–3.

Keynejad, R.C., Dua, T., Barbui, C. and Thornicroft, G. (2017) WHO Mental Health Gap Action Programme (mhGAP) intervention guide: a systematic review of evidence from low and middle-income countries, *Evidence Based Mental Health*, 21, 1, 30–4.

Khalid, A. (2009) 'Subordinate' negotiations: indigenous staff, the colonial state and public health. In Pati, B. and Harrison, M. (eds) *The Social History of Health and Medicine in Colonial India*, pp 45–73. London & New York: Routledge.

Kleinman, A. (2009) Global Mental Health: a Failure of Humanity, *The Lancet*, 374, 603–4.

Kirmayer, L.J. and Pedersen, D. (2014) Toward a new architecture for global mental health, *Transcultural Psychiatry*, 51, 6, 759–76.

Latour, B. and Woolgar, S. (1979) *Laboratory Life: The Construction of Scientific Facts*. Princeton: Princeton University Press.

LeBlanc, S. and Kinsella, E.A. (2016) Toward epistemic justice: a critically reflexive examination of 'Sanism' and implications for knowledge generation, *Studies in Social Justice*, 10, 1, 59–78.

Lingard, B. (2011) "Policy as Numbers: Ac/Counting for Educational Research", *Australian Educational Research*, 38, 355–82.

Lund, C., Tomlinson, M., De Silva, M., Fekadu, A., et al. (2012) PRIME: a programme to reduce the treatment gap for mental disorders in five low- and middle-income countries, *PLOS Medicine*, 9, 12, e1001359.

Maes, K. (2017) *The Lives of Community Health Workers: Local Labour and Global Health in Urban Ethiopia*. London and New York: Routledge.

Merry, S.E. (2016) *The Seductions of Quantification*. Chicago & London: University Of Chicago Press.

Metzl, J. (2009) *The Protest Psychosis: How Schizophrenia Became a Black Disease*. Boston: Beacon Press.

Mills, C. (2014) *Decolonizing Global Mental Health: The Psychiatrization of the Majority World*. London and New York: Routledge.

Mills, C. (2018) 'Invisible problem' to global priority: the inclusion of mental health in the sustainable development goals (SDGs), *Development and Change*, 49, 3, 843–66.

Mills, C. and Hilberg, E. (2018) The construction of mental health as a technological problem in India, *Critical Public Health*. https://doi.org/10.1080/09581596.2018.1508823.

Mol, A. (2002) *The Body Multiple: Ontology in Medical Practice*. Durham: Duke University Press.

Münster, D. (2015) farmers' suicide and the moral economy of agriculture: victimhood, voice, and agro-environmental responsibility in South India. In Broz, L. and Münster, D. (eds) *Suicide and Agency*, pp 105–25. London & New York: Routledge.

Nissen, N. and Risør, M.B. (2018) *Diagnostic Fluidity: Working with Uncertainty and Mutability*. Tarragona: Publicacions de la Universitat Rovira i Virgili.

Orr, J. (2006) *Panic Diaries: A Genealogy of Panic Disorder*. Durham & London: Duke University Press.

Patel, V. (2012) Global mental health: from science to action, *Harvard Review of Psychiatry*, 20, 1, 6–12.

Patel, V., Collins, P.Y., Copeland, J., Kakuma, R., et al. (2011) The movement for global mental health, *The British Journal of Psychiatry*, 198, 2, 88–90.

Perspectives (2009) *Harvesting Despair: Agrarian Crisis in India*. Delhi: Perspectives.

Petersen, I., Lund, C. and Stein, D.J. (2011) Optimizing mental health services in low and middle-income countries, *Current Opinion in Psychiatry*, 24, 4, 318–23.

Pickersgill, M.D. (2013) Debating DSM–5: diagnosis and the sociology of critique, *Journal of Medical Ethics*, 40, 521–5.

Porter, T.M. (1995) *Trust in Numbers: The Pursuit of Objectivity in Science and Public Life*. Princeton: Princeton University Press.

Rose, N. (1999) *Powers of Freedom: Reframing Political Thought*. Cambridge: Cambridge University Press.

Rose, D. (2017) Service user/survivor-led research in mental health: epistemological possibilities, *Disability & Society*, 32, 6, 773–89.

Russo, J. and Sweeney, A. (2016) *Searching for a Rose Garden: Challenging Psychiatry, Fostering Mad Studies*. Monmouth: PCCS Books.

Sarin, A. and Jain, S. (2012) The census of india and the mentally ill, *Indian Journal of Psychiatry*, 54, 1, 32–6.

Spitzer, R.L. and Endicott, J. (1968) Diagno: a computer program for psychiatric diagnosis utilizing the differential diagnostic procedure, *Archives of General Psychiatry*, 18, 746–56.

Stoler, A.L. (2002) Colonial archives and the arts of governance, *Archival Science*, 2, 87–109.

Strathern, M. (1992) *Reproducing the Future: Anthropology, Kinship and the New Reproductive Technologies*. New York: Routledge.

Summergrad, P. (2016) Investing in global mental health: the time for action is now, *The Lancet Psychiatry*, 3, 5, 390–1.

Sunder Rajan, K. (2017) *Pharmocracy: Value, Politics, and Knowledge in Global Biomedicine*. Durham: Duke University Press Books.

Timmermans, S. and Berg, M. (2003) *The Gold Standard: The Challenge of Evidence-Based and Standardization in Health Care*. Philadelphia: Temple University Press.

UN Human Rights Council (2017) *Report of the Special Rapporteur on the Right of Everyone to the Enjoyment of the Highest Attainable Standard of Physical and Mental Health*, 35th Session. A/HRC/ 35/21. Geneva: UN General Assembly. Available at: https://reliefweb.int/sites/reliefweb.int/files/ resources/G1707604.pdf (Last accessed 18 January 2018).

Ussher, J.M. (2017) A critical feminist analysis of madness: pathologising femininity through psychiatric discourse. In Cohen, B.M.Z. (ed) *Routledge International Handbook of Critical Mental Health*, pp 72– 8. London & New York: Routledge.

Weisz, G., Cambrosio, A. and Cointet, J.-P. (2017) Mapping global health: a network analysis of a heterogeneous publication domain, *BioSocieties*, 12, 4, 520–42.

White, R.G. and Sashidharan, S.P. (2014) Towards a more nuanced global mental health, *The British Journal of Psychiatry*, 204, 6, 415–7.

WHO (2008) mhGAP evidence & research – Mental Health Gap Action Programme. WHO. Available at: http://www.who.int/mental_health/evidence/mhGAP/en/ (Last accessed 6 January 2018).

WHO (2009) Mental Health Gap Action Programme (mhGAP) guidelines for interventions on mental, neurological and substance use disorders. WHO mhGAP guideline process. WHO. Available at: http://www.who. int/mental_health/mhgap/evidence/mhgap_guideline_process_2009.pdf (Last accessed 19 December 2018).

WHO (2012) Mental health and human rights—a hidden emergency. Available:http://www.who.int/menta l_health/policy/quality_rights/en/index.html (Last accessed 27 January 2012).

WHO (2014). Preventing suicide: a global imperative. WHO. Available at: http://apps.who.int/iris/bitstrea m/10665/131056/1/9789241564779_eng.pdf?ua=1 (Last accessed 15 January 2018).

WHO (2015) WHO mhGAP guideline update. Available at: http://www.who.int/mental_health/mhgap/ guideline_2015/en/ (Last accessed 6 January 2018).

WHO (2016) mhGAP Intervention Guide – version 2.0. WHO. Available at: http://www.who.int/mental_ health/mhgap/mhGAP_intervention_guide_02/en/ (Last accessed 6 January 2018).

WHO (2017a) mhGAP training manuals. WHO. Available at: http://apps.who.int/iris/bitstream/10665/ 259161/1/WHO-MSD-MER-17.6-eng.pdf (Last accessed 18 January 2018).

WHO (2017b) mhGAP forum 2017 – summary report. WHO. Available at: http://www.who.int/mental_ health/mhgap/mhGAP_forum_report_2017.pdf (Last accessed 18 January 2018).

WHO (2017c) WHO releases mhGAP Intervention Guide app. WHO. Available at: http://www.who. int/mental_health/mhgap/e_mhgap/en/ Last accessed 6 January 2018).

WHO (2018) WHO Mental Health Gap Action Programme (mhGAP). WHO. Available at: http://www. who.int/mental_health/mhgap/en/ (Last accessed 6 January 2018).

WHO Global Health Observatory Data (2014) Psychiatrists and nurses (per 100 000 population). WHO. Available at: http://www.who.int/gho/mental_health/human_resources/psychiatrists_nurses/en/ (Last accessed 18 January 2018).

Whooley, O. (2017) The DSM and the spectre of ignorance: psychiatric classification as a tool of professional power. In Cohen, B.M.Z. (ed) *Routledge International Handbook of Critical Mental Health*, pp 179–85. London & New York: Routledge.

Whyte, S.R., van der Geest, S. and Hardon, A. 2003. *Social Lives of Medicines*. Cambridge & New York: Cambridge University Press.

Sociology of Health & Illness Vol. 41 No. S1 2019 ISSN 0141-9889, pp. 176–192
doi: 10.1111/1467-9566.12900

Algorithmic assemblages of care: imaginaries, epistemologies and repair work

Nete Schwennesen

Department of Anthropology & Centre for Medical Science and Technology Studies, Department of Public Health, Copenhagen University, Copenhagen, Denmark

Abstract   In the past decade, the figure of the algorithm has emerged as a matter of concern in discussions about the current state of the healthcare sector and what it may become. While analytical focus has mainly centred on 'algorithmic entities', the paper argues that we have to move our analytical focus towards 'algorithmic assemblages', if we are to understand how advanced algorithms will affect health care. Departing from this figure, the paper explores how an algorithmic system, designed to 'take on' the role of a physiotherapist in physical rehabilitation programmes in Denmark, was designed and made to work in practice. On the basis of ethnographic fieldwork, it is demonstrated that the algorithmic system is a fragile accomplishment and outcome of negotiations between the imaginaries embedded in its design and the ongoing adjustments of IT workers, patients and professionals. Drawing on recent work on the fragility and incompleteness of algorithms, it is suggested that the algorithmic system needs to be creatively 'repaired' to build and maintain enabling connections between bodies in-motion and professionals in arrangements of care. The paper concludes by addressing accountability for the workings of algorithmic systems in medical practice, suggesting that such questions must also be discussed in relation to encounters between algorithmic imaginaries, health professionals and patients, and the various forms of 'repair work' needed to enable algorithmic systems to work in practice. Such acts of accountability cannot be understood within an ethics of transparency, but are better thought of as an ethics of 'response-ability', given the need to intervene and engage with the open-ended outcomes of algorithmic systems.

Keywords: STS (Science and technology studies), algorithms, repair work, care arrangements, accountability, ethnography

Introduction

In the past decade, the figure of the algorithm has emerged as a new matter of concern (Latour 2004) in discussions about the current state of the healthcare sector and what it may become. While the increasing capacity to produce and store 'big data' has for long been depicted as the revolutionising driver behind a more effective and evidence-based healthcare sector (Prainsack 2017), the role of algorithms – the coded instructions through which data are filtered, sorted and processed – has recently attracted attention (Ruckenstein and Schüll 2017). It has been argued that datasets in themselves do not bring transformative value to data and the healthcare

Digital Health: Sociological Perspectives, First Edition.
Edited by Flis Henwood and Benjamin Marent.

sector; rather, it is the algorithmic processing of data (Obermeyer and Emanuel 2016). This emphasis on the role of algorithms in the realisation of a more efficient and evidence-based healthcare sector has been followed by an increased interest in the design of algorithmic systems, to 'take on' professional tasks in clinical practice and care, such as predictive diagnosis and the selection and application of treatment regimens (Burt and Volchenboum 2018).

The distribution of tasks to algorithmic systems and their role in medical treatment and decision-making has been widely debated. On the one hand, medical scientists and policymakers are enthusiastic about the promise of efficiency and better care generated by the design of advanced algorithms in medical practice. This vision is particularly attractive to the many countries worldwide which face the challenge of demographic ageing and a rise in the number of people with chronic diseases (European Commission 2015). Reflecting those hopes and visions, medical algorithms have become objects of investment in a global market (Gartner 2016), and political declarations are being made about boosting research and competitiveness in the field (European Commission 2018). On the other hand, scholars working in the interdisciplinary field of 'critical data studies' (Iliadis and Russo 2016) have raised concerns about the power and agentic capabilities of algorithms in health and other fields (Beer 2017, Cheney-Lippold 2011, Dourish 2016, Gillespie 2014, Introna 2016, Lustig *et al.* 2016, Ziewitz 2016). The concept of 'algorithmic authority' has been suggested to describe how algorithms increasingly have come to shape both individual lives and large-scale social, economic and political processes, while at the same time operating through complex processes of calculation which are often dispersed and not directly amenable to scrutiny (Cheney-Lippold 2011, Lustig *et al.* 2016, Pasquale 2015, Shirky 2009). As the philosopher Frank Pasquale argues, while we may know what goes into the computer and what the outcome is, we know nothing about what happens to data during processing; this process is black-boxed (Pasquale 2015, 21).

The delegation of professional tasks to algorithmic systems constitutes a new 'geography of responsibility' in the contemporary healthcare sector, in which patients and professionals are expected to engage in the production of data and simultaneously respond to various forms of digital feedback (Schwennesen 2016, 2017). While medical researchers, politicians and critical digital data studies scholars have started to take notice of algorithms and their introduction into healthcare practices, little is yet known about how the introduction of advanced algorithmic systems may come to reconfigure medical practice and the relationship between patient and professional. As Ruckenstein and Schull argue, we still need more rigorous accounts of the actual reality of 'datafication of health' as it takes shape in diverse practices, and twists in unforeseen directions (Ruckenstein and Schüll 2017).

In the following, I focus on the configuration of an algorithmic system and how it interacts with patients and professionals in the field of physical rehabilitation. I begin from an ethnographic study on the design and use of an algorithmic system – a smart phone application with five wearable sensors – designed for use in physical rehabilitation in Denmark. The technology embodies the vision of designing an intelligent 'virtual trainer', which can act as a stand-in for a 'real' physical trainer when the patient is doing her home training (Ruttkay and Welbergen 2008), and operates through the algorithmic processing of patients' movement data. The study follows the process of designing and introducing the algorithmic system into physical rehabilitation programmes in a Danish municipality, asking: What are the imaginaries and relations that enable the algorithmic system to come into being? What are the processes through which algorithmic authority is produced, negotiated or sometimes broken down? I trace those relationships and entanglements through three empirical sites: the production and design of the algorithmic system; the interaction between algorithms and patients; and the relational encounters between algorithms, patients and professionals in arrangements of care.

The notion of the algorithm as an apparatus which is both powerful and inscrutable at the same time has come to structure current discussions on algorithms and their role in the contemporary healthcare sector (Beer 2017, Neyland 2016). In these discussions there has been a tendency to detach the algorithm from its surroundings, and to treat it as a technical and impartial form of knowledge. For instance, media scholar Cheney-Lippold, discussing the social impact of algorithms in Internet marketing, argues that algorithms work as a new mode of control, increasingly regulating our lives and telling us 'who we are, what we want and who we should be' (Cheney-Lippold 2011). Likewise, Steiner argues that algorithms have invaded and almost run our lives (Steiner 2013). He states that we are facing an algorithmic revolution, in which algorithms will displace humans in a number of fields, warning that 'algorithms can and will do strange things, when left alone' (Steiner 2013, 3). Similarly, more enthusiastic proponents emphasise the capacity of advanced algorithms to 'revolutionise' medical diagnosis and prognosis in the 21st century (Obermeyer and Emanuel 2016). In turn, both enthusiastic proponents of the capacities of algorithms to direct the healthcare sector towards greater efficiency and better care, as well as critical digital health scholars focusing on the algorithm as an invisible regulatory power, share an understanding of the entity of the algorithm as a powerful force, capable of acting on its own. In this paper, I challenge the proposition of the algorithm as an entity that possesses transformative power in and of itself. By exploring the socio-material entanglements whereby the algorithmic system is made and enabled to work in practice, I illustrate that agency or authority does not inhere in the algorithm itself. Rather, its agentic capabilities are produced through associations made between social and material agencies, such as algorithmic imaginaries, policies, sensors, smartphones, IT workers, private companies, municipalities, physiotherapist and patients. Exploring how these agencies are connected together through the three sites, allows us to see how algorithms and their effects are emergent, malleable and contingent, as they are made, negotiated and transformed through various socio-technical relationships. By drawing on recent work on the fragility and incompleteness of data and algorithms (Jackson 2014, Pink et al. 2018, Tanweer et al. 2016) I illustrate how the algorithmic system needs to be adjusted and creatively 'repaired' to build and maintain meaningful connections that may enable a productive relationship between the system and bodies undergoing rehabilitation. I conclude by discussing who or what we should hold accountable for how algorithmic systems come to work in medical practice. While algorithmic accountability has most often been discussed in relation to questions such as transparency (the need for disclosure of the factors that influence decisions being made by algorithms) and bias (the norms and values embedded in algorithms which might have unfair and discriminatory effects), I suggest that we also have to discuss questions of accountability in relation to the actual and concrete encounters between algorithms, health professionals and patients, and the various forms of 'repair work' needed to enable algorithmic systems to work in practice.

From algorithmic entities to algorithmic assemblages

In order to provide an analytical framework which allows for contingency and emergence, I draw on STS in my analysis of the configuration of the algorithmic system. This directs attention away from the algorithm itself, towards the heterogeneous socio-material assemblages through which the algorithmic system is produced and designed and made to work in practice. The notion of the assemblage refers here to the ongoing flow through which social and material agencies make connections with one another and come to constitute the agential capacities of an entity (Bennett 2009, Latour 2005, Wahlberg 2018). It relies on a constructivist ontology, which states that entities (algorithms, patients, professionals) are not distinct and definable, but are fundamentally inter-twined with each other in socio-material networks, gaining their specific qualities through these relations (Barad 2007, Latour 1999, Mol 2002). That is, no a priori assumptions about the existence of certain entities are made from the outset. A controversial tenet, therefore, is that agency is not to be considered a property of any pre-given entity (algorithms or humans) but an effect of relational associations consisting of both human and non-human actors (Barad 2007, Latour 1999). As such, everything that can be observed to cause an effect on the course of a situation or an event can be conceived of as an actor (Latour 1999, 124). The question of algorithmic power or authority hence must be considered an effect of the connections established between various human and non-human elements in the algorithmic assemblage; it is the emergent interactional encounters between the elements which decide the function of the algorithm and its agentic capabilities.

Working with the analytical framework of 'algorithmic assemblage' rather than 'algorithmic entity' enables exploration of the ongoing processes through which heterogeneous elements such as algorithmic imaginaries, policies, sensors, smartphones, IT workers, companies, physiotherapists and patients form connections with one another in a range of sites and temporalities. From this perspective, the algorithm is but one element of the broader socio-technical assemblage in which it is embedded. In my analysis, I combine this analytical approach with theories on the mutual constitution of bodies and technologies in the field of health and telecare (Langstrup 2013, Mol 2000, Oudshoorn 2008, Pols 2012); social studies of self-tracking devices (Kristensen and Ruckenstein 2018, Lomborg et al. 2018, Lupton 2013, Schüll 2016); recent studies on bodily sense-making and engagements with data (Lupton 2018, Lupton and Maslen 2018); and studies that have pointed to the fragility and incompleteness of data and algorithms (Jackson 2014, Pink et al. 2018, Tanweer et al. 2016).

The Danish Case: Digitalisation of the public sector in Denmark

Denmark is a welfare state in the Scandinavian tradition, with a tax-based, universal healthcare system. Like many countries in the world, Denmark faces the challenge of demographic ageing due to the increasing longevity of life; it is expected that the cost of care for elderly citizens and those with chronic diseases will rise significantly in the future (Danish Government 2016). As a potential solution to the 'problem' of demographic ageing in the Danish welfare state, the Danish government has increasingly invested in the development of public–private innovative partnerships, with the aim of transforming its know-how on care services into the design of innovative welfare technologies. This transformation is being promoted by several political strategies and initiatives. A recent, highly profiled initiative was the establishment of the SIRI Commission, whose leading officials and experts were to explore the potential for using artificial intelligence in healthcare services (Siri Commission 2018). Under the heading, 'Health and the good life is what we aim for – data and artificial intelligence is the means', the commission recommended that Denmark in the future should become a specialised 'hub' for experimentation with, and development of, new digital technologies in health, and suggested a number of initiatives aimed at reaching this goal (Siri Commission 2018). By exploring and investing in the development of new digital welfare solutions, the intention was not only to make care work more efficient by making those products available for use by the Danish welfare state but also to export them to a global market, thereby providing the basis for an economically sustainable welfare state in the future. These strategic and political acts can be seen as elements in a broader socio-technical imaginary (Jasanoff and Kim 2015) of a future Danish welfare state, in which high-tech solutions and processes of automatisation are positioned as 'curators' of its sustainability. The desirable future, in this case, is a transformation of the Danish welfare state, which was previously 'fuelled' by its agricultural economy, to a nation sustained by the export of high-tech digital welfare solutions. This collective vision both serves to justify new investments in new digital technologies and reaffirms the state's capacity to act as a responsible servant of the public good; it is currently being materialised through the launch of an ambitious dgitalisation strategy in the public sector. Physical rehabilitation has been mentioned as particularly well suited to further digitalisation, and municipalities have been encouraged to invest in new digital technologies in this field (Danish Government 2013). Following this call, several municipalities in Denmark have invested in the algorithmic system, and it is now being offered to patients who are referred to municipal physical rehabilitation units after hip replacement surgery.

Method and background

The present work is based on an ethnographic study of the production and use of the algorithmic system at a rehabilitation centre in a municipality in Denmark. The algorithmic training system consists of a smartphone with an app and five wireless sensors equipped with elastic rubber bands, which the patient wears during home training: two on each leg and one on the back. The sensors are virtually connected to the smartphone and produce data on bodily movement that serve as input to the algorithmic system. The sensors monitor the movement of the different parts of the body where they are placed (upper leg, lower leg, back), and measure the angles between them. The data on bodily movement are translated and transformed into immediate digital feedback to the patient, with the aim of guiding and motivating the patient during training. The data appear as text messages (e.g. 'keep up the good work') and visual images (between one and three stars) on the smartphone interface, and a digital voice correcting the patient's movement (e.g., 'lift your knees to a higher position'). In addition, an avatar on the interface of the smartphone imitates the patient's movement.

The patient's movement data flow through a digital system, to which both therapist and patient have access. The system calculates the number of exercises which have been performed at home, and indicates with a colour code the quality of those movements: exercises evaluated as not good enough are marked in red, exercises evaluated as good in green and exercises evaluated as in between are in yellow. In order to make the rehabilitation process most efficient, the system is programmed to progress automatically with new and more demanding routines when a number of exercises have been performed correctly.

On the company's homepage, the system is presented as an 'intelligent trainer', which enables supervised and flexible home training. This image of the system as a competent proxy for a 'real' physiotherapist is reflected in the ways in which the technology is implemented in the arrangement of physical rehabilitation. Although patients were previously offered group-based training sessions at the rehabilitation centre for one hour twice a week, patients who want to use it are only offered one session per week. The assumption is that the technology is able to guide the patient at home, which to a certain extent can substitute for training with a 'real' physiotherapist. Thus, responsibility for guidance and professional supervision is partly delegated to the algorithmic system, and patients are expected to actively engage in the process of generating and responding to data on bodily movement.

For 6 months in 2016–2017, I followed thirty people undergoing physical rehabilitation who had been offered the use of the technology, attending weekly 1-hour training sessions and physiotherapist–patient conversations about the technology, and engaging in informal conversations with physiotherapists and patients. Additionally, I interviewed sixteen patients in their

homes and observed their home training with the technology. I also interviewed five physiotherapists who were primarily responsible for the training session with users, a health consultant who was engaged in the process of developing the technology and an IT worker who was
responsible for the algorithmic system. Extensive field notes were taken in clinical encounters
at the rehabilitation centre and during home training, which were written up immediately after
leaving the site. Subsequently, field notes were analysed across sources and sites. Interviews
were transcribed and general themes were identified across the field notes and the transcripts,
with a focus on the imaginaries and relationships influencing the design of the algorithmic system and its functioning in physical rehabilitation arrangements.

Analysis

*Transferring expertise from health professionals to algorithmic codes: Designing the
algorithmic system*
The algorithmic system was designed with the intention that it would act as a proxy for the health
professional in its interaction with patients. Through algorithmic transformation of movement
data into digital feedback (oral, textual and visual), the vision was to create a device which was
able to interact with patients. The process whereby the algorithmic system was designed reflects
this vision of substitution as it relied on the idea that human expertise can be transferred from
humans to algorithmic codes. The developers describe the development of the design as a bot-
tom-up process. Professionals were at first invited to identify all the parameters that they saw as
important in their assessment of whether or not particular exercises were sufficiently carried out.

> HC: With each exercise, we were at first just sitting and writing everything down: 'What do
> we look at in a squat? We look for knee flexion in both legs; we look at how far one
> goes down in hip flexion; is the weight evenly distributed on both sides?' All the
> things we'd like to know, we wrote down – and then we sort of had the developers
> take a look at what the system can then say something intelligent about. And what it
> can't say anything about.

This process of identifying parameters for professional assessment of different exercises was
followed by one of selection and prioritisation of specific parameters. Professionals were asked
to sort and prioritise the parameters that they found most important:

> HC: As physiotherapists, we had to sit down and be pretty tough in setting priorities in rela-
> tion to the kind of parameters feedback should be given on ... I mean, I think we've
> sometimes sat down with 20 to 25 and ended with 4 to 5. So we have actually cut it
> down quite a bit. You could say that there has also been a natural selection, because, I
> mean, of course we started just by writing everything down: 'What am I looking at in
> this exercise?' right? And with the sensor set-up we have – for this target group it's on
> the legs – then it's only the lower extremities that we can say anything about. So for
> example, if there were some parameters that dealt with what one does with the arms or
> something else, then of course, we could say, 'The sensors can't say anything about
> that.' So of course, that was automatically discarded.

What comes to the fore here is that specific parameters for assessment of bodily movement
were not only decided by the physiotherapists' professional assessment of what it takes to do
an exercise well but also by the capabilities of the algorithmic system and the sensors. The
set-up, with its sensors on the lower extremities of the body, is not able to measure the

movement of the upper part of the body, and some parameters were excluded because of the sensors' inability to process data on them. Hence, the specific parameters that went into the algorithmic system were not decided by professional expertise alone, but were regulated by the technological ability to produce data on identified parameters.

In addition to the process of selecting the parameters that serve as input data for the algorithmic system, physiotherapists also had to suggest where to draw the lines between 'good', 'bad' or 'in between' bodily movement in relation to the parameters. These evaluative boundaries express three different intervals of angles between monitored body parts, and were contested among the physiotherapists:

> HC: Every exercise has been made with three levels, and there we have sort of sat around and had these very loud discussions about how many degrees it takes before it's accepted as a good performance. And then we've sometimes had to adjust it downwards, because we've found out that we may have been a bit too tough in relation to what the target group was actually capable of. And other times it's been the other way around: we've had to dial up some of the parameters because it's been too easy to carry it out. And actually, we still do that on an ongoing basis here now: the more municipalities, the more users we get on board, that's where we get some feedback on how well it fits the target group, right? So it's kind of an ongoing process.

The selected intervals of angles between body parts being measured serve as input data to the algorithmic system, and decide whether the patient will receive corrective or encouraging feedback. The distinction between 'good' or 'bad' bodily movement not only divides movement into different categories; these divisions are also attached to a valuation of the quality of bodily movement. By deciding on the particular intervals of angles between 'good' and 'bad' bodily movement, the physiotherapists enact a performative 'agentic cut' (Barad 2007) through which bodily movement is evaluated and assessed. Barad uses this concept to emphasise that apparatuses of knowledge production are not objective observers, but must be considered as productive and part of the very phenomenon they seek to measure (Barad 2007, 115). From this point of view, it is the algorithms and the created boundaries between 'good' and 'bad' bodily movement which articulate the body as moving 'well' or 'poorly'. While the algorithmic processing of patient movement data is built on a vision of professional substitution, the algorithmic articulation of bodily movement does not correspond to professional expert assessments. Tellingly, the health consultant emphasised that the algorithmic apparatus represents a limited version of professionalism, one which conflicts with a more holistic approach in which bodily movement is assessed in relation to the movement of the body as a whole.

In opposition to a view of algorithms as a fixed way of ordering and processing data, data processing emerges through a temporal flow of knowledge production, through which digital feedback is created. An IT worker describes the algorithmic system as a complicated process of calculative steps, consisting of predefined rules for how to proceed to the next step, through which input data are transformed into feedback. Hence, the system can be described as a sequence of calculative steps with defined criteria for whether or not to move forward to the next calculative step.

> IT worker: It's sort of like having a recipe [sic] for a computer, with a list of instructions that the computer follows.... in our system, we have the sensors that tell us about whether the angles are this way or that way, and then a number appears based on that. In an exercise, you can then say that, ok, we have a start position and an end position, and then the system receives various inputs underway that determine if some defined conditions have

been met, if the end position has been reached. When it then says that, then it jumps to the next step and waits until the input indicates that you have met the conditions for a start position, et cetera.

What comes to the fore here is that the action of the algorithmic system has a temporal flow which decides the 'doing' of the algorithm. The 'doing' of the algorithm is constituted by the calculative steps embedded in the algorithmic system, rather than in particular parameters or codes themselves. Specific rules were added to the temporal flow of the algorithmic system, based on assumptions about human behaviour and motivation (at least 15 seconds between corrections, only repeated 'bad' movements will trigger a correction, the same correction can only occur twice etc.). These rules reflect the attempt to add sensitivity to the algorithmic processing of data in order to keep patients motivated during training and provide a balance between judgement and re-enforcement, which is expressed below:

HC: At least 15 seconds need to pass before it mentions a new correction, so you have time to take it in, right? Then you can also have the situation where it'll only be in the next set that you get that correction. And again, we've also placed a message into the sensors saying that if this is not a recurring mistake, then it's not important. I mean, if it's something you do several times, then it's a mistake that needs fixing. But if it's because you just happened to lose your balance, then it's not a mistake to be fixed. So in that way, we've tried to make it fit as much as possible with real life, because you'll often find yourself making maybe a single mistake and then you don't need to be beaten over the head and told 'remember to distribute the weight equally across both legs', because you know to remember to do that ... There's also something about the same correction only being able to appear two or three times, because, if you keep getting the same correction, it can become irritating for the patient. There are also the voiced corrections that are played while doing the movement. When you are done with the exercise, there is a written correction, and there is only room for one on the screen, and it will always be the one that you have had the hardest time doing well. And then you might say, in reality there could be three messages, but there, for the sake of user friendliness, we have said that it should be the one they have had the toughest time with ... There are, after all, tolerance thresholds for patients in relation to how many corrections one can receive without becoming demotivated, so it's a fine line to walk.

In addition to the stricter focus on professional assessment of bodily movement (as illustrated in the previous section), sentient rules were added to the algorithmic processing of data, to 'sensitivise' the digital feedback the patient receives during training. As the health consultant says, this is to 'make it fit as much as possible with real life'. In real life, interaction between physiotherapist and patient is not only regulated by strict professional assessments and corrections of bodily movement but also by human empathy and care. As she further points out, choosing the level of corrective feedback to the patient is a 'fine line to walk', so that the patient does not lose the motivation to continue with the training.

There is clear inspiration here from the growing self-tracking industry, which offers individuals various forms of tracking devices designed to monitor and measure health and behaviour (e.g. Fitbit, Vivofit, Endomondo, Apple Watch etc.). Anthropologist Natasha Schüll, in her study on self-tracking technologies, offers a detailed account of how they are designed to govern users through real-time 'micro-nudging' (Schüll 2016). Nudging is a strategic method for guiding human behaviour and decision-making in a specific direction through positive reinforcement, in contrast with other ways of achieving compliance, such as legislation or enforcement (Sunstein and Thaler 2008). As Schull shows, many self-tracking technologies today operate within a gamified logic designed to keep users on their platforms through real-time nudging (Schüll 2016). This new 'behavioural-informatics mode of regulation' is designed to 'hook' the user into engaging in a constant state of data production. Similarly, the algorithmic processing of data is designed with foundations in human anticipations and assumptions about human behaviour and how to keep patients 'hooked' when they are training at home.

While the algorithmic system is founded on a socio-technical imaginary of the possibility of replacing professional work with advanced algorithmic codes, it is clear that the process of transferring professional expertise to algorithmic codes is not straightforward. The making of the algorithmic system and the digital feedback it creates are outcomes of a complicated process involving a variety of human (physiotherapists, IT workers) and non-human (algorithmic imaginaries, policies, sensors, parameters, computers) and various judgements and assumptions about patient motivation and behaviour. Moreover, the algorithmic system is not a final and clear cut entity, but is better understood as a temporal sequence of actions and decision-making, designed with the intention of keeping the patient 'hooked' during training. The complex character of the algorithmic system was described by an IT worker using the analogy of 'spaghetti' to illustrate the tangled and opaque connections between parameters, algorithms and codes that make up the system, thus emphasising that an algorithmic system is a messy and fragile accomplishment, rather than a closed and stable system of calculation. In the following section, we see what happens when this specific form of bodily valuation and articulation interacts with patients and professionals in real-time arrangements of care.

Producing and interacting with digital feedback during home training
The algorithmic system consists of a daily training programme which the patient must complete at home. Most patients welcome the possibility of supervised training in their homes as promised by the technology. After undergoing hip replacement surgery, many find it difficult to move around in everyday life, and travel back and forth between home and rehabilitation centre are experienced as a hassle. Free transportation is offered by a municipal transportation agency; however, this would often involve many hours of waiting. Hence, for most patients, training with the technology was perceived as a means to greater flexibility and independence in their movement towards recovery.

Like telecare applications for chronic disease management, the technology promises 'care at a distance' (Langstrup 2013, Oudshoorn 2008, Pols 2012) by mobilising the home as a new space for care. Moving care from institutions to the homes of patients in need of care demands the emplacement of various objects and activities in everyday life (Langstrup 2013). In this case, patients had to rearrange the home to allow for physical training, often explaining how they had to move furniture and the bed around to make enough space. Moreover, before every training session, smartphones and sensors had to be calibrated, which involves a careful spatial re-arrangement of the body, the smartphone and the sensors. A distance of at least three meters between the smartphone and the five sensors, along with a specific angle between them, were required for successful calibration. During calibration, a digital voice guides the patients on how to move the body correctly. During the process of calibration, a relation between the sensors, the body and the smartphone is established, which serves as input data for the algorithmic processing of movement data. In order for the calibration to be successfully completed, the body, the sensors and the smartphone must be carefully arranged; the sensors must be located at specific places on the body, the distance and angle between the body with the sensors and the smartphone must be correct, and so on. In many cases the patients experienced problems:

> Lena: It's all about whether it calibrates [correctly]. That's the key. Something went wrong the last time I used it, and it looked like one of my legs was a little bent on my

phone avatar. Now, I place the phone on the floor when I start. That helps. If I instead place it on the table, then when I get up from the chair, the avatar's body goes into the floor instead of up, and then it doesn't count my exercises and makes the avatar on the phone look odd.

This patient experienced problems when she placed the smartphone on the table, but found that if she placed the smartphone on the floor, the calibration could proceed successfully. This process of tinkering with the elements in this new socio-technical arrangement of physical rehabilitation (body, sensors, smartphone, chair), illustrates the need for arranging and putting human and non-human actors 'in place', for the system to be able to produce and process data on bodily movement.

If calibration proceeds successfully, the algorithmic system guides the patient through the exercises with a digital voice which counts the exercises when a movement is registered in the system as input data; it then tells the patient what kind of exercises will ensue:

> Digital voice: One, Two. Three. Four. Five. Six. Seven. Eight. Nine. Ten. You have now completed the first set. Take a small break before continuing with the next set. Switch to your left side. One. Two. Three. Four. Five. Six. Seven. Eight. Nine. Ten. Switch to your right side.

During and after a set of exercises, the patient receives various forms of feedback (as described above): stars on the smartphone interface indicating the overall quality of a sequence of exercises; digital text messages communicating encouragement and a digital voice giving immediate corrective feedback. In many ways, the interaction between the technology and the patients resembles the relationship between a patient and a health professional. The patients trust the competence of it and try to obey the corrective feedback they receive. They are emotionally affected by its responses: pleased when it gives positive feedback and frustrated when it communicates corrections. In their analysis of relational encounters between medical technologies and users, Pols and Moser argue that affective ties to technologies can be created when the technology promises something which is of great value to the user (Pols and Moser 2009). The algorithmic system promises a flexible pathway to 'efficient recovery' after hip replacement surgery, which is a value shared by patients, professionals and municipal administrators. Through the mechanism of the affective relationship that develops in its interaction with the patients, the patients adapt and react to the technology in order to obtain the value (efficient recovery) that it promises.

This process of affective attachment is generated by a relationship of trust in the technology and its ability to act as a competent stand-in for a health professional; the patients believe that following the training programme and acting according to its feedback provides the most efficient route to recovery. This trust is reinforced through its anthropomorphised digital voice. In interviews, when discussing their encounters with the technology during training, patients describe it as a human being, and ascribe a gender to it.

However, over time, the relationship between the technology and patients often became more ambivalent. Many patients felt that the corrections they received from the system were sometimes not logical, or were difficult to understand:

Digital voice: Keep the knee stretched.
Rose:　　　My knee's already stretched, see? I can't stretch it more than this, can I?
Nete:　　　No.
Rose:　　　I get so mad at him.

Digital voice:	Four. Five. Six. Seven. Eight. Nine. Ten. You have now completed the second set. Take a small break before continuing with the next set. Switch to your left side. One. Keep the knee stretched.
Rose:	Just look – I'm stretching it as much as I can.
Nete:	Yes, I see that.
Rose:	Isn't that absurd?
Digital voice:	One, two, three, four, five, six, seven. Eight. Nine. Ten. Switch to your right side.

The patients experienced a gap between expectations of the technology as a competent stand-in for the physiotherapist, and the behaviour of it as the exact opposite; this generated frustration, anger and a feeling of being trapped, with no possibility of satisfying the technology:

Ruth: You think you're doing everything properly, and you do them [the exercises] believing you're doing it right; you try to correct yourself, and then you think, 'Damn it, he still won't shut up. This is just too much,' you start to think.

| Nete: | So you get mad at the voice? |
| Ruth: | … I start to think, 'All right, now he's really annoying me and he needs to stop,' [laughs] because we've just discussed it, or, well, we haven't discussed it, but I heard him the first time. |

This tension between initial high expectations, and actual experience of the technology as a less competent stand-in for the physiotherapist, opened up a space where questions of authority, trust and responsibility were negotiated. In encounters between digital feedback and bodily movement, patients appeared, as we have seen, not only as knowing or perceiving bodies but also as sensing bodies. Recent work on digital meaning-making in the context of self-tracking emphasises the role of the body in processes of making sense of data (Lupton 2018). This work has emphasised the 'liveliness' of data, whose meaning is grasped as a result of encounters between bodily senses and digital data in everyday lives, thereby pointing towards an ongoing tension between sensory, affective and digital input in and around the activity being tracked (Kristensen and Ruckenstein 2018, Lomborg *et al.* 2018, Lupton 2018, Pink *et al.* 2017). The training programme and the speed with which it progressed over time occasionally clashed with the speed of bodily recovery. In some situations, this tension created what was described by health professionals as 'over-compliant' bodies: bodies that gave authority only to the algorithmic system, rather than to the sensing body itself. These patients could experience severe pain and possible bodily regression, rather than progression.

For other patients the tension opened up a space of potential creativity and improvisation, where the authority of the system was negotiated in relation to bodily sensations and pain. This generated a transformation of the relationship between the system and patients, whereby the technology came to occupy a liminal space somewhere between a competent, trusted physiotherapist and a thing without any meaning.

Carla: Well, we all know that it is just an algorithm, it is just a machine, it is not a human being.

The liminal character of the algorithmic system would not only change the technology but also the patient and how she related to the digital feedback. In some situations patients started to exercise without using it; some even hired a private physiotherapist to guide their training progress. In these situations, the algorithmic system was not able to uphold its authority and became a worthless object without any meaning. Other patients decided to continue to do their physical training with the technology; however, they would increasingly take on responsibility for the training. In these trajectories, patients would not become emotionally affected by the systems digital feedback; they would skip exercises experienced as particularly painful, take a break when sensing pain (even though it encouraged progression) and adjust the daily training programme according to their other physical activities. When patients took on the responsibility of acting as a competent trainer in this way, it also deprived the algorithmic system of authority.

The various forms of encounters between algorithms, devices and patients illustrate the liveliness of algorithms, as algorithms are articulated and incorporated into everyday lives (Lupton 2018). Lupton uses the notion of liveliness to account for the situated and emergent articulation and sense-making of algorithms and data, as patients negotiate between their sensory and affective knowledge of their bodies and the knowledge generated by algorithms (Lupton 2018). I suggest that we might think of this tension between bodily sensing and digital feedback, and the creativity and improvisation involved in the ongoing sense-making of data, as instances of 'broken data' and 'repair work'. Pink and colleagues introduce these metaphors to account for the materiality of data, and the incomplete and fractured character of digital data, when data are made sense of in everyday encounters (Pink *et al.* 2018). I suggest that we might see patients' negotiations with digital feedback as examples of 'repair work' which sustains and enables the algorithmic system to work in practice.

Interacting with algorithms in fragile arrangements of care
Research on telecare illuminates how the introduction of communication technologies to existing care arrangements constitutes new 'geographies of responsibilities', redistributing expectations, roles and tasks between healthcare professionals and patients, as well as between humans and machines (Pols 2012, Schwennesen 2017). Hence, the algorithmic system enters a relationship between patient and health professional that contains expectations and roles that each party is expected to undertake. The algorithmic system was designed with the intent that it should work as a substitute for physiotherapists, something emphasised by its anthropomorphic appearance and digitally voiced feedback. Like the patients, however, physiotherapists experienced a gap between the planned substitution and their actual experience when working with it. While they saw the technology as an element which could bring fun and entertainment to physical rehabilitation programmes, possibly encouraging patients' motivation, they saw it as an incompetent version of a physiotherapist:

> I think technology will never be able to replace a physiotherapist. It can't, I don't think it can .... I think it's a fine alternative that may suit some people who'd find it fun and something they can incorporate into their life, so I think those options should exist. So, I'm certainly an advocate for technology, but there's also something about it that makes me think – well, I don't know how to explain it. I also think there's something wrong about it. I mean, I feel that a computer's basically a computer, you know? And like I told you as well, it's uncomprehending, which is basically because it's only been programmed to act according to certain standards. So it's not intelligent as such; it's just been programmed by humans to do what it does. What I might sort of feel sometimes is a bit, well [sigh]. I mean, it's because it doesn't understand that the human body can vary considerably between people, so even though the technology has been designed by people who understand that, there are still some difficulties; there can still be some problems it doesn't understand. For example, it keeps correcting an exercise that the patient can't do any differently, because there may be some purely anatomical issues.

The notion of the technology as an incompetent version of a physiotherapist expressed here, also came to the fore in interactions between patients and professionals during the weekly one-hour training session at the rehabilitation centre, when patients often asked questions related to the ambiguous feedback they received during home training. When they complained about the technology and its lack of responsiveness, health professionals often replied that it was 'thick-headed', 'not very bright' or 'not able to deal with complex detail'. In doing so, the health professionals de-authorised the system, and gave authority to the patients to judge for themselves when to obey the feedback and when not. However, for many patients, this was not experienced as a considered response to their experienced problems.

> Sandra: When I tell them that it hurts, they just tell me that I am training too much. Well, yes, I am training too much, but what do they want me to do? I just follow the exercise program . . . . The program doesn't take my specific body into account, and I can't adjust the training program myself. I am not educated in this; this is the first time I try it . . . . I don't think that the physiotherapists take responsibility for this.

As this quote shows, some felt they were left alone with the impossible task of deciding for themselves when not to follow the feedback, how much pain they should accept before stopping the exercises, how often to train and so on, which, as we saw in the previous section, caused frustration and, in many cases, a loss of trust. During sessions at the centre, patients raised many questions and doubts about their experience with the technology at home, calling for alternative assessments of their bodily movements by the physiotherapists. Most physiotherapists found this new type of 'inquisitive patient' difficult to handle, but engaged occasionally in the production of alternative feedback, as expressed by the physiotherapist below:

> They have a lot of questions – 'Is this wrong or right?'; 'This part is hurting, what does that mean?' – a lot of questions, also in relation to the technology. 'That machine is constantly complaining, even though I feel like I'm doing it right'; 'Am I doing this right?' And that is when we occasionally delve into it and the conversation goes something like, 'Exercise 3, that's a pelvic lift, how do you do that? It says I should lift more.' And then we look at it and assess the exercise and say, 'That looks great. If you do it like that at home, that would be really good. Sometimes you kind of have to ignore what he's saying, you know?'

By allowing for the production of alternative feedback, a competitive relationship between algorithmic system and the physiotherapists was established, which delegated authority to patients to respond selectively to the digital feedback. This supported the patients in becoming better able to take a more critical position on the feedback they received during training at home, and to engage in the necessary 'repair work' that would allow for a more productive relationship with the system. Physiotherapists also emphasise the problem of 'over-compliant' bodies, and their sense of responsibility about identifying those who may be training too much with the technology. The physiotherapist below explains that she would recommend 'over-compliant bodies' to engage in 'repair work' by skipping some of the exercises or only doing the exercise programme every other day. She also stresses, however, that she finds it difficult to get a feeling for all the patients in this new arrangement of care, where they only see patients once a week instead of twice.

> [W]e also have to make sure they don't exercise too much. . . . If it leads to them being in greater pain than before, then we simply have to ask them to only do the exercises every other day or skip some of the exercises if they find them painful to do. It's a little more difficult to get a sense of how the person is doing when you only see them once a week – to have a sense of how things are going otherwise, to follow up on everything. It's easier if

you see them twice a week; then we're better able to follow up on what we've talked about previously, because there's a lot we have to remember if we only see them once a week. And they also have so many questions, after all, and sometimes it's a bit 'woah', so it's a little hard to control … . [I]t's different if you see them twice a week. Then the questions are more spread out, and they're not always so full of questions.

The sense that it was difficult to get a feeling for every patient during the weekly one-hour training session was combined with a sense that the initial intention of cost-efficiency – of being able to save time by reducing the number of weekly training sessions – was not experienced as an overall gain in time. Even though the number of weekly training sessions was reduced, they had the sense that the saved time was used up on all the extra work needed to make the arrangement function in practice, such as introducing the system to the patients, checking up on patients' movement data before the training session and so on.

We don't get more time just because we only see them once a week. They also need to be introduced to the technology. That's an hour you have to put aside for that. And we still have to put time aside to check how they are doing at home. I try to put time aside to do that once a week, but it's difficult … . It's hard to find time for that during some periods. And that's when I have to push it down the priority list, to be honest. Anything that doesn't directly concern the patient gets pushed down the priority list.

Not unlike the invisible work that patients and professionals carried out, in Oudshoorn's study on cardiac telemonitoring technology, this repair work took time and introduced new work for patients and professionals (Oudshoorn 2008). In opposition to the anticipated imaginary, that more advanced algorithmic systems, will lead to more efficiency and better care, the metaphors of 'broken data' and 'repair work' invite us to make visible and reflect on the work that is needed to make these algorithmic arrangements work in practice.

Conclusions

In this paper, I have unpacked the set of relations that enable an algorithmic system to come into being, examining how it is made and remade in three empirical sites: the production and design of the algorithmic system itself; the interaction between algorithms and patients and the relational encounters between algorithms, patients and professionals in arrangements of care. In opposition to singular understandings of algorithms and the contemporary imaginary of algorithms as revolutionising forces in themselves – commonly held among enthusiastic proponents and critics alike – I have illustrated that algorithms do not inherently possess agency or authority. Rather, their agentic capabilities are produced through situated connections being made between various socio-material actors, such as algorithmic imaginaries, policies, sensors, smartphones, IT workers, private companies, municipalities, physiotherapists and patients. By studying the anticipations that go into the design of an algorithmic system, and the negotiations and lively 'repair work' appearing in encounters between algorithms, patients and professionals, it becomes clear that algorithms are not just the creations of IT workers or programmers, or the effects they create based on certain input, they also consist of the imaginaries that shape our thinking about what we can expect from them, and what patients and professionals make of them in concrete interactions. As we have seen, the algorithmic system is only one element in a broader apparatus through which bodies and movements are articulated and evaluated in physical rehabilitation, and cannot be understood merely as a technical, objective or impartial mode of operation or form of knowledge; algorithmic systems are fragile accomplishments and not objects that can meaningfully be studied as units in themselves. Imposing the metaphor of 'broken' data on situations where digital feedback emerged in unanticipated forms, or caused pain, enabled me to understand the work needed to uphold the algorithmic system as 'repair work' – undertaken by both patients and professionals – in order to align arrangements with patients' bodily progression.

As algorithms are emergent and constantly unfolding across time and space, their outcomes must be considered as always local and situated. Working in conjunction with an algorithmic system designed to take on professional tasks, whether as a patient or a professional, implies sensing, learning and becoming intimate with it in order to build and maintain meaningful connections that enable a productive relationship between the system and particular bodies. How patients and professionals interacted with the system, and what form such repair work took in this study, subtly changed and was reshaped through the engagement with algorithmic processing of movement data over time. This means that, if we are to understand how algorithms affect medical practice and relationships between patients and professionals, we have to replace singular ethnographic snapshots of interactions and entanglements with in-depth accounts of the ongoing practical and sense-making 'repair work' which enables the systems to work over time.

The analytical move from algorithmic entity to algorithmic assemblages has implications for how we can think about accountability in relation to algorithms. Algorithmic accountability has most often been discussed in relation to the need for transparency and disclosure of the values, decisions and normativities that go into the creation of algorithmic systems, and their bias and potential discriminatory effects (Pasquale 2015). Such questions of accountability rely on an understanding of algorithms as a stable mode of knowledge production, and do not take into account what happens when algorithmic systems come to interact with patients and professionals in arrangements of care. To conclude, I suggest that we also have to discuss questions of algorithmic accountability in relation to actual and concrete ongoing encounters between algorithmic imaginaries, algorithmic systems, health professionals and patients, and the various forms of 'repair work' needed to enable algorithmic systems to work in practice. As we have seen in this paper, such 'repair work' is necessary if bodies are to be made to move and be affected by the algorithmic system explored here, in ways which generate bodily progression and recovery, rather than broken bodies. Such acts of accountability cannot be understood within an ethics of transparency, but are better thought of as an ethics of 'response-ability' (Martin *et al.* 2015) directed towards the need for intervening and engaging with the open-ended nature of the possible outcomes of algorithmic systems. This requires an algorithmic system and a wider arrangement of care which makes itself available to respond to the various ways in which particular bodies are moved and affected by the system, without knowing ahead of time what form such a response might take.

Address for correspondence: Department of Anthropology & Centre for Medical Science and Technology Studies, Department of Public Health, Copenhagen University, Copenhagen, Denmark. E-mail: ns@anthro.ku.dk

Acknowledgements

Thank you to all the patients and professionals who accepted to be part of this study. Thanks also to Klaus Hoeyer, Ayo Wahlberg and Henriette Langstrup who commented on earlier versions of the paper and to two anonymous reviewers who provided valuable comments. The study was supported by the Nordea Foundation.

References

Barad, K. (2007) *Meeting the Universe Halfway: Quantum Physics and the Entanglement of Matter and Meaning*. Durham, NC: Duke University Press.

Beer, D. (2017) *The Social Power of Algorithms*, pp 1–13. Information, Communication and Society.

Bennett, J. (2009) *Vibrant Matter: A Political Ecology of Things*. Durham, NC: Duke University Press.

Burt, A. and Volchenboum, S. (2018) How health care changes when algorithms start making diagnosis. *Harvard Business Review*. Available at https://hbr.org/2018/05/how-health-care-changes-when-algo rithms-start-making-diagnoses (Last accessed 8 May 2018).

Cheney-Lippold, J. (2011) A new algorithmic identity: soft biopolitics and the modulation of control, *Theory, Culture & Society*, 28, 6, 164–81.

Danish Government. (2013) Strategy for digital welfare 2013-2020. Available at http://www.digst.dk/Ser vicemenu/English/Policy-and-Strategy/Strategy-for-Digital-Welfare (Last accessed 27 January 2018).

Danish Government. (2016) Et stærkere og mere trygt digitalt samfund - Den fællesoffentlige digitaliser-ingsstrategi 2016-2020. Available at https://digst.dk/media/12811/strategi-2016-2020-enkelt-tilgaengelig. pdf (Last accessed 27 January 2018).

Dourish, P. (2016) Algorithms and their others: algorithmic culture in context, *Big Data & Society*, 3, 2. https://doi.org/2053951716665128

European Commission. (2015) Innovation for active & health ageing. Available at https://ec.europa.eu/ research/innovation-union/pdf/active-healthy-ageing/ageing_summit_report.pdf (Last accessed 27 Febru-ary 2017)

European Commission. (2018) Declaration of Cooperation on Artificial Intelligence. Available at http:// digiczech.eu/wp-content/uploads/2018/04/Annex-I-AI-Declaration-latest-version.pdf (Last accessed 24 September 2018)

Gartner. (2016) *Advanced Analytics Are at the Beating Heart of Algorithmic Business*. Gartner report.

Gillespie, T. (2014) The relevance of algorithms. In Gillespie, T., Boczkowski, P., Foot, K. (eds.) *Media Tech-nologies: Essays on Communication, Materiality, and Society*, pp. 167–94. Cambridge, MA: The MIT Press.

Iliadis, A. and Russo, F. (2016) Critical data studies: an introduction, *Big Data & Society*, 3, 2. https:// doi.org/2053951716674238.

Introna, L.D. (2016) Algorithms, governance, and governmentality: on governing academic writing, *Science, Technology, & Human Values*, 41, 1, 17–49.

Jackson, S.J. (2014) *11 Rethinking Repair*. Media technologies: Essays on communication, materiality, and society, pp 221–39.

Jasanoff, S. and Kim, S.H. (eds) (2015) *Dreamscapes of Modernity: Sociotechnical Imaginaries and the Fabrication of Power*. Chicago, IL: University of Chicago Press.

Kristensen, D.B. and Ruckenstein, M. (2018) Co-evolving with self-tracking technologies, *New Media & Society*, 20, 3624–40.

Langstrup, H. (2013) Chronic care infrastructures and the home, *Sociology of health & illness*, 35, 7, 1008–22.

Latour, B. (1999) *Pandora's Hope: Essays on the Reality of Science Studies*. Cambridge, MA: Harvard University Press.

Latour, B. (2004) Why has critique run out of steam? From matters of fact to matters of concern, *Critical inquiry*, 30, 2, 225–48.

Latour, B. (2005) *Reassembling the Social: An Introduction to Actor-Network-Theory*. Oxford, UK: Oxford University Press.

Lomborg, S., Thylstrup, N.B. and Schwartz, J. (2018) The temporal flows of self-tracking: checking in, moving on, staying hooked. *New Media & Society*, 20, 4590–607.

Lupton, D. (2013) Quantifying the body: monitoring and measuring health in the age of mHealth tech-nologies, *Critical Public Health*, 23, 4, 393–403.

Lupton, D. (2018) How do data come to matter? Living and becoming with personal data, *Big Data & Society*, 5, 2. https://doi.org/2053951718786314.

Lupton, D. and Maslen, S. (2018) The more-than-human sensorium: sensory engagements with digital self-tracking technologies, *The Senses and Society*, 13, 190–202.

Lustig, C., Pine, K., Nardi, B., Irani, L., *et al.* (2016) Algorithmic authority: the ethics, politics, and economics of algorithms that interpret, decide, and manage. In *Proceedings of the 2016 CHI Conference Extended Abstracts on Human Factors in Computing Systems (CHI EA '16)*, (pp. 1057–62). https://doi.org/10.1145/2851581.2886426.

Martin, A., Myers, N. and Viseu, A. (2015) The politics of care in technoscience, *Social Studies of Science*, 45, 5, 625–41.

Mol, A. (2000) What diagnostic devices do: the case of blood sugar measurement, *Theoretical medicine and bioethics*, 21, 1, 9–22.

Mol, A. (2002) *The Body Multiple: Ontology in Medical Practice*. Durham, NC: Duke University Press.

Neyland, D. (2016) Bearing account-able witness to the ethical algorithmic system, *Science, Technology, & Human Values*, 41, 1, 50–76.

Obermeyer, Z. and Emanuel, E.J. (2016) Predicting the future—big data, machine learning, and clinical medicine, *The New England journal of medicine*, 375, 13, 1216.

Oudshoorn, N. (2008) Diagnosis at a distance: the invisible work of patients and healthcare professionals in cardiac telemonitoring technology, *Sociology of Health & Illness*, 30, 2, 272–88.

Pasquale, F. (2015) *The Black box Society: The Secret Algorithms That Control Money and Information*. Cambridge, MA: Harvard University Press.

Pink, S., Ruckenstein, M., Willim, R. and Duque, M. (2018) Broken data: conceptualising data in an emerging world, *Big Data & Society*, 5, 1. https://doi.org/2053951717753228

Pink, S., Sumartojo, S., Lupton, D., Heyes, L.B.C., *et al.* (2017) Mundane data: The routines, contingencies and accomplishments of digital living, *Big Data & Society*, 4, 1. https//doi.org/2053951717700924.

Pols, J. (2012) *Care at a Distance: On the Closeness of Technology*. Amsterdam, Netherlands: Amsterdam University Press.

Pols, J. and Moser, I. (2009) Cold technologies versus warm care? On affective and social relations with and through care technologies, *ALTER-European Journal of Disability Research/Revue Européenne de Recherche sur le Handicap*, 3, 2, 159–78.

Prainsack, B. (2017) *Personalized Medicine: Empowered Patients in the 21st Century?* New York City, NY: NYU Press.

Ruckenstein, M. and Schüll, N.D. (2017) The datafication of health, *Annual Review of Anthropology*, 46, 261–78.

Ruttkay, Z. and Welbergen, H. (2008) Elbows higher! Performing, observing and correcting exercises by a virtual trainer. International Workshop on Intelligent Virtual Agents, Springer Berlin Heidelberg.

Schüll, N.D. (2016) Data for life: wearable technology and the design of self-care, *BioSocieties*, 11, 3, 317–33.

Schwennesen, N. (2016) Et omsorgsfuldt (selv) bedrag?: Om brug af robotter der imiterer mennesker i ældreplejen, *Gerontologi*, 32, 1, 28–33.

Schwennesen, N. (2017) When self-tracking enters physical rehabilitation: from 'pushed'self-tracking to ongoing affective encounters in arrangements of care, *Digital Health*, 3. https://doi.org/2055207617725231.

Shirky, C. (2009) A speculative post on the idea of algorithmic authority. *Clay Shirky*.

Siri Commission. (2018) Health and the good life is what we aim for – data and artificial intelligence is the means. Siri Commission. Available at https://ida.dk/sites/default/files/sundhed_og_det_gode_liv_da ta_og_kunstig_intelligens_siri-komissionen_januar_2018.pdf (Last accessed 1 October 2018)

Steiner, C. (2013) *Automate This: How Algorithms Took Over our Markets, our Jobs, and the World*. London, UK: Penguin.

Sunstein, C. and Thaler, R. (2008) Nudge. *The politics of libertarian paternalism*. New Haven.

Tanweer, A., Fiore-Gartland, B. and Aragon, C. (2016) Impediment to insight to innovation: understanding data assemblages through the breakdown–repair process, *Information, Communication & Society*, 19, 6, 736–52.

Wahlberg, A. (2018) *Good Quality: The Routinization of Sperm Banking in China*. Berkeley, CA: University of California Press.

Ziewitz, M. (2016) Governing algorithms: Myth, mess, and methods, *Science, Technology, & Human Values*, 41, 1, 3–16.

Sociology of Health & Illness Vol. 41 No. S1 2019 ISSN 0141-9889, pp. 193–209
doi: 10.1111/1467-9566.12881

The datafication of reproduction: time-lapse embryo imaging and the commercialisation of IVF

Lucy van de Wiel ⓘ

Department of Sociology, University of Cambridge, Cambridge, UK

Abstract   The 21st century has witnessed the emergence of *in silico* reproduction alongside the familiar *in vitro* reproduction (e.g. IVF), as increasingly large and automatically-generated data sets have come to play an instrumental role in assisted reproduction. The article addresses this datafication of reproduction by analysing time-lapse embryo imaging, a key data-driven technology for embryo selection in IVF cycles. It discusses the new forms of knowledge and value creation enabled by data-driven embryo selection and positions this technology as a harbinger of a wider datafication of (reproductive) health. By analysing the new ways of seeing embryos with '*in silico* vision,' the 'data generativity' of developing embryos and the patenting of embryo selection algorithms, I argue that this datafied method of embryo selection may not just result in more or less 'IVF success,' but also affects the conceptualisation and commercialisation of the assisted reproductive process. In doing so, I highlight how the datafication of reproduction both reflects and reinforces a consolidating trend in the fertility sector—characterised by mergers resulting in larger fertility chains, online platforms organising fertility care and expanded portfolios of companies aiming to cover each step of the IVF cycle.

Keywords: reproductive health, reproductive rights, reproductive technology, IVF, time-lapse embryo imaging, datafication

Recent years have seen an intensification of the datafication of reproduction, as increasingly large and automatically generated data sets have come to play an instrumental role in the technological reproduction of human life. This development is evident at all stages of the reproductive process, whether in fertility apps for timing conception, genomic fertility testing or the use of quantified visual data for embryo selection in IVF (*in vitro* fertilisation). The emergence of *in silico* reproduction alongside the familiar *in vitro* reproduction (e.g. IVF) follows from an understanding that an increasing number of aspects of reproduction can be 'measured and monitored and treated as technical problems with technical solutions' (Kitchin 2014, p. 181). It concerns not simply the use of data, which has long been part of technologised reproduction, but the attempted optimisation, automation and standardisation of assisted reproductive processes in ways that rely on, generate and analyse large data sets with novel computational technologies, including predictive analytics and machine learning.

One of the major changes in assisted reproduction today is the introduction of data technologies in the fertility lab with the aim of improving, automating and standardising previously manual processes. Yet in spite of the growing scholarship on digital health, the datafication of assisted reproduction remains surprisingly understudied. As the so-called 'data revolution' is transforming health care at large (Kitchin 2014), it is pertinent to focus on assisted reproduction in particular because it is a relatively unregulated sector in which bioinnovations – including data-centric ones – are introduced rapidly. Such innovations are relevant beyond their clinical (in)efficacy given the culturally specific and politically charged nature of reproductive processes and their reconceptualisation and reconfiguration in the face of new reproductive technologies (Franklin 2013).

One key influential reproductive data technology is time-lapse embryo imaging, a new data-intensive method of embryo selection used for deciding which embryos will be implanted in the womb in IVF. This embryo selection method displaces the embryologist's manual appraisal of embryos under the microscope by continuously filming them in the incubator, quantifying the visual information and predicting their viability through algorithmic analyses. Hailed as the 'greatest breakthrough in IVF in 25 years,' and criticised for its rapid introduction in the absence of 'high level evidence of improved live birth rates, safety and cost effectiveness' (Armstrong *et al.* 2015a,b, Harper *et al.* 2017, Walsh 2013a), time-lapse embryo imaging is now widely available in fertility clinics worldwide and is changing the face of IVF.

Major players in the fertility industry – including pharmaceutical giant Merck and biotechnology company Vitrolife – have heavily invested in time-lapse imaging and distribute systems to clinics across the globe. Although the HFEA, the UK's fertility regulator, advises that there is 'certainly not enough evidence to show that time-lapse imaging improves birth rates,' demand for this technology is growing (HFEA 2018). For example, Vitrolife reported almost $100 million net global sales of time-lapse technologies in 2017, while the first quarter of 2018 has already secured $30 million net sales after the company received regulatory approval for its *Embryoscope* system in China, one of the world's largest fertility markets (BusinessWire 2011; Vitrolife 2018a). As fertility clinics invest in time-lapse imaging, more intended parents will be confronted with the question of whether to include this add-on in their IVF cycles – often at an increased cost.

This article focuses on the new forms of knowledge and value production emerging with this data-driven time-lapse method of embryo selection and situates them in the techno-economic dynamics of an emerging global reproductive data infrastructure. It is written from the conviction that, in order to understand contemporary socio-technological changes in human reproduction, we have to take into account the rationalities, power relations and global institutional configurations in the 'reproductive-industrial complex' from which these bioinnovations emerge (Vertommen 2017). In doing so, this project seeks to not simply present a case study of one particular reproductive technology, but approaches the rise of time-lapse embryo imaging as a lens onto the dynamics underlying the introduction of data-driven bioinnovations in (reproductive) health care more broadly.

Adopting Vertommen's genealogical method for the analysis of emerging bioeconomies, this article characterises the datafication of reproduction by analysing the genealogy of data-driven embryo selection in the contemporary global fertility sector (2017, pp. 286–7). Through a case study approach, which Feagin *et al.* (1991, p. 1) define as an 'in-depth, multifaceted investigation [that is] conducted in great detail and often relies on the use of several data sources,' I approach time-lapse selection as 'an instance of [the] broader phenomenon' of datafied reproduction. Transposing Bal's (2002) method of cultural analysis to this critical case study, I analyse time-lapse embryo imaging by close reading key discursive objects that organise the marketisation of this technology – including patents, financial reports, direct-to-consumer advertisements and online platforms – in dialogue with influential conceptual frameworks in reproductive sociology and critical data studies.

This study builds on the work on the commercialisation and conceptualisation of prenatal life and fertility technologies in the field of reproductive sociology, notably by scholars such as Sarah Franklin (2013), Charis Thompson (2013) and Marcia Inhorn (2015). It provides an update on Deborah Spar's (2006) analysis of the fertility market in *The Baby Business* by focusing on a newer, data-driven technology that allows for a characterisation of more recent changes in the IVF sector, including its ongoing expansion and consolidation, the rise of private equity investments, the significance of patenting and the commercialisation of reproductive data. These focus points align with a surge of scholarship in science and technology studies concerned with the relation between reproduction, cellular life and capital. Notably, the work on 'biovalue' and 'biocapital' by Sarah Franklin (2013), Catherine Waldby and Robert Mitchell (2006), Cori Hayden (2003) and Sunder Rajan (2006) analyses the transformation of biological substance into 'generative forms of capital through which further commodities and value are created' (Murphy 2017, p. 13). Drawing on Melinda Cooper's characterisation of the self-generative capacities of stem cells and finance, it analyses the generative relations between embryogenesis, capital and biodata emerging with data-driven IVF (2008). It brings this work into dialogue with data studies by drawing on Van Dijck and colleagues' (2016), Hogle's (2016) and Kitchin's (2014) critical readings of the governance implications of 'datafication.' In doing so, it introduces in the field of reproductive sociology a focus on the 'data revolution' in global IVF, which is fundamentally changing the mechanisms through which we can conceive, control and commercialise reproduction at large.

In this way, I examine how the development and distribution of server-connected embryo selection apparatuses is remaking assisted reproduction by introducing 'emergent reproductive data infrastructures,' 'new reproductive bioeconomies of data sharing' and an 'expansion of the scope of reproductive risk through predictive analytics' by focusing on three aspects. Firstly, I propose reproductive data technologies such as time-lapse embryo imaging introduce an '*in silico* vision,' an algorithmic way of seeing through historical data sets that makes previous populations visible as the basis for future predictions. Secondly, I examine several controversies surrounding the patents and proprietary algorithms of embryo development and discuss how they reveal an ongoing renegotiation of the locus and ownership of expert knowledge and medical authority. Thirdly, by situating this technology in the institutional context of consolidating fertility, biotech and pharmaceutical companies, I address how time-lapse embryo imaging brings together self- and automated tracking, data infrastructures and social media in contemporary practices of technologically assisted reproduction. In doing so, I argue that this datafied method of embryo selection may not just result in more or less 'IVF success,' but also affects the conceptualisation and commercialisation of the assisted reproductive process and impacts the very coming into being of prenatal life.

In silico vision

Since its 2013 introduction in the UK, time-lapse embryo imaging has been promoted by major fertility clinics as an alternative, and superior, form of embryo selection. Whereas conventional selection relies on once-daily assessment of *in vitro* embryos under the microscope, time-lapse embryo imaging enables the embryos to remain undisturbed in the incubator and be photographed every 5–20 minutes. The visual data derived from these images are matched against predictive parameters to assess embryo quality. Emerging in the wake of an increasingly public visual interface with prenatal life, e.g. through imagery of IVF and fetal ultrasound, both of which have had a profound impact on public and private imagination of the reproductive process, the resulting time-lapse embryo videos add yet another visual dimension to the encounter with early human life on screen (Duden 1993, Franklin 2013). For example, a downloadable embryo video is part of the IVF package at CARE, the UK's largest fertility group, and Genea clinics live-stream images of developing embryos from the incubator to intended parents' iPads. Yet beyond another mode of medical imaging that brings the embryo into view, these embryo videos introduce an '*in silico* vision,' an algorithmically assisted way of seeing that makes the embryo legible, and its viability calculable, in new ways.

The advent of routine time-lapse imaging in the fertility clinic reconfigures the visual recognition of embryonic developmental stages. Rather than requiring manual observation, automated tracking algorithms record a number of visual aspects of development (e.g. cell division or cell quantity). In this process, a multiplicity of parameters recording specific visual aspects of the cells may be combined to ascribe a unique quantified value to each embryo (Merck 2015). In turn, the time-lapse system matches the resulting visual data against historical data about previous cohorts of embryos to give a prediction of embryo viability. The viability outcomes are automatically layered onto the embryo videos with numerical scores, colours or superimposed words ('high' or 'low'). Data analysis thus plays a key role in watching embryos in time-lapse embryo imaging as a means of not only making them visible, but rendering their viability legible, calculable and manageable.

The move from daily examinations under the microscope to time-lapse embryo imaging then introduces a data-assisted way of seeing, or '*in silico* vision' in the embryological work flow. Now touching the screen instead of the petri dish, time-lapse embryo imaging allows embryologists to observe, record and compare cellular behaviours that occurred in the petri dish in their absence – both in the incubated embryo cohort and those historical populations that preceded them. Tracking algorithms can record key developmental markers and provide suggestions for manual annotation (Vitrolife 2015a). They likewise detect activities 'beyond what the human eye is capable of measuring' by recording, for example, changes in the embryo's textural granularity (Merck 2015). In each of these ways, the introduction of *in silico* vision into the IVF lab presents an alternative mode of 'authorised seeing' alongside the embryologist's medical gaze through the microscope (Foucault 1973, Jasanoff 2017).[1]

With *in silico* vision, 'assisted seeing' through data correlations integrates calculation and observation with the aim of detecting regularity in temporally and spatially disperse embryo cohorts. This approach entails an epistemological shift in knowledge production about embryos, which is becoming a new standard as the popularity of these time-lapse systems grows.[2] The marketing of time-lapse imaging positions *in silico* vision as a superior method of non-invasive embryo observation that allows for 'a more objective analysis' (Vitrolife 2018b). Although the epistemic fallacies underlying such claims to observational objectivity have been demonstrated,[3] I here follow Sheila Jasanoff's approach of not attempting an 'inquiry into the validity of particular data claims,' but exploring 'how power works in re-representing things that happen in the world in the form of data points' (2017, p. 2). The claim to a 'more objective analysis' is in line with what Jasanoff calls a 'view from nowhere' – in contrast with views from everywhere and somewhere – as the ideal-type of a 'disinterested purity of science.' This regime of seeing aligns with the problematic notion that 'data' can 'sanitize the world of observation,' erasing from view the observational standpoints and associated political choices underlying the compilation of authoritative information (Jasanoff 2017, p. 12).

However, as manual observation and assessment is supplemented by automated and datafied methods, there is not an erasure, but in fact a multiplication of observational standpoints as the embryologist ceases to be the sole observer and decision-maker in embryo selection. *In silico* vision denotes a more networked model of knowledge production that creates new forms of dependency in attaining 'more objective' visions of prenatal life that are enmeshed with attendant data-centric forms of commodification. Essential components of *in silico* vision – the system itself, its interfaces, the data sets it generates and the algorithms with which they are analysed – may now be owned by corporate actors, thereby positioning embryo selection as a significant nexus of power relations and capital flows in contemporary IVF.

This paper examines the power relations at work in the establishment of *in silico* vision and the widespread introduction of data-driven embryo selection, as a particular organisation between those that produce, analyse and claim ownership of embryo data is built into the very means of seeing prenatal life. These concerns are vividly articulated through the controversies surrounding the patenting of data-driven embryo selection systems.

Patenting data-driven embryo selection

The patenting of time-lapse imaging systems brought embryo development into the realm of private property and thereby provoked controversy in the scientific and bioethics community. Because these patents include temporal parameters of embryo development, they provoked discussions about the patentability of natural phenomena. This section addresses the institutional and regulatory contexts from which the patenting of embryonic development emerges and their significance in rendering embryo development generative and valuable in new ways. It thereby highlights how the datafication transition in IVF raises fundamental questions about the conceptualisation and commercialisation of prenatal life as data-driven embryo selection becomes a means for creating new forms of capital accumulation.

Between 2011 and 2013, both US and European patent offices issued patents covering the timing of cellular development as 'predictive parameters' in embryo selection to Stanford University, with exclusive licensing to Auxogyn (now Progyny), the company that produced the *Eeva* test. The patents describe the association of 'good developmental competence' with cellular temporal markers, such as a 'duration of first cytokinesis [...] between 0 and 30 minutes' and a 'time interval [...] between the resolution of cytokinesis 1 and the onset of cytokinesis 2 [of] 8–15 hours' (Baer *et al.* 2011, Wong *et al.* 2012, 2013). Rather than only describing the technicalities of the embryo selection method, the patents thus also include the temporal specifics of embryo development as part of the patented intellectual property.

Consequently, the question arose to what extent the timing of embryo development is a natural phenomenon, and therefore unpatentable, or an essential part of a new, patentable invention. Jacques Cohen, chief Editor of *Reproductive BioMedicine Online*, led a scholarly response to the Auxogyn patents and wrote a plea against 'patenting time and other natural phenomena' in this journal:

Claiming cell cycle timing or duration as an invention that merits a patent would strike most students of developmental biology as an unlikely proposition but researchers at Stanford University have successfully done exactly that! The first three cell cycles in the human embryo developing *in vitro* are now owned by a corporation. (Cohen 2013a, p. 109)

He argues that 'the length of the cell cycle is not an invention and its key role in development is not a new observation; it is an indisputable and well-known fact of nature' that has been described since the late 19th century. A precedent of patenting temporal phenomena, he claims, will have long-term problematic effects (2013a, p. 109). In response, Stanford professor and inventor of the patent Renee Reijo Pera claimed that the patents cover the 'assays intended to distinguish optimal [and suboptimal] embryos for transfer in IVF' and therefore entail a method rather than a natural phenomenon (2013).

In the ensuing riposte between Reijo Pera and Cohen, the former argues that the 'diagnosis of embryo viability' does not address a 'naturally occurring phenomenon' because there is 'no need to distinguish quality amongst as many as 5–10 embryos (or even more) in natural conception; and in nature women simply do not conceive outside of the body' (2013, p. 113). Cohen responds that no studies have supported the premise that *in vivo* and *in vitro* cell cycles are fundamentally different processes; in fact it is their close resemblance that has resulted in the birth of over 5 million children from IVF. 'Arguing that those processes were somehow not natural (and therefore patentable),' he suggests, 'may instigate an entirely different discussion, not unlike those that engaged the opponents of IVF in its early days' (Cohen 2013b, p. 115).

The uncertainty surrounding the patentability of embryo development in the context of time-lapse embryo imaging is another iteration of an ongoing renegotiation of legal ownership of human biological substances, and the data derived from them. In *Bioinformation* (2017), Bronwyn Parry and Beth Greenhough describe the difficulties of differentiating between 'discoveries' from 'inventions' in the context of biotechnologically reworked material, such as isolated DNA or immortalised cell lines. A series of legal rulings have determined that intellectual property rights to human biologicals can be claimed even if they are derived from human bodies, 'because bringing them into the world was deemed an act of manufacture or invention, not just discovery' and the patents would recompense corporations for their expended labour (Parry and Greenhough 2017, p. 74).

Yet it is important to recognise that in the case of time-lapse embryo imaging, the legal establishment of embryo development as patentable property occurs in response to purportedly 'non-invasive' data-driven technologies. Time-lapse embryo imaging does not isolate or reconfigure the embryo in any way that is directly instrumentalised – as is the case for previously patented synthesised DNA or immortalised stem cell lines. Rather, it introduces new ways of extracting and analysing data from embryos and thereby repositions certain temporal parameters of embryo development as instruments for selection. It is, then, its manifestation in time as potential data points that can be instrumentalised in algorithm development and algorithmic analysis that denaturalises and re-technologises the embryo and its divisions. We may consider how the broader trend of datafication in health care, and the attendant patenting of data-driven health technologies, has re-ontologising effects, as it brings more previously natural bodily phenomena in the realm of patentable inventions by virtue of their changing relationships to the expanding data sets and algorithmic instruments that record and analyse them.

Returning to Pera-Reijo and Cohen's discussion, the latter's response does not address another, possibly more interesting aspect of Pera-Reijo's justification of patenting the embryonic cell cycle, namely the political bioeconomies of embryo research and its clinical translations. Pera-Reijo explains the patent application followed the Republican 1996 Dickey–Wicker Amendment, which ceased US federal funding for human embryo research that resulted in the destruction of embryos, including those donated by IVF patients (2013).[4] This restriction has resulted in scientists such as Pera-Reijo searching non-federal funding from for-profit partners, who would invest private capital in embryo research that could be translated into clinical benefits. She states that 'without patents to protect the inventions made in this process, it would be nearly impossible to attract the investment finance needed to move a technology from the research and development phase, through clinical trials, through the regulatory process and ultimately to commercialization' (Reijo Pera 2013, pp. 113–4). Conservative politics, informed by a widespread anti-abortion sentiment in the United States, thus played a key role in enlisting embryo research within a capitalist logic that requires a redefinition of embryo development as invention.

Beyond the question of whether the patent is legitimate, what is at stake in these developments is the marketisation of evolving data and algorithms used for data-driven embryo selection. While Cohen's critique focused primarily on fixed temporal specificities of prenatal development, these and later time-lapse imaging patents describe temporal markers as more dynamic variables. For example, the same patent quoted above identifies 'first cytokinesis, the second cleavage division and synchronicity of the second and third cleavage divisions' as parameters that

> can be measured automatically using the cell tracking algorithms and software previously described. The systems and methods described can be used to diagnose embryo outcome with key imaging predictors and can allow for the transfer of fewer embryos earlier in development. (Wong *et al.* 2013)

Rather than fixing specific temporal values of these parameters, it is precisely a more dynamic model which combines ongoing automated tracking, data generation and algorithmic analysis that underlies a data-driven approach to 'diagnos[ing] embryo outcome with key imaging predictors' (Wong *et al.* 2013). Reframed as diagnosis, this claim to predicting embryonic developmental potential is highly marketable in an IVF process that is characterised by uncertainty at each step of the way.

Yet the key transformative aspect of this dynamic, data-driven embryo selection remains underdiscussed in the patenting debate; it follows less from questions on the nature of the embryo and more from time-lapse systems' introduction of the *data-generativity* of embryos. Cellular generativity was at the heart of the patenting of stem cells, through which, Cooper argues, 'the self-regeneration of life will coincide with the self-valorisation of value' (2008, p. 147). The patenting of embryo development similarly points to a mode of cellular generativity that coincides with value production. The incubated embryo's data-generativity propels not only clinical and scientific knowledge production, but also the emergence of future life, as the data flows drawn from time-lapse embryos can be repurposed as tools for future selections. Once datafied as both tool and object of selection, the incubated developing embryo enters the realm of economic valuation neither, in the first instance, as an exchangeable commodity, nor as the materially and commercially self-accumulative stem cell line (Cooper 2008, p. 148), but rather as a generative node in an ongoing automated process of data and algorithm production that anticipates and, potentially, enables future reproduction.[5] In other words, what is at stake in the datafication of embryo development is the transmutation of enmeshed knowledge, reproductive and capital value emerging from the data-generativity of prenatal life.

The algorithmisation of embryo development

At the heart of the valuation of data-driven embryo selection is the emergence of new software and algorithmic products, which produce new forms of datafied biocapital. As Pottage remarks, it has not only been patenting but 'the adroit exploitation of trademarks and branding strategies,' that has spurred the growing popularity of particular time-lapse embryo imaging systems. Of all the embryology technologies used in fertility labs, time-lapse embryo imaging is one of the few that is branded and directly marketed to patients (Pottage 2018). The specific software and algorithms developed on the basis of the data-generativity of previous embryo populations have moreover become products in their own right that are integral to the knowledge production and commercialisation strategies in data-driven embryo selection.

The datafication of embryo selection converts numerous variables of embryo development into quantified data and this phenomenon enables the emergence of new reproductive bioeconomies of data sharing between different actors and institutions in the fertility sector. In the field of critical data studies, concerns have been raised about the 'big data divide,' or the 'exacerbation of power imbalances in the digital era resulting from the differential access to data.' Critical reflection on datafication, it is suggested, requires considering 'the asymmetric relationship between those who collect, store and mine large quantities of data, and those whom data collection targets' (Andrejevic 2014, p. 1673).

When IVF cycles become data-generating, different organisations in the fertility sector become data-rich in new ways. When using these technologies, the fertility clinic takes up a new role of gathering sizeable data sets on developing embryos in routine clinical practice and, in some cases, using these to develop in-house algorithms. While many clinics have R&D activities, the ongoing data collection at the scale that time-lapse systems introduce is unprecedented, as is the introduction of algorithmic products to render this data legible. Time-lapse system producers, likewise, are gaining access to uniquely large, privately held data sets about embryo development. For example, Vitrolife, producer of the popular *EmbryoScope* system, has access to embryo development profiles and implantation outcomes from over 30,000 embryos. Embryologists and IVF clinics worldwide have contributed to this data set since 2009, thus reportedly creating 'the world's largest database of embryo development with known clinical outcome' (Montag 2015, Vitrolife 2015a). Emerging from a market-driven context, time-lapse embryo imaging systems are thus instrumental in the creation of asymmetric relations of private reproductive data ownership, diverging significantly from a public health-approach to open data sharing that characterised the early history of IVF in the 1970s and 1980s.

Rather than inherently valuable, these large-scale data sets extracted from developing embryos only acquire value when 'data are collated, curated, interpreted and otherwise acted upon' (Lezaun 2013, p. 481). This work of rendering embryo data valuable in both reproductive and monetary terms is one of the new forms of labour emerging with datafication that becomes visible through the marketisation of algorithmic software for embryo selection. CAREfertility, the UK's largest fertility group, for example, has developed its own proprietary algorithms for embryo selection using the *Embryoscope*. Beyond the potential for improving reproductive outcomes in their reproductive cycles, this process itself has become part of its communication to patients:

> Our scientists are world-leaders in time-lapse technology, and our CAREmaps technique is really highly developed; we've innovated models that can help us choose the best embryo more reliably, allowing us to see whether each has a low, medium or high chance of success. (CAREfertility 2018)

Rather than only promoting time-lapse embryo imaging itself, the CARE website specifically markets its proprietary CAREmaps (morphokinetic algorithms to predict success) as the key to IVF success. The datafication of embryo selection thus creates novel algorithmic products, which reflect both the new forms of bioinformatical labour in the fertility clinic and new forms of value production both through the branding of technological innovation and a promise of increased IVF success that comes with an additional price tag.

At the level of the producer, the labour of collecting and instrumentalising embryo data likewise yields software products. Vitrolife's 'largest database' of known implantation data (KID) is translated into a valuable asset through its *KIDScore* tool. Along with Vitrolife's *EmbryoScope*, clinics can purchase this software package, which consists of algorithms that measure the 'implantation potential' of the embryos in the incubator and provides a 'morphokinetic score' between 1 and 5 to embryologists, who can then 'select the embryos ranked high with better chances of implanting and becoming a child' (Vitrolife 2015b). The rival system *Eeva* similarly is coupled with the *Xtend Algorithm* software package, which was developed on the basis of multi-centre reference data on file at producer Progyny (Merck 2015). *KIDScore* and *Xtend Algorithm* assign scores to the embryos to indicate which is more likely to survive. Given that these algorithmic tools rely on large sets of known implantation data, this practice newly aligns the generation of biodata with the generation of biocapital. Social scientist Linda Hogle argues that a 'tidal wave of efforts to extract value from health data has accompanied the big data phenomena, leading to considerable investments by pharmaceutical, medical device and health risk management companies' – and, in this case, leading to algorithmic products in their own right (2016, p. 386).

The development of Vitrolife's and Merck's algorithmic products relies on the presence of existing networks of data connectivities between pharmaceutical, biotechnological and fertility companies, given that *KIDScore* and *Xtend* were developed on the basis of data sets sourced from IVF clinics across the world. The (contested) claim that such networked embryo data collection is feasible with these time-lapse systems is itself a key element in the marketisation of these algorithmic products. After all, their selling point is not simply the promise of improved pregnancy rates, but an improved workflow in the lab. Vitrolife emphasises that *KIDScore* is easy to use and requires annotation of only a limited number of variables, which its predictive analytics method anticipates. It thereby enables a 'high level of consistency in embryo scoring in your clinic' (Vitrolife 2015b). Echoing Jasanoff's (2017) 'view from nowhere' regime of sight, this discursive framing of the software points to 'an overarching principle of inter-changeability' underlying the promise of datafication in IVF, which applies not only to intra-clinic, but also inter-clinic variability (Lezaun 2013, p. 481). It is this principle that motivates the claim that 'KIDScore is universal to all clinics and can be used immediately without acquiring your own data first' (Vitrolife 2015b). The upholding of a model of universality and interchangeable standardisation is both a key driver and an effect of the datafication of embryo selection. Similarly, it is part of a marketing strategy to extend automated embryo selection to more clinics, while being in and of itself a condition of emergence for the networked repro-ductive bioeconomies of data sharing and data ownership emerging with data-driven IVF.

As a result, the datafication of embryo selection entails at once the clinical introduction of integrated apparatuses for reproductive data generation, the creation of connected networks of data sharing, and the production of biocapital out of biodata by means of algorithmisation – all of which combine in a system that is marketed directly to patients and fertility clinics. The large-scale redistributions of embryo data between fertility companies that produce and use time-lapse embryo imaging not only create new forms of value, but also reorder institutional relationships as lines between research and clinical practices are blurred. What is at stake in these developments is that data asymmetries between clinical, pharmaceutical and biotechno-logical organisations reflect and reconfigure the power dynamics in the fertility sector, which I will discuss in the next section.

Consolidation and reproductive data infrastructures

The datafication of reproduction is not only transformative in its own right, it is but also indicative of how the broader IVF market is being reshaped. The growing popularity of time-lapse embryo imaging is situated within an expanding, and increasingly consolidating, fertility sector. The move towards consolidation is manifest in the merging of fertility clinics into larger chains, the growing influence of online platforms in organising fertility care and the portfolio expansion of pharmaceutical and biotechnological companies to include a wider range of fertility products and incorporate each step of the fertility journey. The institutional genealogy of time-lapse embryo imaging gives insight into, and emerges from, these consolidating developments in the global fertility industry.

Consolidating fertility groups: mergers and acquisitions

As the global fertility market is growing steadily and is estimated to exceed $21 billion by 2020, fertility clinics are increasingly merging into larger chains (Maida 2016). Trends of reproduction later in life, greater awareness and acceptance of fertility treatments, increasing privatisation in the UK and increasing insurance coverage in the US have been suggested as drivers in this expansion (De Martino and Shapiro 2017, Williams *et al.* 2017). Whereas new freezing technologies (e.g. egg freezing) preserve reproductive potential and expand IVF's target group with fertile women, new data technologies predict reproductive potential and expand the IVF cycle with additional treatments (add-ons such as time-lapse embryo imaging).

The growth in the sector has been characterised by an ongoing 'merger and acquisition cycle' as large fertility groups expand their international reach. For example, Australian market leader Virtus Health, the world's first publically listed fertility business, operates 46 IVF clinics, after having completed four acquisitions in 2016–2017 and expanding to Ireland, Denmark and Singapore. Likewise, Abu Dhabi-based NMC Health acquired both EUVITRO in Spain in 2015 ($162 million) and Fakih IVF Group in the United Arab Emirates ($207 million) (Williams *et al.* 2017). In the UK, CARE Fertility is the largest provider of IVF and has a steadily expanding chain of fertility clinics across the country and in Ireland (CHR 2015). The 2017 merger of Spanish IVI and US RMNAJ has created the world's largest fertility group, reaching around €300 m revenue (Pedrós and González 2017).

The datafication of reproduction is situated within these consolidating developments in the fertility sector. Given the significant price tag of time-lapse embryo imaging systems, transitioning to this data-driven method of embryo selection is more feasible for larger clinics. Aided by economies of scale, larger, consolidated clinics are typically early adopters of these high-investment systems. For example, abovementioned Fakih IVF announces on its homepage that it was the first to introduce the *EmbryoScope* in the AUE. As Madeira and Carbone (2016, p. 112) report, the high cost of lab equipment is frequently mitigated through group discounts if they are purchased by a larger fertility organisation. Likewise, CAREfertility (2018), the largest UK fertility group, writes in a large header on its website that they 'were the first UK clinic to introduce time-lapse embryo imaging.' Promoting these technologies to (potential) patients and the wider public, CAREfertility was at the centre of high-profile media exposure of time-lapse embryo imaging, which included televised BBC news reports on purportedly the 'biggest breakthrough in IVF in 25 years' (Walsh 2013b).

This association between consolidation and high-investment innovations gains another dimension in the context of datafication. Because time-lapse imaging generates data streams with each IVF cycle, larger centres with more annual cycles have the benefit of gaining larger data sets on embryo development. Depending on whether this data is thought to be clinic-specific or sufficiently standardised to be comparable amongst different branches, these data sets can attain biovalue as a means to do research and develop algorithms for embryo selection derived from in-house IVF cycles.

By rendering the IVF cycle both data-driven and data-generative, time-lapse embryo imaging introduces an infrastructural change in the organisation of assisted reproduction. Beyond adding another 'add-on' to an increasingly wide array of treatment options for IVF patients, the server-connected time-lapse imaging systems establish a wider reproductive data infrastructure to facilitate embryo selection in which the machines function as generative nodes. No longer confined within the walls of the IVF lab, embryo selection becomes a process that is differently dispersed across time and space as collected embryo data may be shared with patients, embryologists or manufacturers. The practices of data sharing across these new infrastructures differ as some clinics only use a local area network and keep their data in-house, while others share and receive embryo data with other organisations. The new pathways for (automated) embryo data sharing that emerge with the introduction of time-lapse embryo imaging enable new forms of connectivity between actors in the fertility industry – whether through the live-streaming of embryo videos from the incubator to the intended parents' iPad or through downloads of updated parameters for embryo selection from the manufacturer into the local time-lapse system. Even if not all pathways for data sharing built-in to the system are necessarily in use, the introduction of time-lapse systems facilitates automated embryo data exchanges between the manufacturer, the patient and the incubator in the IVF lab. The resultant key shift is that the direction and scope of embryo data flows are constrained by the clinic's decision-making rather than primarily logistic in nature.

The spatial dispersal of the embryo selection process enabled by time-lapse systems particularly suits the spatial dispersal of consolidated fertility companies that expand their geographical reach through mergers and acquisitions. The connectivity built-in to the time-lapse systems offers a means of bridging the distances between clinics within a single group by streamlining embryo selection protocols and practices and by sharing embryo data to build proprietary data sets. The alignment of in-house reproductive data infrastructures and the organisational model of consolidated fertility companies may thus widen the gap associated with data and financial asymmetries between smaller and larger organisations. In the case of time-lapse embryo imaging, consolidation and datafication thus appear to function as mutually reinforcing conditions of co-emergence. Larger clinics facilitate the introduction of the apparatuses while the connected and automated method materialised in the machine facilitates coordinating clinical processes across different labs and clinics.

Platformising fertility: consolidating across technological domains

The institutional genealogy of time-lapse embryo imaging highlights a wider trend of 'platformisation' (Van Dijck *et al.* 2016). Here the online fertility platform, rather than the fertility clinic, comes to function as a key organising principle of fertility care. A case in point is the *Eeva* test, which was first produced by Auxogyn, a biotechnological company which attained exclusive licensing for the technology through the abovementioned Stanford patent. In 2014, Auxogyn merged with *FertilityAuthority*, a 'patient-matching technology platform' and self-reportedly the world's largest fertility web portal with 1 million monthly visitors, which had itself acquired the leading global FertileThoughts.com social network in 2010 (Fertility Authority 2015). The resulting Progyny, *Eeva's* producer and self-described 'digital health company,' is organised around the online platform as the point of access to a network of clinics and a variety of in-house services, including IVF Advantage (fertility loans), Eggbanxx (egg freezing) and Progyny corporate fertility insurance.[6] In this platformised approach to fertility care, Progyny's mission is to be 'the go-to source for all fertility solutions' (Mack 2016). It thus brings digital health to assisted reproduction by combining investments in a data-driven embryo selection technology with a digital reproductive health platform that integrates branded biotechnological, clinical, financing, insurance and communication services.

By integrating previously separate fertility services under its online umbrella, the company disrupts the conventional clinic-based delivery of fertility care and introduces new treatment rationales for reproductive decision-making through its online and offline channels in line with its diverse portfolio. For example, the *Eeva* test had its own website, was the subject of expert advice on the *FertilityAuthority* platform and was introduced in moderator-initiated discussions on the *FertileThoughts* forum. It was also included in Progyny's corporate fertility benefit package, which covered treatment plans for employees that 'start with egg or embryo freezing, include testing of the embryo to reduce miscarriage, and include a single embryo transfer (SET) that when coupled with the healthiest embryo, result in the fastest track to success' (McCarthy 2016). The *Eeva* test is thus embedded in a broader reframing of the reproductive process through Progyny's mission to 'combine service, science and data to optimise the clinical outcomes of fertility treatments' (Progyny 2017). Egg freezing is included as a means to avoid the risk of future involuntary childlessness and optimise a potential IVF procedure with higher quality eggs. The inclusion of data-driven embryo selection approaches is rationalised as a condition for successful single embryo transfer to avoid multiple births.

Progyny's vision thus promotes a treatment rationale that expands the scope of IVF both by encouraging younger fertile women to pre-emptively undergo infertility treatment and by increasing the number of treatment steps in each cycle to optimise clinical outcomes. This reframing of the reproductive process entails both the financialisation of reproductive risk and its proposed mitigation through a highly technologised and revenue-generating set of treatments. Progyny's pre-emptive treatment rationale of avoiding reproductive and financial risk thus normalises a high-tech IVF treatment course for a larger group of potential candidates, which may be reached through both online platforms and their employers' HR departments, and unambiguously represents reproductive and data technologies as the best risk-mitigating strategies to 'ensure that anyone who wants to have a child, can have one' (Progyny 2017).

Consolidating the whole IVF journey
The increasing prevalence of time-lapse embryo imaging also intersects with a consolidating trend of vertical integration of the fertility industry, as those companies producing reproductive data technologies expand their portfolios to cover the 'entire IVF journey.' All of the major companies producing time-lapse imaging apparatuses – Genea, Progyny, Merck and Vitrolife – explicitly voice this ambition in their marketing and investment materials. Vitrolife's presents its various products – laboratory instruments, culture media, imaging technologies, etc – as an integrated portfolio to 'maximise success every step of the way' (Vitrolife 2018c). Likewise, upon introducing its Geri time-lapse system, Merck announced that 'With an Extended Fertility Technologies Portfolio Merck now Covers all IVF Steps' (Merck 2016). After various acquisitions and alliances since 2013, Merck and Vitrolife, a pharmaceutical and biotechnological company, currently distribute all four major time-lapse embryo imaging systems. In line with the ambition to cover every stage of the IVF process, the 'add-on' technology of time-lapse embryo imaging provides an opportunity to expand the treatment steps per cycle and popularise new forms of standardisation within assisted reproduction.

Vitrolife produces both the *Primovision* system and, after acquisition of its former producer Fertilitech in 2014, the *Embryoscope*. Vitrolife specialises in IVF culture media and disposables, such as pipettes and dishes. The inclusion of time-lapse embryo imaging in their business model has proven to be highly successful and sales of these machines have increased each quarter since 2014 (Vitrolife 2018a). They estimate that 10% of IVF centres in the world and over half of UK clinics use their time-lapse embryo imaging machines (Vitrolife 2017, p. 3). These high figures indicate that a growing number of patients and professionals will encounter the option to include these machines as part of their IVF cycles. As the company seeks to cover every step of the reproductive process, the IVF cycle overlaps with the 'value chain' of Vitrolife products (Axelsson 2016, p. 6). The added step of data-driven embryo-selection technology affirms the wider trend of the 'value per cycle increasing through better technologies,' an effect that is intensified by a related trend of more cycles following a single 'oocyte pick-up' (Axelsson 2016, p. 16). Addressing investors, the company specifically makes the business case for time-lapse embryo imaging as a high-tech marketing tool and as a means to increase income per cycle, given that the cost (€50–€200) is significantly lower than the standard selling price (€400–€1000) per treatment (Ramsing 2016, p. 11). In considering digital reproductive health, it is important to highlight that the emergence of new digital subjectivities, knowledges and networks is situated in a rapidly growing global fertility sector; its rationality of expansion is a key driver of the increasing datafication of reproduction.

Another major player in the fertility sector is Merck, a multinational pharmaceutical company with approximately 50,000 employees in 70 countries, which is a leading distributor of the fertility drugs used in IVF cycles. Recently biosimilars to Merck's major fertility drugs for IVF ovarian stimulation have been introduced (Allahbadia and Allahbadia 2016, Winstel *et al.* 2017). At this time, the company is also expanding its portfolio to include time-lapse embryo imaging by partnering with both Genea, which produces the *Geri* system, and abovementioned Progyny, which produces the *Eeva* test. Investments in these data-driven systems are part of its broader strategy to 'cover all IVF steps' and develop 'from a drug provider to an integrated fertility partner' (Wenzel 2017). Alongside this ambition, a key goal of the Global Fertility Alliance, of which Merck is a founding member, is to promote 'standardisation and automation in *in vitro* fertilisation (IVF) clinics' (GFA 2018). Investments in automated and standardised embryo selection through data-driven technologies that materialise these principles align with this wider goal.

The blurring of the lines between clinical and capitalist rationales in these global reproductive bioeconomies is foundational to the datafication of reproduction and raises concerns about the implications of the concomitant corporatisation of IVF. The valuation of time-lapse embryo imaging follows not only from the commodification of add-on treatments, algorithms and selection apparatuses, but it is also a materialisation of an expansive drive within global IVF enabled by standardisation, automation and data-generativity. Alongside a critique that IVF becomes overly shaped by corporate interests is a concern that the specific corporatisation of data-driven embryo selection may both enlist fertility clinics and patients in treatment rationales that require even more investment per cycle and create technological lock-ins that make clinics beholden to particular platforms, thereby potentially intensifying data and financial asymmetries within assisted reproduction (Kitchin 2014, pp. 181–2).

Conclusion

The data-driven selection of embryos with time-lapse embryo imaging has primarily been discussed in terms of its clinical efficacy, but its introduction reflects and reconfigures a range of practices within the contemporary fertility sector. As Sarah Franklin (2013) has argued for IVF, time-lapse embryo imaging provides a lens onto the reconceptualisation and recommodification of prenatal life when data technologies and reproductive technologies meet.

The datafication of embryo selection shifts clinical practice by introducing a new treatment option that renders embryo viability visible and calculable by means of an algorithmically assisted way of seeing. With the introduction of this '*in silico* vision' in the embryological workflow, IVF cycles do not only produce babies, but also sizable data sets on embryo development. As data flows of embryos are shared – or withheld – between embryologists, corporations and patients, embryo selection becomes a more networked and commercialised activity in which different actors have a stake.

The establishment of emergent reproductive data infrastructures through the introduction of growing numbers of time-lapse embryo imaging systems raises questions about who may access and who can claim ownership of this embryo data. The patenting of this process highlights how the embryos' data-generativity may be repurposed as a method for selection, how observable characteristics of embryo development are transformed into private property, and how the development of bioinnovations is increasingly reliant on funding from for-profit partners. The sizable data sets about embryogenesis collected through this system provide the basis for the creation of new algorithmic products for embryo selection by biotechnological and pharmaceutical companies. This process of turning biodata into biocapital relies on reproductive data infrastructures, through which new data and power asymmetries between different actors in the fertility sector are construed and consolidated.

What is remarkable about the commercialisation of time-lapse technologies is the way in which strategies of patenting, direct-to-consumer branding, privately held data accumulation, its algorithmisation into selection tools and ownership of the whole IVF supply chain are combined into a total system for data-driven embryo selection. This multipronged move towards datafication, and the concomitant promise of automation, standardisation and data/capital accumulation in a more networked mode of embryo selection, both reflects and reinforces a consolidating trend in the fertility sector – characterised by mergers resulting in larger fertility chains, online platforms adopting a key role in the organisation of fertility care and the portfolio expansion of pharmaceutical and biotechnological companies to cover each step of the IVF cycle.

In the context of this Special Issue I therefore want to emphasise that the emergence of new digital subjectivities, knowledges and networks in digital reproductive health are situated in a rapidly growing global fertility sector; its rationality of expansion is a key driver of the datafication of reproduction. What is at stake, then, in the enmeshed forms of biocapital and biodata that emerge with the datafication of (reproductive) health care is not only the increase or decrease of pregnancy rates, but numerous conceptual, epistemological and institutional shifts that lie at the foundation of both contemporary technologised reproduction and the future reconfigurations of the relation between biomedicine and society. It is, in other words, crucial to understand data-driven IVF as not a peripheral phenomenon, but as a harbinger of how power relations between networks of social and corporate actors can be built-in to the institutional infrastructures that deliver digital health.

Address for correspondence: Lucy van de Wiel, Department of Sociology, University of Cambridge, 16 Mill Lane, Cambridge CB2 1SB, UK. E-mail: lvdw2@cam.ac.uk

Acknowledgements

The research on which this article is based was supported by the Wellcome Trust (Grant 209829/Z/17/Z) and the Alan Turing Institute. I would like to thank the anonymous peer reviewers and the members of the Reproductive Sociology Research Group (ReproSoc) at the University of Cambridge for their feedback.

Notes

1 For a discussion of the medical gaze in relation to the prenatal imagery produced in time-lapse embryo imaging, see Van de Wiel (2017, 2018).

2   Time-lapse embryo imaging is widely used in scientific studies in developmental biology. The tripling
    of citations on time-lapse embryo imaging from 447 to 1358 between 2013 and 2017 gives an indica-
    tion of the impact of this technology on the field. Citation report generated at Thomson Reuter's Web
    of Science '([time-lapse OR "time lapse"] AND [IVF OR ICSI OR "embryo selection"]).'
3   See Fox Keller (1996).
4   See Thompson (2013) for a detailed discussion of the Dickey–Wicker Amendment (pp. 79–84).
5   See Franklin (2013) for a discussion of the 'retooling' of reproductive substance in processes of
    'bioindustrialisation' (p. 64).
6   With a network of over 455 clinics and a focus on servicing Fortune 500 companies, Progyny is cur-
    rently the leading fertility benefits provider in the US.

References

Allahbadia, G.N. and Allahbadia, A. (2016) Recombinants versus biosimilars in ovarian stimulation.
In Allahbadia, G.N. and Morimoto, Y. (eds) *Ovarian Stimulation Protocols*, pp 71–7. New Delhi:
Springer.

Andrejevic, M. (2014) Big data, Big questions, *International Journal of Communication*, 8, 17.

Armstrong, S., Arroll, N., Cree, L.M., Jordan, V., *et al.* (2015a) Time-lapse systems for embryo incuba-
tion and assessment in assisted reproduction, *Cochrane Database Systematic Review*, 2, CD011320.
https://doi.org/10.1002/14651858.cd011320.pub2.

Armstrong, S., Vail, A., Mastenbroek, S., Jordan, V., *et al.* (2015b) Time-lapse in the IVF-lab: how should
we assess potential benefit?, *Human Reproduction*, 30, 3–8.

Axelsson, T. (2016) *Kapitalmarknadsdag 20 September 2016*. Gothenburg, Sweden: Vitrolife.

Baer, T.M., Behr, B., Loewke, K.E., Reijo-Pera, R.A., *et al.* (2011) Imaging and evaluating embryos,
oocytes, and stem cells. Patent US7963906 B2. Washington: U.S. Patent and Trademark Office.

Bal, M. (2002) *Travelling Concepts in the Humanities: A Rough Guide*. Toronto: University of Toronto
Press.

BusinessWire. (2011) Vitrolife is the first company in china to receive regulatory approval for an entire
IVF culture media portfolio. BusinessWire. Available at https://www.businesswire.com/news/home/
20110505005795/en/Vitrolife-Company-China-Receive-Regulatory-Approval-Entire (Last accessed 25
August 2018).

CAREfertility. (2018) CAREmaps. CARE Fertil. Available at https://www.carefertility.com/treatments/
embryology-treatments/caremaps/ (Last accessed 5 April 2018).

CHR. (2015) The "industrialization" of infertility care. Cent. Hum. Reprod. Available at https://www.ce
nterforhumanreprod.com/fertility/the-industrialization-of-infertility-care/ (Last accessed 22 January
2018).

Cohen, J. (2013a) On patenting time and other natural phenomena, *Reproductive BioMedicine Online*,
27, 109–10.

Cohen, J. (2013b) Patenting time: a response to Professor Reijo Pera's argument that the cell cycle of an
embryo developing in vitro is not natural, *Reproductive BioMedicine Online*, 27, 115.

Cooper, M.E. (2008) *Life as Surplus: Biotechnology and Capitalism in the Neoliberal Era*. Seattle:
University of Washington Press.

De Martino, M. and Shapiro, L. (2017) *Conceiving the Next Phase of Growth for Private IVF Clinics*.
London: Candesic.

Duden, B. (1993) Visualizing "life," *Science and Culture*, 3, 562–600.

Feagin, J.R., Orum, A.M. and Sjoberg, G. (1991) *A Case for the Case Study*. Chapel Hill and London:
UNC Press.

Fertility Authority. (2015) Join the country's largest fertility directory network. Fertil. Auth. Available at
https://www.fertilityauthority.com/advertise-us (Last accessed 31 July 2015).

Foucault, M. (1973) *The Birth of the Clinic: An Archaeology of Medical Perception*. London: Routledge.

Fox Keller, E. (1996) The biological gaze. In Bird, J., Curtis, B., Mash, M., Putnam, T., Robertson, G. and Tickner, L. (eds) *Futurenatural: Nature, Science, Culture*, pp 107–21. London; New York: Routledge.

Franklin, S. (2013) *Biological Relatives: IVF, Stem Cells, and the Future of Kinship*. Durham: Duke University Press.

GFA. (2018) Overview of the GFA. Glob. Fertil. Alliance. Available at http://www.globalfertilityalliance. org/index.php/about-the-gfa/overview (Last accessed 4 February 2018).

Harper, J., Jackson, E., Sermon, K., Aitken, R.J., *et al.* (2017) Adjuncts in the IVF laboratory: where is the evidence for "add-on" interventions?, *Human Reproduction*, 32, 485–91.

Hayden, C. (2003) *When Nature Goes Public: The Making and Unmaking of Bioprospecting in Mexico*. Princeton: Princeton University Press.

HFEA. (2018) Treatment add-ons. Hum. Fertil. Embryol. Auth. Available at https://www.hfea.gov.uk/trea tments/explore-all-treatments/treatment-add-ons/ (Last accessed 10 June 2018).

Hogle, L.F. (2016) Data-intensive resourcing in healthcare, *BioSocieties*, 11, 372–93.

Inhorn, M.C. (2015) *Cosmopolitan Conceptions: IVF Sojourns in Global Dubai*. Durham: Duke University Press.

Jasanoff, S. (2017) Virtual, visible, and actionable: data assemblages and the sightlines of justice, *Big Data & Society*, 4. https://doi.org/10.1177/2053951717724477.

Kitchin, R. (2014) *The Data Revolution*. Los Angeles: Sage.

Lezaun, J. (2013) The escalating politics of "Big Biology," *BioSocieties*, 8, 480–5.

Mack, H. (2016) Progyny rebrands, launches new website for fertility health services. MobiHealthNews. Available at http://www.mobihealthnews.com/content/progyny-rebrands-launches-new-website-fertility- health-services (Last accessed 3 February 2018).

Madeira, J. and Carbone, J. (2016) Buyers in the baby market: toward a transparent consumerism, *Washington Law Review*, 91, 71–107.

Maida, J. (2016) Global fertility services market to exceed USD 21 billion by 2020, according to technavio. BusinessWire. Available at https://www.businesswire.com/news/home/20160420005059/en/ Global-Fertility-Services-Market-Exceed-USD-21 (Last accessed 22 January 2018).

McCarthy, R. (2016) Progyny to present at 34th annual J.P. Morgan Healthcare conference. PRWeb. Available at http://www.prweb.com/releases/2016/01/prweb13155994.htm (Last accessed 28 January 2018).

Merck. (2015) The Eeva™ test. Merck. Available at https://www.professionalsinfertility.com/en_GB/our- fertility-news-technology/the-eeva-test.html (Last accessed 3 February 2018).

Merck. (2016) With an extended fertility technologies portfolio Merck now covers all IVF steps. Merck Group. Available at http://www.merckgroup.com/en/news/fertility-technologies-portfolio-17-11-2016. html (Last accessed 26 August 2018).

Montag, M. (2015) How a decision support tool based on known implantation data can enhance embryo selection. Vitrolife. Available at http://blog.vitrolife.com/togetheralltheway/how-a-decision-support-tool- based-on-known-implantation-data-can-enhance-embryo-selection (Last accessed 2 February 2018).

Murphy, M. (2017) *The Economization of Life*. Durham and London: Duke University Press.

Parry, B. and Greenhough, B. (2017) *Bioinformation*. Cambridge, UK: Polity Press.

Pedrós, R. and González, M. (2017) IVI's expansion plan. IVI. Available at https://ivi-fertility.com/notes/ ivi-arrives-at-america-hand-in-hand-with-rmanj-and-consolidates-as-the-largest-group-of-assisted-reprod uction-in-the-world/ (Last accessed 22 January 2018).

Pottage, A. (2018) Dignity again, *Reproductive BioMedicine Online*, 36, 285–7.

Progyny. (2017) Progyny named to the 2017 CNBC disruptor 50 list. Progyny. Available at http://www. rmanj.com/wp-content/uploads/2015/04/RMANJ_Infertility-In-America-SurveyReport-_04152015.pdf (Last accessed 28 January 2018).

Ramsing, N. (2016) Clinical relevance of time-lapse. Vitrolife. Available at http://www.vitrolife.com/ Global/Corporate/Investors/CMD%202016-09/CEO%20presentation.pdf (Last accessed 2 April 2018).

Reijo Pera, R.A. (2013) More than just a matter of time, *Reproductive BioMedicine Online*, 27, 113–4.

Spar, D.L. (2006) *The Baby Business: How Money, Science, and Politics Drive the Commerce of Conception*. Boston: Harvard Business Press.

Sunder Rajan, K. (2006) *Biocapital: The Constitution of Postgenomic Life*. Durham: Duke University Press.

Thompson, C. (2013) *Good Science: The Ethical Choreography of Stem Cell Research*. London; Cambridge: MIT Press.

Van de Wiel, L. (2017) Cellular origins: a visual analysis of time-lapse embryo imaging. In Lykke, N. and Lie, M. (eds) *Assisted Reproduction Across Borders: Feminist Perspectives on Normalization, Disruptions and Transmissions*, pp 288–301. New York and Abingdon: Routledge.

Van de Wiel, L. (2018) Prenatal imaging: egg freezing, embryo selection and the visual politics of reproductive time. *Catalyst: Feminism, Theory, Technoscience*, 4, 2, 1–35.

Van Dijck, J., Poell, T. and Waal, M. (2016) *De Platformsamenleving*. Amsterdam: Amsterdam University Press.

Vertommen, S. (2017) From the pergonal project to Kadimastem: a genealogy of Israel's reproductive-industrial complex, *BioSocieties*, 12, 282–306.

Vitrolife. (2015a) KIDScore™ D3 & D5 decision support tool. Vitrolife. Available at http://www.vitrolife.com/en/Products/EmbryoScope-Time-Lapse-System/KIDScore-decision-support-tool-/ (Last accessed 2 February 2018).

Vitrolife. (2015b) KIDScore decision support tool. Vitrolifetube. Available at https://www.youtube.com/watch?time_continue=74&v=tPtR81sBbzI (Last accessed 3 February 2018).

Vitrolife. (2017) *Interim Report January–June 2017 (Interim Report)*. Gothenburg, Sweden: Vitrolife. Available at http://mb.cision.com/Main/1031/9804468/401074.pdf (Last accessed 8 February 2018).

Vitrolife. (2018a) *Interim Report January–March 2018 (Interim Report)*. Gothenburg, Sweden: Vitrolife.

Vitrolife. (2018b) Vitrolife – EmbryoScope time-lapse system. Vitrolife. Available at https://www.vitrolife.com/en/products/time-lapse-systems/embryoscope-time-lapse-system/ (Last accessed 25 August 2018).

Vitrolife. (2018c) Vitrolife – IVF journey. Vitrolife. Available at https://www.vitrolife.com/en/ivf-journey/#. Last accessed 26 August 2018.

Waldby, C. and Mitchell, R. (2006) *Tissue Economies: Blood, Organs, and Cell Lines in Late Capitalism*. Durham: Duke University Press.

Walsh, F. (2013a) IVF "may be boosted by time-lapse embryo imaging." BBC. Available at http://www.bbc.com/news/health-22559247 (Last accessed 24 February 2015).

Walsh, F. (2013b) Time-lapse imaging "improves IVF." BBC. Available at http://www.bbc.com/news/health-22559247 (Last accessed 24 February 2015).

Wenzel, D. (2017) Fertile ground: why Merck is investing in fertility treatment centres, *European Pharmaceutical Review*.

Williams, E., Surowiak, M. and Szymanski, M. (2017) *Fertility Clinics, Q1 2017*. Boston: Capstone Partners.

Winstel, R., Wieland, J., Gertz, B., Mueller, A., et al. (2017) Manufacturing of recombinant human follicle-stimulating hormone Ovaleap® comparability with Gonal-f®, and performance/consistency, *Drugs in R&D*, 17, 305–12. https://doi.org/10.1007/s40268-017-0182-z.

Wong, C.C., Loewke, K.E., Baer, T.M., Reijo-Pera, R.A., et al. (2012) Imaging and evaluating embryos, oocytes, and stem cells. Patent US8337387 B2.

Wong, C.C., Loewke, K.E., Baer, T.M., Reijo-Pera, R.A., et al. (2013) Imaging and evaluating embryos, oocytes, and stem cells. Patent EP2430454 B1.

Index

Digital Health: Sociological Perspectives, First Edition.
Edited by Flis Henwood and Benjamin Marent.
Chapters © 2019 The Authors. Book Compilation © 2019 Foundation for the Sociology of Health & Illness/John Wiley & Sons Ltd.